T0336790

Life-Threatening Effects of Antipsychotic Drugs

Life-Threatening Effects of Antipsychotic Drugs

Edited by

Peter Manu
Hofstra Northwell School of Medicine, Hempstead, NY, United States;
South Oaks Hospital, Amityville, NY, United States

Robert J. Flanagan
King's College Hospital, London, United Kingdom

Kathlyn J. Ronaldson
Monash University, Melbourne, VIC, Australia

AMSTERDAM • BOSTON • HEIDELBERG • LONDON
NEW YORK • OXFORD • PARIS • SAN DIEGO
SAN FRANCISCO • SINGAPORE • SYDNEY • TOKYO
Academic Press is an imprint of Elsevier

Academic Press is an imprint of Elsevier
125 London Wall, London EC2Y 5AS, United Kingdom
525 B Street, Suite 1800, San Diego, CA 92101-4495, United States
50 Hampshire Street, 5th Floor, Cambridge, MA 02139, United States
The Boulevard, Langford Lane, Kidlington, Oxford OX5 1GB, United Kingdom

Copyright © 2016 Elsevier Inc. All rights reserved.

No part of this publication may be reproduced or transmitted in any form or by any means, electronic
or mechanical, including photocopying, recording, or any information storage and retrieval system,
without permission in writing from the publisher. Details on how to seek permission, further information
about the Publisher's permissions policies and our arrangements with organizations such as the
Copyright Clearance Center and the Copyright Licensing Agency, can be found at our website:
www.elsevier.com/permissions.

This book and the individual contributions contained in it are protected under copyright by the Publisher
(other than as may be noted herein).

Notices
Knowledge and best practice in this field are constantly changing. As new research and experience
broaden our understanding, changes in research methods, professional practices, or medical treatment
may become necessary.

Practitioners and researchers must always rely on their own experience and knowledge in evaluating
and using any information, methods, compounds, or experiments described herein. In using such
information or methods they should be mindful of their own safety and the safety of others, including
parties for whom they have a professional responsibility.

To the fullest extent of the law, neither the Publisher nor the authors, contributors, or editors, assume
any liability for any injury and/or damage to persons or property as a matter of products liability,
negligence or otherwise, or from any use or operation of any methods, products, instructions, or ideas
contained in the material herein.

British Library Cataloguing-in-Publication Data
A catalogue record for this book is available from the British Library

Library of Congress Cataloging-in-Publication Data
A catalog record for this book is available from the Library of Congress

ISBN: 978-0-12-803376-0

For Information on all Academic Press publications
visit our website at https://www.elsevier.com/

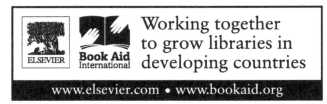

Working together
to grow libraries in
developing countries

www.elsevier.com • www.bookaid.org

Publisher: Nikki Levy
Acquisition Editor: Nikki Levy
Editorial Project Manager: Barbara Makinster
Production Project Manager: Julie-Ann Stansfield
Designer: Matthew Limbert

Typeset by MPS Limited, Chennai, India

Contents

3.   Pulmonary Embolism

*Peter Manu, Christopher Hohman, James F. Barrecchia
and Matisyahu Shulman*

4.   Orthostatic Hypotension

James J. Gugger and Megan J. Ehret

Part II
Hematological Complications of Treatment With Antipsychotic Drugs

5.   Severe Neutropenia and Agranulocytosis

John Lally and Robert J. Flanagan

Part III
Antipsychotic-Related Pathology of the Digestive System

6. Gastrointestinal Hypomotility and Dysphagia

Robert J. Flanagan and Kathlyn J. Ronaldson

7. Liver Failure

Katie F.M. Marwick

8. Pancreatitis

Peter Manu, Matisyahu Shulman and Kathlyn J. Ronaldson

Part IV
Major Neurological and Neuromuscular Adverse Effects of Antipsychotic Drugs

9. Seizures

Tilman Steinert and Walter Fröscher

10. Neuroleptic Malignant Syndrome

Julie Langan Martin and Daniel J. Martin

Part V
Metabolic Complications of Antipsychotic Drug Treatment

12. Type 2 Diabetes Mellitus

*Davy Vancampfort, Richard I.G. Holt, Brendon Stubbs,
Marc De Hert, Katherine Samaras and Alex J. Mitchell*

Part VI
Other Life-Threatening Effects of Antipsychotic Drugs
13.   Interstitial Nephritis and Interstitial Lung Disease
Kathlyn J. Ronaldson

Part VII
Clinical and Forensic Challenges in the Use of Antipsychotic Drugs
14.   The Benefits of Antipsychotic Drugs: Symptom Control and Improved Quality of Life
Jian-Ping Zhang

List of Contributors

James F. Barrecchia Zucker Hillside Hospital, Glen Oaks, NY, United States

Dan Cohen Mental Health Services North-Holland North, Heerhugowaard, The Netherlands; University of Groningen, Groningen, The Netherlands

Anca Dan Colentina Hospital, Bucharest, Romania

Gheorghe-Andrei Dan Colentina Hospital, Bucharest, Romania; Carol Davila University of Medicine and Pharmacy, Bucharest, Romania

Marc De Hert University Psychiatric Center University of Leuven, Kortenberg, Belgium

Megan J. Ehret Fort Belvoir Community Hospital, Fort Belvoir, VA, United States

Robert J. Flanagan King's College Hospital, London, United Kingdom

Walter Fröscher Ulm University, Ulm, Germany

James J. Gugger Johns Hopkins School of Medicine, Baltimore, MD, United States

Christopher Hohman Zucker Hillside Hospital, Glen Oaks, NY, United States

Richard I.G. Holt University of Southampton, Southampton, United Kingdom

John Lally King's College London, London, United Kingdom

Julie Langan Martin University of Glasgow, Glasgow, United Kingdom

Peter Manu Hofstra Northwell School of Medicine, Hempstead, NY, United States; South Oaks Hospital, Amityville, NY, United States

Daniel J. Martin University of Glasgow, Glasgow, United Kingdom

Katie F.M. Marwick University of Edinburgh, Edinburgh, United Kingdom

Alex J. Mitchell University of Leicester, Leicester, United Kingdom

Kathlyn J. Ronaldson Monash University, Melbourne, VIC, Australia

Katherine Samaras Garvan Institute of Medical Research, Sydney, NSW, Australia

Matisyahu Shulman Zucker Hillside Hospital, Glen Oaks, NY, United States

Tilman Steinert Ulm University, Ulm, Germany

Brendon Stubbs King's College London, London, United Kingdom; Maudsley NHS Foundation Trust, London, United Kingdom

Davy Vancampfort University Psychiatric Center University of Leuven, Kortenberg, Belgium

Jian-Ping Zhang Hofstra Northwell School of Medicine, Hempstead, NY, United States

Foreword

The Art and Science of Balance: Managing the Efficacy and Safety of Antipsychotic Drugs

With the serendipitous discovery of chlorpromazine as the first "major tranquillizer" over six decades ago, a new class of "antipsychotics" was born. After predominant use for psychosis and agitation associated with different psychiatric and medical conditions, antipsychotic medications became used much more widely about two decades ago. This more widespread use of anti-psychotics coincides with the development of a new "class" of antipsychotics, the so-called "atypical" or second-generation antipsychotics that had less of the neuromotor adverse effects of the so-called "typical" or first-generation antipsychotics, but that also affected more extra-dopaminergic neurotransmitter targets. In fact, nowadays, antipsychotics are being used the most for nonpsy-chotic conditions, including motor tics, stuttering, behavioral dysregulation and impulsivity, nonpsychotic aggression, irritability, mania, depression, anxiety, insomnia, obsessions and compulsions, eating disorders, etc.

It is clear that the heterogeneous class of medications that is still called antipsychotics is efficacious for severe mental disorders and their various symptoms that are often highly impairing. However, as with all medications, these molecules can also have adverse effects. Clinically, efficacy and safety need to be balanced. In the medical literature, adverse effects are often given a second place to the exploration and description of efficacy. However, for many psychiatrically ill patients, concerns about tolerability and safety trump efficacy considerations. Similarly, clinicians' ability to effectively use medi-cations is limited by their propensity to cause relevant side effects. Although there are articles, chapters, and, even, books that focus on adverse effects, the book *Life-Threatening Effects of Antipsychotic Drugs* is the first of its kind.

While the title could sound alarmist, the clear intention of this impressive volume is not to warn against the use of antipsychotics. The deliberation about the use, choice of agent, and duration of treatment is a clinical decision. Rather, the book's seven sections populated by 16 chapters and written by experts in the respective areas, aim to thoroughly educate about the possibility and nature of severe and potentially life-threatening adverse effects of antipsychotics. The book and its chapters tell clinicians that these adverse effects, although fortunately generally rare, do exist and that clinicians need to be equipped to identify and deal with them in order to provide optimal care. Detailed knowledge about the serious adverse events covered in this book should not lead clinicians to stop using antipsychotics when they are needed, but should rather lead to a more informed and judicious use of antipsychotics. Clinicians should not be intimidated by the described potentially life-threatening adverse effects, but rather be as educated as possible about how to prevent, identify, and manage them. Patients' and families' participation in shared decision making also needs to be informed by such knowledge as appropriate.

Any drug effect results from an interaction between the pharmacodynamic and pharmacokinetic properties of the medication, the clinician prescribing the medication in a certain way, the individual patient receiving the medication, and specific circumstances at the time. Most individual risk can be anticipated, monitored, and managed. However, there are also idiosyncratic reactions, interactions with other medications and unpredictable outcomes. The best way to deal with the unknown is to educate oneself as much as possible about the known around it. In this spirit, *Life-Threatening Effects of Antipsychotic Drugs* will help clinicians to be less surprised and caught off guard, feel equipped about what and when to ask and to monitor in order to catch signs of developing adverse effects early, how to manage adverse events appropriately, and when to refer to other specialists as needed. Having read or consulted this authoritative book will help clinicians optimize the benefit-to-risk ratio for their patients who require acute or ongoing antipsychotic treatment.

Clearly, despite the scholarship and clinical wisdom contained in each chapter of *Life-Threatening Effects of Antipsychotic Drugs*, a lot more needs to be learned. Additional research is needed to identify patient level risk factors and to help identify potentially life-threatening adverse effects before they become so serious that they cannot be managed well anymore. Other treatment strategies that can effectively counter potentially serious adverse effects need to be identified, so that they are not life-threatening. Medications need to be developed devoid of the described risks. While there will hopefully be additional knowledge added over the next years to come, *Life-Threatening Effects of Antipsychotic Drugs* summarizes what we know to date, providing clinicians with tools to improve their care of patients treated with antipsychotics.

Christoph U. Correll and John M. Kane

Preface

Medical deteriorations can have major adverse consequences for psychiatric patients. They interrupt behavioral interventions and may require the discontinuation of psychotropic drug treatment. When they occur in a psychiatric hospital ward, such deteriorations prolong the length of stay and can add considerable expense to the episode of mental illness. They may also prove fatal even when the conditions are rapidly diagnosed and treated. Most of the time, the life-threatening somatic disorders encountered in psychiatric practice are due to exacerbations of established conditions, such as coronary artery disease, chronic obstructive pulmonary disease, or liver cirrhosis. However, some of the cases represent adverse effects of psychotropic drugs. In this category, the greatest concern is represented by the antipsychotic drugs, molecules that bind to numerous receptors in the brain and elsewhere and may lead to many organ-specific or systemic complications.

The deaths occurring in persons taking antipsychotic drugs belong to four categories: homicides or suicides; natural deaths not-related to the antipsychotic treatment; overdoses; and adverse effects of medications taken in therapeutic doses. The mechanisms of deaths produced by adverse effects of antipsychotic drugs prescribed, administered and taken in therapeutic dosages are relatively well understood. The antipsychotic-induced delay in myocardial repolarization may lead to a polymorphic ventricular arrhythmia, *torsades de pointes*, which can degenerate into ventricular fibrillation and produce sudden cardiac death. Pump failure and cardiogenic shock may complicate the left ventricular dysfunction of antipsychotic-induced myocarditis. Gas exchange failure and low cardiac output explain the death of patients who developed massive pulmonary thromboembolism, a multifactorial condition to which antipsychotics may contribute directly by creating a hypercoagulable state, and indirectly through decreased mobility, morbid obesity, and inflammatory changes. Patients with drug-induced agranulocytosis, severe gastrointestinal hypomotility, or pancreatitis are at risk of dying from septic shock or from multiple organ failure. Multiple organ failure may also complicate neuroleptic malignant syndrome, rhabdomyolysis, and heat stroke. Postictal arousal failure followed by respiratory arrest is sometimes seen in patients who had a drug-induced seizure. Asphyxia is the mode of death in patients with airway obstruction produced by neuroleptic-related oropharyngeal dysphagia. Finally, in patients with severe drug-induced kidney or liver failure, death may be the outcome of catastrophic bleeding.

The scientific assessment of these potentially fatal drug effects is limited by the lack or prospective, long-term controlled trials and by suboptimal postmortem investigations. Without exception, all of the large-scale epidemiological studies on fatality rates presented in this book have relied on clinical assessments, rather than on complete forensic evaluation that included a careful autopsy and accurate toxicological measurements. Therefore, the prevention of these medical deteriorations has remained the subject of debate, as has the risk of recurrent complications once the antipsychotic drug therapy is restarted.

This book represents the first attempt to describe in detail what is known about life-threatening adverse effects of antipsychotic drugs. Edited by a multidisciplinary team, the chapters describing these adverse effects are based on the best available evidence, presented in a sequence that will allow the readers to learn the epidemiology, pathobiology, clinical features, and principles of management and prevention of these complications in psychiatric settings. Additional chapters highlight the benefits of antipsychotic drugs and propose models for risk—benefit analyses by frontline clinicians. The work is not intended to replace print and electronic resources required for the practice of psychopharmacology, but to offer a sensible framework for dealing with complications that may have devastating consequences on patients, their families, and their physicians.

Peter Manu, Robert J. Flanagan and Kathlyn J. Ronaldson
Editors

Acknowledgments

This book owes its existence to the hard work, talent, and dedication of our contributors, scientists and clinicians from Australia, Belgium, Germany, Great Britain, Ireland, the Netherlands, Romania, and the United States. As the Editors of their work, we extend our thanks and deep appreciation to all for their investment of time together with their insight, knowledge, and discernment. We are also grateful to John Kane and Christoph Correll for their advice during the planning of the book and for providing an illuminating Foreword to it.

Kathlyn Ronaldson is grateful to Professor John McNeil, Head, Department of Epidemiology and Preventive Medicine, Monash University for enabling her access to the resources of the University to complete the work of writing chapters and editing this book.

We acknowledge the valuable suggestions made by the Elsevier's reviewers of our book proposal and the grace and patience with which Julie-Ann Stansfield and her team have worked with us during the production of this book.

Symbols and Conventions

We have used either Système Internationale (SI) symbols for quantities such as g (gram), m (meter), s (second), or symbols accepted for use with SI such as L (liter), min (minute), h (hour), d (day), mo (month), yr (year). We have adopted the superscript notation for use with symbols, e.g., $mg\,L^{-1}$, as this expresses rates, e.g., min^{-1}, and complex units, e.g., $mg\,kg^{-1}\,day^{-1}$, clearly and unambiguously.

For more information on SI, see Flanagan, R.J., 1995. Leading article: SI units—common sense not dogma is needed. Br. J. Clin. Pharmacol. 39, 589–594.

Part I

Cardiovascular Adverse Effects of Antipsychotic Drugs

Chapter 1

Sudden Cardiac Death and Ventricular Arrhythmias

Peter Manu[1,2], Anca Dan[3] and Gheorghe-Andrei Dan[3,4]

[1]*Hofstra Northwell School of Medicine, Hempstead, NY, United States,* [2]*South Oaks Hospital, Amityville, NY, United States,* [3]*Colentina Hospital, Bucharest, Romania,* [4]*Carol Davila University of Medicine and Pharmacy, Bucharest, Romania*

1.1 EPIDEMIOLOGY

Large epidemiological studies of sudden cardiac death (SCD) in persons treated with antipsychotic drugs in the United States have been first performed at Vanderbilt University School of Medicine in Nashville, TN (Ray et al., 2001, 2009).

An early study evaluated retrospectively the relationship between treatment with first-generation antipsychotics and SCD in a cohort of 481,744 of Tennessee Medicaid enrollees aged 15–84 with 1,282,996 person-years of follow-up from Jan. 1, 1988 through Dec. 31, 1993. There were 1487 SCDs, defined as a pulseless condition, fatal within 48 hours of onset, occurring in the absence of other causes of death and consistent with a ventricular tachyarrhythmia. The sample included 26,749 person-years with current antipsychotic use at a dose greater than 100 mg thioridazine equivalent, 31,881 person-years with current use of a lower dose, and 37,881 person-years of antipsychotic use in the past year. Multivariate rate-ratios of SCD were calculated from Poisson regression models that included age, sex, race, calendar year, cardiovascular disease, and medical or surgical hospital admission for noncardiac illness. The magnitude of confounding by smoking was assessed in a secondary analysis of a subsample given a diagnosis of bronchitis or emphysema.

Overall, the cohort had 11.6 SCDs/10,000 person-years of follow-up. Compared with nonusers, current antipsychotic use at doses greater than 100 mg thioridazine equivalent had a rate-ratio of 2.39 (95% confidence

Life-Threatening Effects of Antipsychotic Drugs. DOI: http://dx.doi.org/10.1016/B978-0-12-803376-0.00001-0
© 2016 Elsevier Inc. All rights reserved.

TABLE 1.1 Rate-Ratios of Sudden Cardiac Death in Persons Treated With Conventional Antipsychotics

Drug	Rate-Ratio	95% Confidence Interval
Thiothixene	4.23	2.00−8.91
Chlorpromazine	3.64	1.36−9.74
Thioridazine	3.19	1.32−7.68
Haloperidol	1.90	1.10−3.30

Source: Data from Ray, W.A., Meredith, S., Thapa, P.B., Meador, K.G., Hall, K., Murray K.T., 2001. Antipsychotics and the risk of sudden cardiac death. Arch. Gen. Psychiatry 58 (12), 1161−1167.

interval 1.77−3.22). The corresponding rate-ratios were 1.30 (95% confidence interval 0.98−1.72) for patients taking lower daily doses and 1.20 (95% confidence interval 0.91−1.58) for past treatment with first-generation antipsychotics. Females treated with antipsychotics had a higher rate-ratio (2.97, 95% confidence interval 1.96−4.50) than males (1.91, 95% confidence interval 1.24−2.95). The rate-ratios differed considerably from drug to drug, with the worst being observed for thiothixene and the lowest for haloperidol (Table 1.1). The presence of cardiovascular disease did not change significantly the magnitude of the difference in the risk of SCD between current users and nonusers of antipsychotic drugs. The rate-ratio of SCD between users and nonusers of moderate doses of antipsychotics with comparable cardiovascular disease were 3.18 (95% confidence interval 1.95−5.16) for a mild condition, 2.12 (95% confidence interval 1.08−4.14) for moderate severity, and 3.53 (95% confidence interval 1.66−7.51) for a disorder with high severity.

For the assessment of the risk of sudden death in individuals treated with atypical (second-generation) antipsychotics, the Vanderbilt group evaluated retrospectively 46,089 users of single atypical drugs, 44,218 users of first-generation drugs, and 186,600 matched nonusers in a cohort of Medicaid enrollees in Tennessee from Jan. 1, 1990 through Dec. 31, 2005 (Ray et al., 2009). The study end-point was a sudden pulseless condition interpreted as ventricular tachyarrhythmia, as indicated by death certificates linked to medical records retrievable from an electronic database. Hospital deaths, including those occurring 30 days after discharge were not included, because data regarding drug treatment during the hospital stay could not be ascertained. Also excluded were patients with "a cardiac cause that was not consistent with a ventricular tachyarrhythmia (e.g., heart failure)" (p. 227). A cardiovascular risk score was calculated for each subject from baseline variables, which included recorded diagnoses, prescribed medications, compliance with

TABLE 1.2 Rate-Ratios of Sudden Cardiac Death in Persons Treated With Atypical Antipsychotics

Drug	Rate-Ratio	95% Confidence Interval
Clozapine	3.67	1.94–6.94
Risperidone	2.91	2.26–3.76
Olanzapine	2.04	1.52–2.74
Quetiapine	1.88	1.30–2.71

Source: Data from Ray, W.A., Chung, C.P., Murray, K.T., Hall, K., Stein, C.M., 2009. Atypical antipsychotic drugs and the risk of sudden cardiac death. N. Engl. J. Med. 360 (3), 225–235.

treatment, and utilization of health care resources. Users and nonusers of antipsychotic drugs were matched at a 1:2 ratio, according to a propensity score designed to adjust for age, gender, and severity of psychiatric illness.

The final sample consisted of 67,824 users and 116,069 nonusers age 30−74 with 1,042,159 person-years of follow-up during which there were 1870 sudden deaths or 1.79 per 1000 person-years. The incidence-rate ratios of SCD were 1.99 for users of typical antipsychotics and 2.26 for individuals treated with atypical antipsychotics. Compared with nonusers, current users of haloperidol had a rate-ratio of SCD of 1.61 (95% confidence interval 1.16−2.24), which was substantially lower than the rate-ratio recorded for thioridazine (3.19, 95% confidence interval 2.41−4.21). The rate-ratios were significantly greater in current users of the four atypical antipsychotics studied as compared with nonusers (Table 1.2). Former users did not show an increase in the rate of SCD. The rate-ratios increased linearly according to the dose for both drug classes, but the trend reached statistical significance only for thioridazine and risperidone. Current use of typical and atypical antipsychotics showed a similar increase in rate-ratios in the analyses of cohorts matched according to the propensity score or year of starting treatment with these drugs.

A similar project was completed at the Center for Clinical Epidemiology and Biostatistics, University of Pennsylvania School of Medicine in Philadelphia (Hennessy et al., 2002; Leonard et al., 2013). The first report contained data produced by a cohort of outpatients enrolled in the Medicaid program in three states (Hennessy et al., 2002). The cohort included patients with schizophrenia treated with haloperidol ($n = 41,295$), thioridazine ($n = 23,950$), risperidone ($n = 22,057$), and clozapine ($n = 8330$). The control subjects were individuals prescribed medications for glaucoma ($n = 21,545$) and psoriasis ($n = 7541$). The study outcomes were culled from the administrative data covering the period 1993−96 and included the diagnoses of cardiac arrest, sudden death of unknown cause, unexplained death occurring within 24 hours from the onset of symptoms, unattended death, ventricular fibrillation, and ventricular flutter. A large number drugs (e.g., lipid lowering medications, antiarrhythmics, thiazide diuretics, calcium channel blockers, and angiotensin converting enzyme inhibitors) and diseases (e.g., heart failure, coronary artery disease, cardiac conduction abnormalities, obesity, and alcohol misuse) were examined as potential confounders. Antipsychotic dosages were transformed in thioridazine equivalents (100 mg thioridazine = 2.5 mg haloperidol = 0.75 mg risperidone = 50 mg clozapine).

The rate of cardiac arrest and ventricular tachyarrhythmia/1000 person-years was 3.4 (95% confidence interval 2.8−4.1) for individuals receiving glaucoma drugs and 1.8 (95% confidence interval 1.1−2.8) for those treated for psoriasis. Medicaid enrollees treated for schizophrenia with antipsychotic drugs had higher rates of cardiac arrest and life-threatening rhythm disturbances (Table 1.3). A linear-dose response relation was observed only for thioridazine. The potential confounders did not change the rate-ratios of the study's end-points for patients taking the four antipsychotics studied.

A comparison of the risk of SCD in patients treated with atypical and typical antipsychotics was later published by the same investigators from the University of Pennsylvania (Leonard et al., 2013). The authors assembled a cohort of Medicaid and dually eligible Medicaid/Medicare beneficiaries in five states (California, Florida, New York, Ohio, and Pennsylvania) and identified 459,614 users of antipsychotic drugs who were 30−75 years of age and produced 221,164 person-years of observation. The end-point was sudden death or life-threatening ventricular arrhythmias (i.e., paroxysmal ventricular tachycardia, ventricular flutter, and ventricular fibrillation) observed in the Emergency Department or during a hospital admission. Treatment with olanzapine was chosen as the referent. The database did not allow the ascertainment of alcohol use and smoking status.

TABLE 1.3 Rates of Cardiac Arrest and Ventricular Arrhythmias in Patients Treated with Antipsychotic Drugs

Drug	Rate/1000 person-years	95% Confidence Interval
Risperidone	5.0	3.7−6.6
Haloperidol	4.2	3.5−5.0
Thioridazine	3.8	3.0−4.7
Clozapine	2.2	1.3−3.4

Source: Data from Hennessy, S., Bilker, W.B., Knauss, J.S., Margolis, D.J., Kimmel, S.E., Reyniolds, R.F., et al., 2002. Cardiac arrest and ventricular arrhythmia in patients taking antipsychotic drugs: cohort study using administrative data. BMJ 325 (7372): 1070.

There were 747 end-point events, for a crude incidence of 3.4/1000 person-years. The incidence of sudden deaths, based on 483 instances, was 2.2/1000 person-years. Compared with olanzapine, the hazard ratios were higher for the typical antipsychotics chlorpromazine (2.06, 95% confidence interval 1.20−3.53) and haloperidol (1.72, 95% confidence interval 1.28−2.31), but lower for quetiapine (0.73, 95% confidence interval 0.57−0.93). The hazard ratios for perphenazine, olanzapine, and risperidone were similar. The risk of sudden death and or major ventricular arrhythmia was highest in patients given their first prescription for chlorpromazine and haloperidol. A dose−response relationship was identified only for haloperidol. The data were compared with the results of the study evaluating the risk of SCD in Medicaid beneficiaries from Tennessee (Ray et al., 2009) by resetting that cohort's reference group from nonusers to olanzapine. The results were contradictory for haloperidol, equivocal for risperidone, and similar for quetiapine.

The risk of SCD in patients treated with antipsychotic drugs was also studied in the Netherlands (Straus et al., 2004), United Kingdom (Jolly et al., 2009; Murray-Thomas et al., 2013), and Taiwan (Wu et al., 2015).

The Dutch study used data retrieved from computer-based medical records of a group of 150 general practitioners for a total of 250,000 patients (Straus et al., 2004). The potential subjects had to be at least 18 years old and to be followed up in the practice for at least 1 year. The outcome variable was a notation in the record using the wording sudden death, unexpected witnessed death, and unwitnessed death in a person last seen in a stable medical condition in the 24 hours preceding the event. Up to 10 age- and gender-matched control subjects were randomly selected from the same practice.

There were 582 sudden deaths and 554 of them were matched with 4463 control subjects. Autopsies were performed in only seven cases. Cases had significantly higher rates of known risk factors for sudden death, such as a history of heart or cerebrovascular disorders, hypertension, diabetes, dyslipidemia, and smoking. Current users of antipsychotic drugs had a substantially higher incidence of sudden death than control subjects (odds ratio 3.3; 95% confidence interval 1.8−6.2). There were no differences between subgroups of patients treated for schizophrenia/schizoaffective disorder or other psychiatric disorders. The risk was increased in patients treated with antipsychotics continuously for more than 90 days and in those receiving more than half of the daily dose equivalents generally used for adults with schizophrenia.

The first UK investigation was a case−control study of persons 20−85 years of age who died from 2003 to 2007 in the Midlands (Jolly et al., 2009). The cases were selected from those referred for forensic evaluation of the cause of deaths occurring in the community. Autopsy findings were used to exclude drug overdoses. Subjects with evidence of coronary atherosclerosis were included in the study if they had no evidence of recent myocardial infarction or plaque rupture. Each case of sudden death was matched with three age-matched control subjects from the same general practice. The odds

TABLE 1.4 Age, Gender-Adjusted Relative Mortality Risk (95% Confidence Interval) in Users of Antipsychotic Drugs, Psychiatric Nonusers, and General Population Control

Groups Compared	Sudden Cardiac Death	Cardiac Mortality
Current users vs psychiatric nonusers	5.76 (2.90−11.45)	1.62 (1.52−1.74)
Current users vs general population	4.45 (2.94−6.73)	1.83 (1.74−1.93)

Source: Data from Murray-Thomas, T., Jones, M.E., Patel, D., Brunner, E., Shatapathy, C.C., Motsko, S., et al., 2013. Risk of mortality (including sudden cardiac death) and major cardiovascular events in atypical and typical antipsychotic users: a study with the general practice research database. Cardiovasc. Psychiatry Neurol. 2013, 247486.

ratios of sudden death were significantly higher in users of typical (3.94, 95% confidence interval 2.05−7.55) and atypical (4.36, 95% confidence interval 2.54−7.51) antipsychotics.

The second UK investigation used the General Practice Research Database which contains medical records of clinicians involved in the care of about 8% of the country's population (Murray-Thomas et al., 2013). A substantial number (40%) of these practices were linked to administrative data repositories of hospital records and death certificates. The study compared 183,392 antipsychotic users with 193,920 persons with psychiatric disorders not using antipsychotics and with 544,726 general population control subjects without a recorded history of psychiatric disorder or exposure to antipsychotics. The primary outcomes were all-cause mortality, cardiac mortality, and SCD. Patients with advanced cardiomyopathies and those with a premortem diagnosis of life-threatening ventricular tachyarrhythmia were excluded.

Current users had a significantly higher rate of SCD and all-cause cardiac mortality than psychiatric nonusers and general population control subjects (Table 1.4). The death rates of specified cardiac cause, that is, diseases of the circulatory system, ischemic heart disease, and heart failure, were similar in users of typical and atypical antipsychotic drugs.

The Taiwanese investigators used prescriptions records to determine the use of antipsychotic drugs and a nationwide insurance database for Emergency Department visits and hospitalization claims to identify individuals with a psychiatric diagnosis and incident of SCD or ventricular arrhythmias from Jan. 2000 to Dec. 2009 (Wu et al., 2015). Patients with a previous hospitalization within 8 weeks prior to end-point and those younger than 16 years of age were not included in the study. The 17,718 cases included 6109 (35.4%) patients with dementia or other organic brain syndrome and 1710 (9.7%) subjects with schizophrenia or other psychoses.

TABLE 1.5 Antipsychotic Drugs Associated With Significantly Higher Adjusted Rate-Ratios of Sudden Cardiac Death/Ventricular Arrhythmias in Psychiatric Patients

Drug	Rate-Ratio	95% Confidence Interval
Clothiapine	2.16	1.03−4.53
Thioridazine	1.78	1.01−3.15
Prochlorperazine	1.69	1.32−2.17
Haloperidol	1.46	1.17−1.83
Risperidone	1.39	1.13−1.72
Quetiapine	1.29	1.07−1.56
Sulpiride	1.26	1.02−1.56

Source: Data from Wu, C., Tsai, Y., Tsai, H., 2015. Antipsychotic drugs and the risk of ventricular arrhythmia and/or sudden cardiac death: a nation-wide cross-over study. J. Am. Heart Assoc. 4, e001568.

A total of 5625 subjects had been prescribed antipsychotic drugs. The group had a risk-rate of SCD or ventricular arrhythmias of 1.53 (95% confidence interval 1.38−1.70) compared with nonusers after adjustment for treatment with antidiabetic, antithrombotic, diuretic, antihypertensive, and lipid-modifying drugs. Significant differences in the adjusted risk-rate of users and nonusers of antipsychotics were observed for four of nine first-generation and three of nine second-generation drugs (Table 1.5). The list of drugs not associated with an excess of sudden deaths/ventricular arrhythmias included chlorpromazine, aripiprazole, clozapine, and ziprasidone.

Two large open-label studies have provided additional information about sertindole, a drug pulled off the market for a presumed association with SCD (Thomas et al., 2010) and ziprasidone, an antipsychotic known to significantly prolong the Q-T interval (QTc) (Strom et al., 2011). The safety of sertindole was evaluated in a head-to-head comparison with risperidone in a multinational, randomized, parallel group study of 9858 subjects with schizophrenia who were followed up for a total of 14,417 person-years (Thomas et al., 2010). Cardiac mortality was significantly higher in the group receiving sertindole (hazard ratio 2.84, 95% confidence interval 1.45−5.55). However, only 3 of the 31 cardiac-related deaths in the sertindole-treated group were considered primary arrhythmias. Ziprasidone was compared with olanzapine in a randomized postmarketing trial that included 18,154 patients with schizophrenia followed for 1 year by unblinded investigators (Strom et al., 2011). The relative risk of nonsuicidal death was 1.02 (95% confidence interval 0.76−1.39).

Pooled data (Salvo et al., 2015) indicate that compared with nonusers, the risk (odds ratio, 95% confidence interval) of SCD is increased for the first-generation antipsychotics thioridazine (4.58, 2.09−10.05) and haloperidol (2.97, 1.59−5.54), as well as for the atypical antipsychotics clozapine (3.67, 1.94−6.94), risperidone (3.04, 2.39−3.86), olanzapine (2.04, 1.52−2.74), and quetiapine (1.72, 1.33−2.23). Taken together, the data indicate that treatment with antipsychotic drugs is associated with a significant, dose-dependent, increase in the risk of sudden death. The strength of the association appears to be similar for first- and second-generation drugs. The inference that the events studied represented SCD due to arrhythmias was disputed by the American Psychiatric Association's Council on Research (Lieberman et al., 2012), which has stated that a retrospective analysis of death certificates (Ray et al., 2009) may have led to an overestimation of the SCD incidence, to an underestimation of the cardiovascular morbidity of users of antipsychotic drugs, and to inadequate control for important confounding variables. The American Psychiatric Association's position is supported by the methodology used to ascertain the sudden arrhythmic death syndrome (Behr et al., 2007), because this diagnosis should be made only in cases with no history of cardiac disease, no identifiable macroscopic cause of death at a complete autopsy, and no abnormal findings on microscopic examination of the heart by a cardiac pathologist.

1.2 PATHOBIOLOGY

Sudden cardiac arrest/death (SCD) is an arrhythmic event precipitated by ventricular tachycardia and ventricular fibrillation (Bayés de Luna et al., 1989). The mechanism is complex and involves the interaction of a modified myocardial substrate (e.g., scar, hypertrophy, or fibrosis) with altered functional properties, such as electrical characteristics and calcium handling (Figs. 1.1 and 1.2). A SCD may occur in the absence of a discernible morphologic substrate when electrical myocardial properties are critically modified by abnormalities of cellular channels responsible for ionic and current flux, which are produced by specific genetic mutations or altered by drugs. In both cases the channel function is either diminished or lost, or is increased. The net result is a critical alteration of the action potential duration (APD) and of the temporal dispersion of myocardial repolarization (Roden, 1998).

1.2.1 Determinants of APD

The APD is the result of many outward and inward cellular currents with specific densities and representation for each myocardial region (Fig. 1.3). The most important electrical characteristic of the myocardial action potential is the presence of the plateau determined by a temporary balance

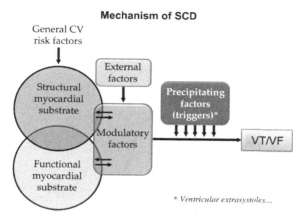

FIGURE 1.1 Mechanism of sudden cardiac death in individuals with altered morphological substrate.

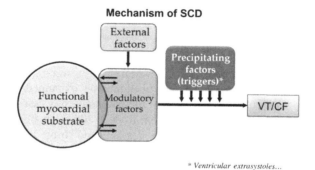

FIGURE 1.2 Mechanism of sudden cardiac death in individuals without morphological abnormalities.

between inward and outward currents. The duration of this plateau and the repolarization process which follows (phase 3 of APD) the plateau (phase 2 of the APD) are the main determinants of the time-length of the action potential. The APD is essential for the coupling of mechanical activity and periodic lack of excitability, but also for electrical synchronization with neighboring regions. The crucial participants of the repolarization process are the potassium slow and fast currents, I_{Ks} and I_{Kr}. Both are subjected to genetic alterations, as in congenital long QT syndromes. I_{Kr} is very sensitive to actions of many drugs. However, it would be simplistic to assume that the important repolarization process is dependent exclusively on these two currents. Instead, it is a highly redundant process involving multiple other known or unknown yet currents, a biological mechanism that has been conceptualized as the *repolarization reserve* (Roden, 2008). The concept

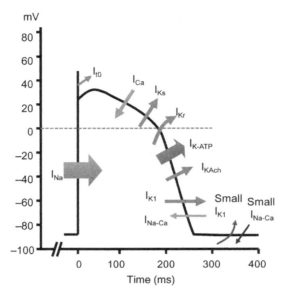

FIGURE 1.3 Main ionic currents responsible for action potential duration.

allows a better understanding of the variability in response to different genetic mutation or drug effects as a phenomenon explained not only by changes in the target channel, but also in the redundant processes responsible for the speed of myocardial repolarization. Roden (2008) has outlined a paradigm shift which had transformed what was believed to be an *idiosyncratic* drug reaction to a purely *syncratic* one (from Greek *idios* meaning peculiar, unique and *krasis* meaning mixture). In the light of this paradigm, individuals exhibiting marked QT prolongation while exposed to a drug which blocks or hampers the I_{Kr} function should be seen as a subpopulation with diminished repolarization reserve (Zipes, 2014). As I_{Kr} is a dominant component of the repolarization reserve, further diminishing of the repolarization reserve could precipitate *torsade de pointes* (TdP), as excessive prolongation of APD is a prerequisite of TdP. An example would be a patient taking a drug with I_{Kr} reducing effect and no obvious APD prolongation in normal state in whom the superimposition of heart failure could lead to development of TdP as heart failure per se diminishes the repolarization reserve through remodeling of the potassium dynamic by influencing the transient outward current (I_{TO}). The repolarization reserve can be reduced indirectly through an increase in sodium current (I_{Na}) leading to an increase in the proportion of depolarizing currents relative to repolarizing currents (Antzelevitch, 2007).

Prolongation of the APD is responsible for the genesis of *triggered activity* which may end in a TdP. The mechanism requires an early afterdepolarization (EAD) positive "spike" of the action potential at the end of phase 2 (induced mainly by an increase in I_{Na}) or during the phase 3 (induced by low I_K), when the cell is partly excitable, which eventually could reach the threshold and evoke a repetitive response. During these processes, the membrane conductance is low and a small calcium current (I_{Ca-L} window) could induce sufficient increase in voltage to reach the threshold (Jalife et al., 2009). This mechanism explains why the fixed combination of verapamil (a calcium channel blocker) with quinidine, known to prolong APD and QT and to induce TdP, is less torsadogenic than quinidine alone. However, localized APD prolongation with consecutive long QT and EAD are not enough to explain initiation and perpetuation of malignant ventricular arrhythmias such as TdP. The additional requirement appears to be a significant increase in the spatial dispersion of myocardial repolarization (Roden, 2008).

1.2.2   Amplification of Myocardial Dispersion of Repolarization

Ventricular myocardium provides an important safety factor against fibrillation (different from atrial myocardium) in that it is depolarized by a homogenous wave from endocardium to epicardium which assumes that adjacent regions are in the same electrical phase (Fig. 1.4a). In fact this homogeneity is not perfect. There are subtle differences between different myocardial layers creating small inhomogeneity of the APD and refractoriness, but these

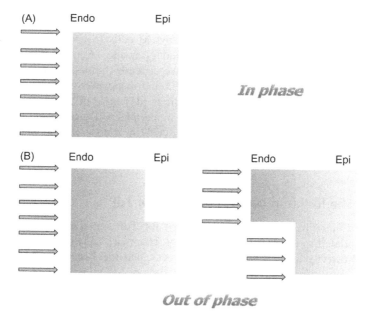

FIGURE 1.4   (a) The homogenous (in phase) and (b) inhomogeneous (out of phase) ventricular activation.

differences are too small to be arrhythmogenic. Structural myocardial abnormalities may create a situation in which adjacent regions are at a different point in the repolarization process, thereby creating the possibility of re-excitation from proximity (Fig. 1.4b). Amplification of transmural dispersion of repolarization together with EAD triggered activity represent the basis for TdP induction observed under QT prolongation conditions (Antzelevitch, 2007).

The mid-myocardial cells, also called M cells, are critical in accentuation of repolarization dispersion. These cells have the ability to prolong more than the neighboring cells, especially in response to slower rate (Anyukhovsky et al., 1999). The repolarizing current I_{Ks} is weak in these cells and counterbalanced by a more pronounced late sodium current when compared with endocardial and epicardial cells. The M cells are particularly sensitive to pathological processes which depress repolarizing currents or increase sodium and calcium depolarizing currents as their APD lengthen more than in epicardial and endocardial cells. These changes induce significant dispersion of repolarization and refractoriness. In the presence of sympathetic stimulation, the shorter APD duration in epicardial and endocardial cells, but not in M cells, augments the transmural repolarization dispersion. Sympathetic stimulation increases the risk for TdP in the case of more homogenous increase in QT, which may occur when the I_{Ks} is impaired. It should be emphasized that there is not always a correlation between QT prolongation and TdP risk as the main arrhythmogenic factor is transmural repolarization dispersion. Amiodarone and pentobarbital increase APD and QT, but decrease the dispersion, primarily in the M cells (Sicouri et al., 1997). Another example is that of quinidine and cisapride (Antzelevitch, 2007). Both drugs block repolarization in a dose-dependent manner and increase QT duration, but at higher dose both APD and dispersion diminish because of inward currents inhibition. Therefore drugs may have different degrees of torsadogenic potential; those increasing in parallel QT and dispersion are most torsadogenic, while those increasing APD in a dose-dependent fashion without parallel increase in dispersion are rarely torsadogenic (amiodarone, ranolazine, pentobarbital).

1.2.3 The Initiation and Perpetuation of TdP

The main electrical abnormalities required for TdP initiation and perpetuation are related to abnormal function of ion channels, APD prolongation and triggered activity, dispersion of refractoriness, and local reentry (Table 1.6). The proximity of regions with longer and shorter APD allow the latter to be reexcited by the former. The local reentry was demonstrated by wedge preparations and was named phase 2 reentry (Antzelevitch, 2008). APD prolongation of the last part of the action potential caused by outward (potassium) currents block, is more torsadogenic than that due to inward

TABLE 1.6 Components of the Torsadogenic Mechanism

Abnormal Function of Ion Channels

1. Loss of function (repolarization currents)
2. Gain of function (inward currents)

APD Prolongation and Triggered Activity

1. Early afterdepolarization
2. Delayed afterdepolarization

Dispersion of Refractoriness

1. Transmural
2. Regional

Local Reentry (Phase 2 Reentry)

sodium currents (Milberg et al., 2007). A triggered activity of early or delayed afterdepolarizations originating in M cells or Purkinje fibers stimulate regions with recovered excitability and tachycardia is subsequently perpetuated by phase 2 reentry. Drugs inhibiting the main inward sodium current I_{Na} change the plateau phase of the action potential and the cell becomes readily excitable from adjacent epicardial, endocardial, or M cells, especially if the APD/QT is already long. The mechanism is similar with that observed in Brugada syndrome where a mutation induces sodium channel loss-of-function.

1.2.4   Drug-Induced Prolongation of QT interval and TdP

Torsadogenic drugs represent approximately 3% of all prescriptions in developed countries (Zipes, 2014). The real incidence of drug-induced long QT interval and TdP is difficult to estimate. One recent report published by the Berlin Pharmacovigilance Center on data from a network of 51 German hospitals (Sarganas et al., 2014) produced an estimate of 2.5 million^{-1} year^{-1} for males and 4.0 million^{-1} year^{-1} for females. The authors point out that prior annual rates based on spontaneous report placed the incidence at 0.26 million^{-1}. This discrepancy is explained by the fact that QT prolongation and TdP have a plurifactorial etiology, such as drug effect and transient electrolyte imbalance.

The incidence of TdP is different for different molecules. For some antiarrhythmic drugs it can reach 1–5%, while for noncardiac drugs the incidence is lower. A well-publicized example is the risk of malignant arrhythmia associated with macrolide antibiotics, which has been estimated to affect 1/8.500 treated individuals with a death rate of 1/30,000 (Viskin et al., 2015). Prediction of TdP based on QT duration is lacking sensibility and specificity. QT interval prolongations to above 500 ms are considered to indicate a significant abnormality, but recent guidelines (Priori et al., 2015) indicate a cutoff value of 480 ms for QTc in repeated 12 channel ECGs. In a majority of cases TdP develops when patients have two or more associated risk factors (Viskin et al., 2015) more often female gender, electrolyte abnormalities, or high drug concentrations (Table 1.7).

Accurate prediction or quantification of risk for TdP is not possible at the present time. Monitored ECGs have shown that drug-induced TdP starts with a short−long−short initiation cycle (i.e., extrasystole−pause−extrasystole), long QTc interval preceding tachycardia, and prominent U wave at the beginning and at the end of tachycardia; the coupling interval is relatively long. The presence of short−long−short cycle(s) is a warning sign for an impending TdP episode.

As discussed, not all drugs that prolong QT are equally torsadogenic. A classification based on the QT prolonging drugs propensity to induce TdP was proposed (Haverkamp et al., 2001). Class A (high torsadogenic) drugs are potent blockers of currents prolonging myocardial repolarization, mainly I_{Kr}. QT prolongation has been documented at therapeutic doses and concentrations, and cases of TdP induced by the drug alone (in the absence of concomitant therapy prolonging repolarization or hypokalemia) have been documented. Class B drugs (medium high torsadogenic potency) prolong myocardial repolarization (i.e., cardiac APD and QT interval) at higher doses or at normal doses with concurrent administration of drugs that inhibit drug metabolism (e.g., by inhibiting the cytochrome P450 metabolism). For this class, the occurrence of TdP seems to require metabolic inhibition and the presence of other risk factors. Class C (low torsadogenic) drugs prolong APD and QT interval at high doses or concentrations that are clearly greater than the therapeutic range. Their effect on repolarization becomes manifest only with overdose or intoxication or in the presence of severe metabolic inhibition. Finally, Class D (torsadogenic potential not clearly established) drugs block repolarizing ion currents in vitro but have not been shown to prolong repolarization in other in vitro models (e.g., papillary muscle fibers or isolated hearts), or the concentrations necessary for this effect were far above the clinical concentrations. Prolongation of the QT interval in humans has not been demonstrated in systematic randomized studies (Haverkamp et al., 2001).

1.2.5 Antipsychotic-Induced QTc Prolongation

The association between treatment with antipsychotic drugs and SCD is generally attributed to these drugs' effect on myocardial repolarization, primarily by blocking the rapidly activating component of the delayed rectifier cardiac potassium current (I_{Kr}), a delay that creates conditions for the emergence of TdP, a polymorphic ventricular tachycardia that may in turn lead to

TABLE 1.7 Risk Factors for TdP Under Drugs Prolonging QT Interval

Condition	Mechanism	Magnitude of Risk
Female gender	Hormonal regulation of repolarization (testosterone effect)	Female/male ratio: 2/1–3/1
Bradycardia and AV block	More susceptibility for pause-dependent abnormal QT prolongation (long-short cycle)	Significant at $<60 \text{ min}^{-1}$
Hypokalemia	Decrease I_{Kr} and/or competitive block of sodium channel; residual I_{Kr} easier to block	Significant at $<3.5 \text{ mEq L}^{-1}$
Hypomagnesemia	Modulation of calcium handling (I_{Ca-L})	Significant when $<1.5 \text{ mEq L}^{-1}$
Recent atrial fibrillation conversion (mainly with QT prolonging drugs)	Post conversion pause and QT remodeling in AF	1–3% with QT prolonging drugs
High drug concentration or rapid infusion of QT prolonging drugs	Dose-concentration effect for QT prolonging drugs; biphase response for cisapride and quinidine	QT can increase with 50 ms with therapeutical dosage
Digitalis	Intracellular calcium overload and DAD; decrease potassium channel trafficking	Exceptional and only with digitalis toxicity
Subclinical genetic LQTS	Abnormal QT prolongation (sensibility) when exposed to I_{Kr} blocking drugs	<10% of congenital LQTS; several mutations described including potassium and sodium channel proteins
Ion channel polymorphism	Minor effect at baseline but leading to TdP with QT prolonging drugs	Several variants described including sodium channel polymorphism S1103Y in 10% Afro-Americans and some rare variants of potassium channel auxiliary proteins
Pharmacokinetic interaction	Interference with drugs metabolized by P450 system and Cyp3A4	Increased concentration when inhibited metabolism to very high in poor metabolizers
Structural abnormalities	Left ventricular hypertrophy, heart failure, left ventricular dysfunction	The importance and magnitude of structural cardiac abnormalities for TdP initiation was not established

Source: After Kannankeril, P., Roden, D.M., Darbar, D., 2010. Drug-induced long QT syndrome. Pharmacol. Rev. 62 (4), 760–781 (Kannankeril et al., 2010); Zipes, D.P., 2014. Cardiac Electrophysiology. From Cell to Bedside, sixth ed. Elsevier, Philadelphia, PA, pp. 1001–1004 and 1101–1102.

ventricular fibrillation (Glassman and Bigger, 2001; Haddad and Anderson, 2002). The blockade of the I_{Kr} is both direct and through the inhibition of the human ether-a-go-go (HERG) gene, which encodes the major protein involved in I_{Kr} (Lee et al., 2006).

The laboratory proof of these effects of antipsychotics has been possible by using two specific animal models. The expression of HERG is assessed in oocytes surgically removed from African clawed frog (*Xenopus laevis*), which are injected with complementary RNA, synthetic transcripts of specific DNA fragments. Solutions of antipsychotics are applied to the cells by continuous perfusion and potassium-filled microelectrodes are used for voltage recordings (Thomas et al., 2003; Choi et al., 2005; Lee et al., 2006). The I_{Kr} activity is measured with voltage clamps in single ventricular myocytes isolated from guinea pig (*Cavia porcellus*) using potassium-filled patch pipettes (Drolet et al., 2001, 2003; Choi et al., 2005; Lee et al., 2006; Morissette et al., 2007).

Using these techniques, significant prolongation of cardiac repolarization by blocking I_{Kr} have been shown for the first-generation drugs pimozide (Drolet et al., 2001) and trifluoperazine (Choi et al., 2005) and for the atypical antipsychotics risperidone (Drolet et al., 2003), clozapine (Lee et al., 2006), and olanzapine (Morissette et al., 2007). HERG blockade was demonstrated for trifluoperazine (Choi et al., 2005), clozapine (Lee et al., 2006), and olanzapine (Morissette et al., 2007). The impact of this effect on the duration of repolarization and risk of ventricular arrhythmia may be attenuated by the concomitant partial blockade of the L-type calcium current, as indicated in guinea pig papillary muscles exposed to risperidone (Christ et al., 2005).

In clinical studies, the myocardial repolarization delay attributable to antipsychotic treatment has been assessed by changes in the heart rate-corrected QTc and their association with TdP and sudden death. The vast literature addressing these issues has been comprehensively reviewed by Hasnain and Vieweg (2014), who concluded that the QTc prolongation–TdP link was not demonstrated in trials of second-generation antipsychotic drugs, that is, in carefully monitored cases receiving standard therapeutic dosages. The analysis of the case reports indicated that the QTc prolongation with/without TdP was most likely to occur when the patients treated with antipsychotic drugs had preexistent risk factors for myocardial repolarization delays and ventricular arrhythmias (Table 1.6). Drug–drug interactions are particularly important and primarily produced cytochrome P450 inhibition (Table 1.8). Of considerable interest is the fact that selective serotonin reuptake inhibitors have been linked to QTc prolongation and TdP in a very limited number of cases (Kogut et al., 2013). Other risk factors, identified in cases of noncardiac drug-induced TdP include bradycardia, recent conversion from atrial fibrillation and ion channel polymorphisms (Marzuillo et al., 2014). A biological gradient has not been demonstrated in a prospective

TABLE 1.8 Examples of Commonly Used Drugs That May Increase the Severity of Myocardial Depolarization Delay Induced by Antipsychotics

Antidepressants
Venlafaxine
Escitalopram
Mirtazapine
Sertraline
Fluoxetine
Imipramine
Clomipramine
Trazodone
Antiinfectives
Trimethoprim/sulfa
Levofloxacin
Azithromycin
Amantadine
Atazanavir
Foscarnet
Ketoconazole
Antiarrhythmics
Sotalol
Dronedarone
Antihypertensives
Nicardipine
Cancer Chemotherapy Drugs
Tamoxifen
Sunitinib
H2-Receptor Antagonists
Famotidine

Source: Adapted from Marzuillo et al. (2014).

study in which plasma levels of ziprasidone, a drug known to produce significant QTc prolongation, were measured on the days electrocardiograms were recorded (Correll et al., 2011) or in a matched case—control assessment of polytherapy with two antipsychotics (Correll et al., 2009).

The correlation between the severity of QTc prolongation and the occurrence of TdP is not strong. For example, in a recent report evaluating the 12 published cases of QTc prolongation during treatment or overdose with quetiapine, there were 4 cases of TdP (Hasnain et al., 2014). The arrhythmia occurred in patients with QTc in the range of 529–720 ms, but three patients with QTc greater than 600 ms (620, 684, and 710 ms) remained arrhythmia-free.

Recent data have questioned the assumption that the mechanism of SCD in patients treated with antipsychotics must involve a lethal ventricular tachyarrhythmia (Teodorescu et al., 2013). The investigation used the Oregon Sudden Unexpected Death Study database collected from 2002 to 2009 to evaluate 509 cases of documented ventricular fibrillation/ventricular tachycardia and 309 instances of pulseless electrical activity. Treatment with antipsychotic drugs was identified as a significant predictor of pulseless electrical activity versus ventricular tachyarrhythmia (odds ratio 2.40; 95% confidence interval 1.2–4.53) after adjusting for age, gender, comorbid conditions, and resuscitation parameters. The explanations proposed for this association include a drug effect on myocardial contractility (Teodorescu et al., 2013), or other antipsychotic-related adverse effects, such as pulmonary embolism and diabetic ketoacidosis (Peacock and Whang, 2013).

1.3 CLINICAL AND LABORATORY FEATURES

The individual who develops chest pain, hypotension, hypoxia, and rales suggestive of pulmonary edema just before dying in the ambulance can be safely assumed to have had an acute coronary event. In many other cases the explanation for the sudden and unexpected death will require careful anatomical, histological, and toxicological assessments. This reality is very poorly captured in death certificates, particularly since ventricular fibrillation or pulseless electrical activity are the final events in any fatality that involves hypoxia, pump failure, metabolic acidosis, or severe electrolyte disturbance.

The majority of sudden and unexpected fatalities in the general population are due to coronary artery disease. The proportion of coronary artery disease as a cause of sudden death was 80% in Hennepin County, Minnesota (Adabag et al., 2010) and 63% in Ireland (Downes et al., 2010). Many of these deaths occur in patients without a clinical documentation of heart disease. In autopsies of adult hospital patients who were presumed to have died of cardiac arrhythmia in Pittsburgh, Pennsylvania, 53% had histological evidence of myocardial infarction (Nichols and Chew, 2012). Similar findings were reported in a prospective study of individuals without history of cardiac disease autopsied in 83 coroner's jurisdictions in England, in whom death was ascribed to acute ischemic changes in more than half of the subjects (Bowker et al., 2003). Other structural and functional heart disorders have

TABLE 1.9 Cardiac Abnormalities Leading to Sudden Death

Structural Disorders

Coronary artery disease

Hypertrophic and/or dilated cardiomyopathy

Right ventricular cardiomyopathy

Aortic stenosis

Myocarditis

Functional Disorders

Long QT syndrome

Brugada syndrome

Preexcitation syndromes

Catecholaminergic polymorphic ventricular tachycardia

Idiopathic ventricular tachycardia

also been found to lead to sudden death (Priori et al., 2001) in the general population, but have not been prospectively evaluated in patients treated with antipsychotic drugs (Table 1.9).

1.4   PREVENTION AND MANAGEMENT

Antipsychotic-induced repolarization abnormalities (prolonged QTc) must be considered in the assessment of the potential for SCD and electrocardiograms must be performed prior to the initiation of antipsychotic treatment for at-risk groups of patients (Table 1.10). At-risk patients with electrocardiographic findings suggesting an increased risk for TdP (Table 1.11) should not be given antipsychotic drugs without clearance from a cardiology consultant and correction of reversible abnormalities, such as electrolyte disturbance or drug—drug interactions.

The available data suggest that a substantial decrease in the prevalence of SCD in patients with severe mental illness can be obtained through programs aimed at the primary prevention of coronary artery disease and secondary prevention of myocardial infarction. In the Framingham Heart Study, from 1950 to 1999, such programs have proven their effectiveness among individuals without psychotic disorders by decreasing the risks of sudden death and nonsudden mortality related to coronary artery disease by 49% and 64%, respectively (Fox et al., 2004). Meaningful reductions will require early detection and treatment of coronary and diabetogenic risk factors in

TABLE 1.10 Indications for Performing Electrocardiograms in Prior to Starting Treatment With Antipsychotic Drugs

Family history of sudden death

Family history of unexplained death before age 40

Family history of QTc prolongation

History of QTc prolongation or abnormal EKG

History of documented arrhythmias

History of symptoms suggestive of arrhythmias (syncope, seizures, dizzy spells, palpitations)

History of cardiovascular disease (coronary artery disease, stroke or transient ischemic attacks, cardiomyopathy, aortic aneurysms, peripheral arterial insufficiency)

History of diabetes mellitus

Age 65 or older

Risk factors (2 or more) for coronary artery disease (hypertension, dyslipidemia, smoking, age 50 or older, family history of coronary artery disease)

Current treatment with drugs known to prolong QTc

Increased risk of hypokalemia and/or hypomagnesemia (e.g., diuretic drugs, recent episodes of diarrhea or vomiting, dehydration)

TABLE 1.11 Electrocardiographic Findings Suggesting Increased Risk of *Torsade de Pointes*

QTc >500 ms

QT dispersion >100 ms (difference between the longest and shortest QT interval in a 12 lead EKG)

Abnormal T waves (long peak-to-end, T alternans)

Large U waves

psychiatric settings, but provider, patient, and system level barriers exist and must be addressed (De Hert et al., 2011), particularly with regard to the access and quality of medical care.

REFERENCES

Adabag, A.S., Peterson, G., Apple, F.S., Titus, J., King, R., Luepker, R.V., 2010. Etiology of sudden death in the community: results of anatomical, metabolic, and genetic evaluation. Am. Heart. J. 159 (1), 33–39.

Antzelevitch, C., 2007. Ionic, molecular, and cellular bases of QT-interval prolongation and torsade de pointes. Europace 9 (Suppl. 4), iv4–15. Available from: http://dx.doi.org/10.1093/europace/eum166.

Antzelevitch, C., 2008. Drug-induced spatial dispersion of repolarization. Cardiol. J. 15 (2), 100–121.

Anyukhovsky, E.P., Sosunov, E.A., Gainullin, R.Z., Rosen, M.R., 1999. The controversial M cell. J. Cardiovasc. Electrophysiol. 10 (2), 244–260.

Bayés de Luna, A., Coumel, P., Leclercq, J.F., 1989. Ambulatory sudden cardiac death: mechanisms of production of fatal arrhythmia on the basis of data from 157 cases. Am. Heart. J. 117 (1), 151–159.

Behr, E.R., Casey, A., Sheppard, M., Wright, M., Bowker, T.J., Davies, M.J., et al., 2007. Sudden arrhythmic death syndrome: a national survey of sudden unexplained cardiac death. Heart 93 (5), 601–605.

Bowker, T.J., Wood, D.A., Davies, M.J., Sheppard, M.N., Cary, N.R., Burton, J.D., et al., 2003. Sudden, unexpected cardiac or unexplained death in England: a national survey. QJM 96 (4), 269–279.

Choi, S.Y., Koh, Y.S., Jo, S.H., 2005. Inhibition of human ether-a-go-go-related gene K^+ channel and IKr of guinea pig cardiomyocytes by antipsychotic drug trifluoperazine. J. Pharmacol. Exp. Ther. 313 (2), 888–895.

Christ, T., Wettwer, E., Ravens, U., 2005. Risperidone-induced action potential prolongation is attenuated by increased repolarization reserve due to concomitant block of I(Ca,L). Naunyn Schmiedebergs Arch. Pharmacol. 371 (5), 393–400.

Correll, C.U., Frederickson, A.M., Figen, V., Ginn-Scott, E.J., Pantaleon Moya, R.A., Kane, J. M., et al., 2009. The QTc interval and its dispersion in patients receiving two atypical antipsychotics: a matched case-control study. Eur. Arch. Psychiatry Clin. Neurosci. 259, 23–27.

Correll, C.U., Lops, J., Figen, V., Kane, J.M., Malhotra, A.K., Manu, P., 2011. QT interval duration and dispersion in children and adolescents treated with ziprasidone. J. Clin. Psychiatry 72, 854–860.

De Hert, M., Cohen, D., Bobes, J., Cetkovich-Bakmas, M., Leucht, S., Ndetei, D.M., et al., 2011. Physical illness in patients with severe mental disorders. II. Barriers to care, monitoring and treatment guidelines, plus recommendations at the system and individual level. World Psychiatry 10 (2), 138–151.

Downes, M.R., Thorne, J., Tengku Khalid, T.N., Hassan, H.A., Leader, M., 2010. Profile of sudden death in an adult population (1999-2008). Ir. Med. J. 103 (6), 183–184.

Drolet, B., Rousseau, G., Daleau, P., Cardinal, R., Simard, C., Turgeon, J., 2001. Pimozide (Orap) prolongs cardiac repolarization by blocking the rapid component of the delayed rectifier potassium current in native cardiac myocytes. J. Cardiovasc. Pharmacol. Ther. 6 (3), 255–260.

Drolet, B., Yang, T., Daleau, P., Roden, D.M., Turgeon, J., 2003. Risperidone prolongs cardiac repolarization by blocking the rapid component of the delayed rectifier potassium current. J. Cardiovasc. Pharmacol. 41 (6), 934–937.

Fox, C.S., Evans, J.C., Larson, M.G., Kannel, W.B., Levy, D., 2004. Temporal trends in coronary heart disease mortality and sudden cardiac death from 1950 to 1999: the Framingham Heart Study. Circulation 110 (5), 522–527.

Glassman, A.H., Bigger Jr., J.T., 2001. Antipsychotic drugs: prolonged QTc interval, torsade de pointes, and sudden death. Am. J. Psychiatry 158 (11), 1774–1782.

Haddad, P.M., Anderson, I.M., 2002. Antipsychotic-related QTc prolongation, torsade de pointes and sudden death. Drugs 62 (11), 1649–1671.

Hasnain, M., Vieweg, W.V., 2014. QTc interval prolongation and torsade de pointes associated with second-generation antipsychotics and antidepressants: a comprehensive review. CNS Drugs 28 (10), 887–920.

Hasnain, M., Vieweg, W.V., Howland, R.H., Kogut, C., Breden Crouse, E.L., Koneru, J.N., et al., 2014. Quetiapine, QTc interval prolongation, and torsade de pointes: a review of case reports. Ther. Adv. Psychopharmacol 4 (3), 130–138.

Jalife, J., Delmar, M., Anumonwo, I., Berenfeld, O., Kalifa, J., 2009. Basic Cardiac Electrophysiology for the Clinician, second ed. Wiley-Blackwell, Oxford, UK, pp. 167–169.

Kannankeril, P., Roden, D.M., Darbar, D., 2010. Drug-induced long QT syndrome. Pharmacol. Rev. 62 (4), 760–781.

Kogut, C., Crouse, E.B., Vieweg, W.V., Hasnain, M., Baranchuk, A., Digby, G.C., et al., 2013. Selective serotonin reuptake inhibitors and torsade de pointes: new concepts and new directions derived from a systematic review of case reports. Ther. Adv. Drug Saf. 4 (5), 189–198.

Haverkamp, W., Eckardt, L., Mo, G., Wedekind, H., Kirchhof, P., Haverkamp, F., et al., 2001. Clinical aspects of ventricular arrhythmias associated with QT prolongation. Eur. Heart J. 3, K81–K88.

Hennessy, S., Bilker, W.B., Knauss, J.S., Margolis, D.J., Kimmel, S.E., Reyniolds, R.F., et al., 2002. Cardiac arrest and ventricular arrhythmia in patients taking antipsychotic drugs: cohort study using administrative data. BMJ 325 (7372), 1070.

Jolly, K., Gammage, M.D., Cheng, K.K., Bradburn, P., Banting, M.V., Langman, M.J., 2009. Sudden death in patients receiving drugs tending to prolong the QT interval. Br. J. Clin. Pharmacol. 68 (5), 743–751.

Lee, S.Y., Kim, Y.J., Kim, K.T., Choe, H., Jo, S.H., 2006. Blockade of HERG human K$^+$ channels and IKr of guinea-pig cardiomyocytes by the antipsychotic drug clozapine. Br. J. Pharmacol. 148 (4), 499–509.

Lieberman, J.A., Merrill, D., Parameswaran, S., 2012. APA Guidance on the Use of Antipsychotic Drugs and Sudden Cardiac Death. N.Y.S. Office of Mental Health, Albany, NY.

Leonard, C.E., Freeman, C.P., Newcomb, C.W., Bilker, W.B., Kimmel, S.E., Strom, B.L., et al., 2013. Antipsychotics and the risks of sudden cardiac death and all-cause death: cohort studies in Medicaid and dually-eligible Medicaid-Medicare beneficiaries in five states. J. Clin. Exp. Cardiol. Suppl. 10 (6), 1–9.

Marzuillo, P., Benettoni, A., Germani, C., Ferrara, G., D'Agata, B., Barbi, E., 2014. Acquired long QT syndrome: a focus for the general pediatrician. Pediatr. Emerg. Care 30 (4), 257–261.

Milberg, P., Hilker, E., Ramtin, S., Cakir, Y., Stypmann, J., Engel, M.A., et al., 2007. Proarrhythmia as a class effect of quinolones: increased dispersion of repolarization and triangulation of action potential predict torsades de pointes. J. Cardiovasc. Electrophysiol. 18 (6), 647–654.

Morissette, P., Hreiche, R., Mallet, L., Vo, D., Knaus, E.E., Turgeon, J., 2007. Olanzapine prolongs cardiac repolarization by blocking the rapid component of the delayed rectifier potassium current. J. Psychopharmacol. 21 (7), 735–741.

Murray-Thomas, T., Jones, M.E., Patel, D., Brunner, E., Shatapathy, C.C., Motsko, S., et al., 2013. Risk of mortality (including sudden cardiac death) and major cardiovascular events in atypical and typical antipsychotic users: a study with the general practice research database. Cardiovasc. Psychiatry Neurol 2013, 247486.

Nichols, L., Chew, B., 2012. Causes of sudden unexpected death of adult hospital patients. J. Hosp. Med. 7 (9), 706–708.

Peacock, J., Whang, W., 2013. Antipsychotic medications and sudden cardiac arrest: more than meets the eye? Heart Rhythm 10 (4), 531–532.

Priori, S.G., Aliot, E., Blomastrom-Lundqvist, L., et al., 2001. Task Force on sudden cardiac death of the European Society of Cardiology. Eur. Heart J. 22, 1374–1450.

Priori, S.G., Blomström-Lundqvist, C., Mazzanti, A., Blom, N., Borggrefe, M., Camm, J., et al., 2015. 2015 ESC Guidelines for the management of patients with ventricular arrhythmias and the prevention of sudden cardiac death: The Task Force for the Management of Patients with Ventricular Arrhythmias and the Prevention of Sudden Cardiac Death of the Europe. Eur. Heart J. 36 (41), 2793–2867. Available from: http://dx.doi.org/10.1093/eurheartj/ehv316.

Ray, W.A., Meredith, S., Thapa, P.B., Meador, K.G., Hall, K., Murray, K.T., 2001. Antipsychotics and the risk of sudden cardiac death. Arch. Gen. Psychiatry 58 (12), 1161–1167.

Ray, W.A., Chung, C.P., Murray, K.T., Hall, K., Stein, C.M., 2009. Atypical antipsychotic drugs and the risk of sudden cardiac death. N. Engl. J. Med. 360 (3), 225–235.

Roden, D.M., 1998. Taking the 'idio' out of 'idiosyncratic': predicting torsades de pointes. Pacing Clin. Electrophysiol. 21 (5), 1029–1034.

Roden, D.M., 2008. Repolarization reserve: a moving target. Circulation 118 (10), 981–982.

Salvo, F., Pariente, A., Shakir, S., Robinson, P., Arnaud, M., Thomas, S.H., et al., 2015. Sudden cardiac and sudden unexpected death related to antipsychotics: a meta-analysis of observational studies. Clin. Pharmacol. Ther. 99 (3), 306–314. Available from: http://dx.doi.org/10.1002/cpt.250.

Sarganas, G., Garbe, E., Klimpel, A., Hering, R.C., Bronder, E., Haverkamp, W., 2014. Epidemiology of symptomatic drug-induced long QT syndrome and torsade de pointes in Germany. Europace 16 (1), 101–108.

Sicouri, S., Moro, S., Litovsky, S., Elizari, M.V., Antzelevitch, C., 1997. Chronic amiodarone reduces transmural dispersion of repolarization in the canine heart. J. Cardiovasc. Electrophysiol. 8 (11), 1269–1279.

Straus, S.M., Bleumink, G.S., Dieleman, J.P., van der Lei, J., t Jong, G.W., Kingma, J.H., et al., 2004. Antipsychotics and the risk of sudden cardiac death. Arch. Intern. Med. 164, 1293–1297.

Strom, B.L., Eng, S.M., Faich, G., Reynolds, R.F., D'Agostino, R.B., Ruskin, J., et al., 2011. Comparative mortality associated with ziprasidone and olanzapine in real-world use among 18,154 patients with schizophrenia: The Ziprasidone Observational Study of Cardiac Outcomes (ZODIAC). Am. J. Psychiatry 168 (2), 193–201.

Teodorescu, C., Reinier, K., Uy-Evanado, A., Chugh, H., Gunson, K., Jui, J., et al., 2013. Antipsychotic drugs are associated with pulseless electrical activity: the Oregon Sudden Unexpected Death Study. Heart Rhythm 10 (4), 526–530.

Thomas, D., Wu, K., Kathöfer, S., Katus, H.A., Schoels, W., Kiehn, J., et al., 2003. The antipsychotic drug chlorpromazine inhibits HERG potassium channels. Br. J. Pharmacol. 139 (3), 567–574.

Thomas, S.H., Drici, M.D., Hall, G.C., Crocq, M.A., Everitt, B., Lader, M.H., et al., 2010. Safety of sertindole versus risperidone in schizophrenia: principal results of the sertindole cohort prospective study (SCoP). Acta Psychiatr. Scand. 122 (5), 345–355.

Viskin, S., Havakuk, O., Schwaber, M.J., 2015. Pro-arrhythmic effects of noncardiac medications. J. Am. Coll. Cardiol. 66 (20), 2185–2188.

Wu, C., Tsai, Y., Tsai, H., 2015. Antipsychotic drugs and the risk of ventricular arrhythmia and/or sudden cardiac death: a nation-wide cross-over study. J. Am. Heart Assoc. 4, e001568.

Zipes, D.P., 2014. Cardiac Electrophysiology. From Cell to Bedside, sixth ed. Elsevier, Philadelphia, PA, pp. 1001–1004 and 1101–1102.

Chapter 2

Myocarditis and Cardiomyopathy

Kathlyn J. Ronaldson
Monash University, Melbourne, VIC, Australia

2.1 DEFINITIONS

Myocarditis is inflammation of the myocardium (Stevenson and Loscalzo, 2012). Specifically, hypersensitivity myocarditis, an idiosyncratic response to a substance, involves infiltration of myocardial tissue with lymphocytes and mononuclear cells, commonly with a high proportion of eosinophils (Stevenson and Loscalzo, 2012). Despite the proliferation of eosinophils in the heart, hypersensitivity myocarditis is distinct from hypereosinophilic syndrome which is characterized by peripheral eosinophilia (Meth and Sperber, 2006). Levels of circulating eosinophils commonly rise with hypersensitivity myocarditis but not always (Ronaldson et al., 2010). The signs and symptoms of myocarditis are usually nonspecific. Cardiac function may be preserved or the condition may lead to left ventricular systolic dysfunction (Caforio et al., 2013; Ronaldson et al., 2011b.

Cardiomyopathy is a heterogeneous group of diseases of the myocardium (Stevenson and Loscalzo, 2012; Wexler et al., 2009). In hypertrophic cardiomyopathy left ventricular wall thickness is increased, but left ventricular ejection fraction (LVEF) is not diminished, while dilated cardiomyopathy is characterized by increased left ventricular diastolic dimension and decreased systolic function. The threshold for dilated cardiomyopathy is usually a LVEF of 50%. Both dilated and hypertrophic cardiomyopathy may occur together in the one case (Roh et al., 2006; Tanner and Culling, 2003). In the early stages of development, cardiomyopathy is asymptomatic, but as the disease progresses symptoms of heart failure are manifest, particularly exertional intolerance.

Life-Threatening Effects of Antipsychotic Drugs. DOI: http://dx.doi.org/10.1016/B978-0-12-803376-0.00002-2
© 2016 Elsevier Inc. All rights reserved.

2.2 EPIDEMIOLOGY

2.2.1 Causality

A data mining study of antipsychotics using the international database of adverse reactions run by the World Health Organisation found evidence supportive of a causal relationship for cardiac muscle disorders, specifically myocarditis and cardiomyopathy, with only clozapine. Possible, considerably weaker, associations were observed with lithium, chlorpromazine, and fluphenazine (Coulter et al., 2001). Although quetiapine and olanzapine may be considered possible contenders for cardiac muscle disorders, because of the confirmed causal relationship with clozapine and their similar chemical structure, no support for these associations was found in this analysis.

Fourteen years after the data mining study, the evidence of causal associations with myocarditis or cardiomyopathy for other antipsychotics, including quetiapine and olanzapine, remains tenuous. Cases of myocarditis and cardiomyopathy with antipsychotics other than clozapine have been published in the literature. Six published cases of cardiomyopathy and/or myocarditis with quetiapine may be considered limited evidence of a causal association (Wassef et al., 2015; Bush and Burgess, 2008; Coffey and Williams, 2011; Nymark et al., 2008; Roesch-Ely et al., 2002). For other antipsychotics, risperidone, perphenazine, amisulpride, chlorpromazine, haloperidol, and aripiprazole, the published cases represent flimsy evidence (Ansari et al., 2003; Bhatia et al., 2009; Brakoulias et al., 2005; Christoffersen et al., 2011; Marti, 2005; Roussel et al., 2006). That myocarditis or cardiomyopathy may have had other causes and occurred coincidentally on antipsychotic use is an alternative explanation for these cases.

Two studies have contributed data pertinent to this discussion. Kelly et al. (2009) reviewed deaths with autopsy reports among patients taking clozapine or risperidone in the US state of Maryland. They found that 5% of deaths with either drug (3% vs 2%, respectively) were caused by cardiomyopathy and one clozapine-related death was caused by myocarditis. While superficially this result could indicate an equivalent causal relationship for clozapine and risperidone, it must be considered that other risk factors for cardiomyopathy are prevalent among patients with schizophrenia and autopsies were available for only 20% of deaths with risperidone and 32% with clozapine. A further study with 47 reports of cardiomyopathy in the French Pharmacovigilance Database, calculated reporting odds ratios (ORs) of 18.9 (95% confidence interval (CI) 6.9−52.2) for clozapine and 14.7 (4.6−47.1) for olanzapine; no other antipsychotics were implicated (Montastruc et al., 2010). While these associations were significant ($p < 0.01$), they were based on only four and three cases, respectively, meaning the results are statistically unstable, as is also indicated by the width of the CIs.

TABLE 2.1 Reports of Myocarditis or Cardiomyopathy With Selected Antipsychotics in the Australian National Adverse Reaction Reporting Program Held by the Therapeutic Goods Administration (2015)

Drug	Number of Reports/Fatal Outcome			
	All Adverse Events	Myocarditis	Cardiomyopathy	Clozapine Implicated
Clozapine	7583/366	801/24	309/11	
Quetiapine	916/40	8/1	8/1	5/0
Olanzapine	1704/74	7/2	12/2	6/2
Risperidone	1471/43	3/0	4/0	2/0
Amisulpride	301/9	1/0	1/0	0
Aripiprazole	301/5	2/1	0	1/0
Haloperidol	816/25	5/0	4/0	7/0
Chlorpromazine	618/22	4/0	1/0	4/0
Zuclopenthixol	188/8	2/0	1/0	2/0

Among adverse events attributable to clozapine and reported to the Australian Therapeutic Goods Administration, more than 10% were of myocarditis and 4% of cardiomyopathy (Table 2.1) (Therapeutic Goods Administration, 2015). In contrast, for other selected antipsychotics, around 1%, or less, of reports was of myocarditis or cardiomyopathy, and for a substantial proportion of these, clozapine was a suspected medicine.

These data provide a tenuous basis for a causal relationship between antipsychotics, other than clozapine, and cardiac muscle disorders. There are further data in support of the relationship with clozapine which should be examined.

Kilian et al. (1999) published a pivotal Australian report describing 15 cases (5 fatal) of myocarditis and 8 (1 fatal) of cardiomyopathy associated with clozapine. All cases of myocarditis had occurred within the first month after commencing clozapine and the authors calculated a mortality rate from myocarditis for patients commencing clozapine of 0.6 per 1000 person-months, using Australian usage data. In contrast, the global background rate for death from myocarditis was 0.33 per million person-months. The 2000-fold difference in rate was indicative of a causal relationship. The case was strengthened by the previously mentioned analysis by Coulter et al. (2001) which found no evidence that myocarditis or cardiomyopathy may be associated with schizophrenia or that clozapine was being used with other drugs causing these disorders.

Further data supporting the causal case for clozapine and myocarditis are the evidence that it typically develops within the first 4 weeks after commencing clozapine (Haas et al., 2007), with 83% of cases occurring between days 14 and 21 inclusive (Ronaldson et al., 2011b). Further, the risk increases with increasing rate of clozapine dose titration as measured by the total dose taken in the first 9 days of clozapine initiation (Ronaldson et al., 2012d).

Mechanistic evidence of a causal association between clozapine and cardiomyopathy will be presented later in this chapter, suffice it to make two points here. First, Kilian et al. (1999) observed that the incidence of cardiomyopathy was fivefold greater among clozapine recipients in Australia than in the general population. Second, cardiomyopathy may develop as a consequence of myocarditis if the disease does not resolve, but continues subclinically (Caforio et al., 2013; Kilian et al., 1999).

Because of the tenuousness of the evidence for an association with antipsychotics other than clozapine, this chapter will focus on clozapine as the causal agent.

2.2.2   Prevalence and Incidence

2.2.2.1   Myocarditis

The incidence of myocarditis with clozapine is controversial (Cohen et al., 2012; Ronaldson et al., 2015a). Myocarditis is reported to occur at least 10 times more frequently in Australia than elsewhere, with the reported incidence elsewhere being less than 1 in 1000 patients commencing clozapine and in Australia greater than 1 in 100. Ronaldson et al. (2015a) have proposed that the difference in reported incidence is attributable not to a higher event rate in Australia, but a higher case ascertainment rate due to use of a monitoring regimen and a high level of suspicion among psychiatrists, cardiologists, and pathologists, together with a well-subscribed central repository for adverse reaction reports. The authors argued that many cases are missed elsewhere for several reasons which include the confounding of the diagnosis by the nonspecific nature of the signs and symptoms; the critical importance of appropriate investigations being conducted at the time of myocardial involvement; and, the dependence of the diagnosis of fatal cases on the affected area of the myocardium being sampled for histology.

2.2.2.2   Cardiomyopathy

It is more common to determine the prevalence, rather than incidence, of cardiomyopathy, as the usual approach is to conduct a cross-sectional study to ascertain the number with left ventricular impairment among patients stabilized for a range of durations on long-term clozapine. Table 2.2 presents the

TABLE 2.2 Prevalence and Incidence of Cardiomyopathy With Clozapine in Various Studies

Reference	Country	Total Patients	Duration of Clozapine	Prevalence	Incidence	Comment
Reinders et al. (2004)	Australia	94		1%		Diagnosis at autopsy after 0.4 yr
Rostagno et al. (2011b)	Italy	38	5.5 ± 3.1 yr mean ± SD	8%		1 had LVEF < 30%
Murch et al. (2013)	Australia	79	Mean 3.7 yr	1%	0.22/100 patient-yr	All had normal baseline echo
Kidd et al. (2013)	Australia	25	Mean 6 yr; range 1–13.5 yr	12%		3 cases diagnosed at 6, 7, and 9 yr; routine echo
Chow et al. (2014b)	Australia	100	6.8 ± 5.3 yr mean ± SD	9%		All asymptomatic; all had echo
Serrano et al. (2014)	Venezuela	125	4.6 ± 4.5 yr mean ± SD	0		All had echo

Echo, echocardiogram; LVEF, left ventricular ejection fraction; SD, standard deviation; yr, year(s).

prevalence or incidence calculated in six studies, of varying quality, and varying results (0−12%) for prevalence (Chow et al., 2014a; Kidd et al., 2013; Murch et al., 2013; Reinders et al., 2004; Rostagno et al., 2011b; Serrano et al., 2014). Of these studies, only that by Murch et al. (2013) included only patients with normal baseline echocardiography; nine patients screened for the study had a LVEF of less than 50% before commencing clozapine. The patients included by Chow et al. (2014a) had taken clozapine for at least 1 year and all were asymptomatic at the time of echocardiography. These authors found no relationship between duration of clozapine use and factors associated with development of cardiomyopathy.

These data leave the prevalence and incidence of cardiomyopathy in patients on clozapine, without baseline left ventricular impairment, an open question. Separation of the effect of clozapine from contributions from diabetes, obesity, familial factors, and age necessitates the inclusion of a matched control group and/or inclusion of these factors in the analysis. Investigation of the relationship with clozapine exposure time requires exclusion of individuals with left ventricular dysfunction at baseline, as well as larger numbers of participants than in any previous study.

2.2.3 Risk Factors

2.2.3.1 Myocarditis

A case−control study of clozapine and myocarditis included 105 cases and 296 controls, matched by psychiatric unit at which clozapine was commenced and approximately by clozapine start date (Ronaldson et al., 2012d). The purpose of the study was to identify risk factors for myocarditis in patients commencing clozapine. All cases were required to have occurred within the first 45 days of clozapine titration and to meet a case definition involving clinical characteristics and cardiac-specific diagnostic measures, in the absence of other possible confounding factors. Control patients were required to have taken clozapine for at least 45 days, to ensure they had sufficient exposure to develop myocarditis, if they were at risk, and to have documented evidence adequate to exclude myocarditis.

In multivariate analysis, this study found that the risk of myocarditis was increased by 26% for every additional 250 mg clozapine administered during the first 9 days after initiation (OR 1.26; 95% CI 1.02−1.55; $p = 0.03$), increased by 31% for each decade in age (OR 1.31; 95% CI 1.07−1.60; $p = 0.009$), and by concomitant administration of sodium valproate (OR 2.59; 95% CI 1.51−4.42; $p = 0.001$). No statistically significant effects were observed with other medication (Table 2.3). The risk was independent of gender, and increasing body mass index (BMI) had an effect approaching statistical significance (for each 5 kg m^{-2} increment OR 1.18; 95% CI

TABLE 2.3 Adjusted Odds Ratios for the Association of Concomitant Medication With Clozapine-Induced Myocarditis

Concomitant Medication	OR	95% CI	p-Value[a]
Sodium valproate	2.59	1.51−4.42	0.001
Amisulpride	0.96	0.42−2.20	0.92
Aripiprazole	2.52	0.95−6.67	0.06
Benzatropine	1.18	0.64−2.16	0.60
Chlorpromazine	1.05	0.36−3.04	0.93
Flupenthixol	0.96	0.32−2.84	0.94
Haloperidol	0.95	0.34−2.62	0.91
Lithium	1.45	0.56−3.74	0.44
Olanzapine	0.83	0.48−1.44	0.51
Quetiapine	0.88	0.46−1.67	0.69
Risperidone	0.92	0.52−1.63	0.78
Zuclopenthixol	0.46	0.18−1.18	0.11

CI, confidence interval; OR, odds ratio.
[a]Correcting for multiple analyses, 12 concomitant medications, the significance threshold is p = 0.004 (0.05/12).
Source: Ronaldson, K.J., Fitzgerald, P.B., Taylor, A.J., Topliss, D.J., Wolfe, R., McNeil, J.J. 2012d. Rapid clozapine dose titration and concomitant sodium valproate increase the risk of myocarditis with clozapine: a case-control study. Schizophr. Res. 141 (2−3), 173−178.

0.97−1.44; $p = 0.09$). Despite increasing the rate of clozapine metabolism, smoking did not have a statistically significant protective effect (OR 0.71; 95% CI 0.40−1.25; $p = 0.23$).

The mechanism for the interaction with sodium valproate is unknown. There are data in support of valproate inhibiting the metabolism of clozapine and data in support of an inducing effect (Diaz et al., 2008, 2014). To date, all studies of this interaction have been of poor quality; clozapine plasma levels in patients taking clozapine alone were not compared with plasma levels in the same patients when they are taking clozapine plus valproate, and the doses were not standardized or matched. Because of the large number of subjects, probably the most reliable data on this question are those published by Couchman et al. (2010). Means and 90% CIs for clozapine and norclozapine plasma concentrations did not differ between 1184 patients taking clozapine and sodium valproate and 24,000 taking clozapine alone. The interaction observed in the risk factor study may in truth be pharmacodynamic, not pharmacokinetic.

In individuals who have previously taken clozapine without developing myocarditis and who are recommencing it, the risk of myocarditis is small, but not vanishingly small. The OR for these patients was 0.19 (95% CI 0.06−0.66; $p = 0.008$). The study included three cases who were recommencing clozapine, and one of these was fatal (Ronaldson et al., 2011a, 2012d).

2.2.3.2 Cardiomyopathy

No systematic studies have been conducted to assess host- or treatment-related risk factors for clozapine-related cardiomyopathy. Cardiomyopathy occurring in a long-term user of clozapine could have other causes, particularly if the individual is obese and has diabetes mellitus, both of which are common among patients with schizophrenia, especially those taking clozapine since metabolic syndrome associated with clozapine increases both bodyweight and insulin resistance (Fitzsimons et al., 2005; Raja, 2011). A study using the Framingham Heart Study cohort found the risk of heart failure increased by 5% in men and 7% in women for every unit increase in BMI (Kenchaiah et al., 2002), and in another study the prevalence of heart failure increased with duration of obesity (Alpert et al., 2014). Nevertheless, this does not exclude clozapine as a contributing factor in a patient with diabetes and long-standing obesity. Familial cardiomyopathy, heart failure following multiple episodes of myocardial infarction, and heart failure associated with hypertension, sarcoidosis, and autoimmune disease are all possible causes, as well as alcohol abuse and cocaine and methamphetamine use (Wexler et al., 2009). There is also evidence to indicate that persistent tachycardia with clozapine puts the patient at risk of developing cardiomyopathy (see Section 2.4) (Chow et al., 2014a; Umana et al., 2003).

2.3 GENETIC VULNERABILITY

No genetic studies have been conducted of clozapine and myocarditis or cardiomyopathy. Evaluation of the logistic regression model, developed in the case−control study referred to above, as a predictive tool yielded an area under the receiver operating characteristics curve (AUC) of 0.71 (95% CI 0.65−0.76) (Ronaldson et al., 2012d). This limited predictive value indicates that other factors, and these may include genetic polymorphisms, make a major contribution to the risk of developing myocarditis during the period of clozapine initiation.

Single predisposing genetic polymorphisms with strong associations (ORs > 80) have been identified in the human leukocyte antigen (HLA) region of chromosome 6 for some other drug hypersensitivity reactions: hypersensitivity to abacavir (Mallal et al., 2008); Stevens Johnson syndrome with carbamazepine (Chung et al., 2004); severe skin reaction with allopurinol (Hung et al., 2005); and cholestatic hepatitis with flucloxacillin (Daly et al., 2009). In the case of abacavir, all validated cases had the genetic polymorphism, though it was not absent in all controls. For these hypersensitivity reactions, for example, abacavir hypersensitivity, rechallenge reliably results in recurrence of the event, usually with greater severity than in the first instance (Escaut et al., 1999; Hetherington et al., 2001). Since clozapine rechallenge following myocarditis does not always result in recurrence of the adverse effect (Ronaldson et al., 2012b), and since clozapine can be continued in some mild cases of myocarditis apparently without adverse consequence (Ronaldson et al., 2012a), it is unlikely that the event will be attributable to a single predisposing genetic polymorphism. The genetic picture with clozapine and myocarditis is likely to be more complex and possibly closer to that seen recently with clozapine-related agranulocytosis which occasionally does not occur on rechallenge (Manu et al., 2012): two variant HLA alleles were associated, but more than 50% of cases had neither of these variants (Goldstein et al., 2014).

Clozapine-associated cardiomyopathy developing as a consequence of myocarditis would be expected to have the same genetic factors as myocarditis. However, cardiomyopathy developing independently of myocarditis may be associated with risk factors for heart failure, a familial predisposition for cardiomyopathy, or sensitivity to sustained tachycardia with clozapine (Lakdawala et al., 2013). This is yet to be investigated.

2.4 PATHOBIOLOGY

2.4.1 Myocarditis

An IgE-mediated hypersensitivity reaction (type I) mechanism for clozapine-induced myocarditis has been proposed on the basis of time to onset (Kilian et al., 1999). The same group has also suggested that a direct toxic effect involving an inflammatory response in the heart may cause the condition. There is now a greater understanding of immune function, the impact of pro-inflammatory cytokines on tissue, molecular mechanisms which may lead to hypersensitivity myocarditis and factors contributing to heart failure.

Pollmacher et al. (1996) explored the effect of clozapine initiation on pro-inflammatory cytokine concentrations and found that those patients (44%) developing fever (>38°C) also had significantly higher TNF-α, soluble interleukin-2 receptor (sIL-2r) and interleukin-6 (IL-6) at week 2. These observations may be relevant to myocarditis, given that fever frequently occurs with myocarditis and the onset of myocarditis is usually in the third week of clozapine, while agranulocytosis typically occurs later in treatment. In a small randomized controlled trial with 15 patients with schizophrenia initiated on clozapine and 15 on olanzapine, conducted by Kluge et al. (2009), fever occurred in 5 patients in the clozapine group, but none in the olanzapine group. Both clozapine and olanzapine activated plasma TNF-α, but only clozapine had a significant effect on sIL-2r and IL-6, and the relationship between fever and cytokine levels was similar to that found by Pollmacher et al. (1996). In both studies fever was self-limiting, and Kluge et al. (2009) found IL-6 levels had returned to baseline by week 6 of clozapine. IL-6 and TNF-α are potent pyrogens.

Wang et al. (2008) and Abdel-Wahab et al. (2014) have established clozapine dose-dependent associations with cytokines and linked these to the development of myocarditis in mice and rats, respectively. Mice treated with clozapine 25 mg kg^{-1} day^{-1} for 14 days had more than double the TNF-α in heart tissue of control mice (Wang et al., 2008). Coadministration of propranolol significantly attenuated the effect on TNF-α, though not as far as to levels observed with clozapine 10 mg kg^{-1} day^{-1}. Abdel-Wahab et al. (2014) found the pro-inflammatory TNF-α increased in cardiac tissue with clozapine, while the anti-inflammatory interleukin-10 (IL-10) decreased. Administration of captopril reversed both of these effects. Wang et al. (2008) also observed increased epinephrine and norepinephrine concentrations with clozapine administration which were reduced with propranolol. Concentrations did not change from day 7 to day 14, although cardiac injury had reduced by day 14. These findings suggest that hypercatecholaminergia may induce myocarditis via the β-adrenergic system, possibly with downregulation of cardiac β-receptors in response to the effect of clozapine, as indicated by the time-related reduction in cardiac effect.

Together, these studies confirm the immunomodulatory effect of clozapine and they suggest that release of pro-inflammatory cytokines and catecholamines has a role in the development of myocarditis associated with clozapine by acting on the β-adrenergic system. There do not appear to be comparable studies examining the effects of other antipsychotics on cytokines or catecholamines in the early weeks of treatment.

2.4.2 Cardiomyopathy

Pro-inflammatory cytokines may influence the development of cardiomyopathy, although the evidence is weaker. One study investigated pro-inflammatory cytokine levels in long-term users of clozapine in the context of metabolic effects (O'Connell et al., 2014). A small number had very high cytokine concentrations, not seen among the healthy controls, but these patients were not investigated for cardiac function. Rises in cytokines, TNF-α, IL-1, IL-6, and IL-18, are implicated in the pathogenesis of heart failure from any cause and levels tend to correlate with increasing functional class (e.g., New York Heart Failure) (Gullestad et al., 2012; Wrigley et al., 2011).

Besides the effects of cytokines, cardiac factors related to the development of cardiomyopathy have been identified. Clozapine-induced myocarditis also may develop into cardiomyopathy, especially if the insult is sustained, such as if clozapine is not discontinued (Kilian et al., 1999). However, for some time it has been thought that cardiomyopathy in patients on long-term clozapine could develop without myocarditis (Rostagno et al., 2011c; Chow et al., 2014a). One hundred patients who had been taking clozapine for at least a year were found to have significantly lower mean LVEF (Simpson's biplane) and significantly less (i.e., more impaired) two-dimensional global longitudinal strain (GLS) than 21 control patients with schizophrenia who had never used clozapine and than 20 healthy controls (Chow et al., 2014b). The control groups had similar age and gender profiles to the clozapine group. None of the clozapine patients had symptomatic heart disease, yet significant cardiomyopathy (LVEF < 50%) was present in 9% of the group. None of the controls had cardiomyopathy. Nearly half (49%) of the clozapine group had impairment of GLS beyond the 95% CI of the control subjects, and increasing heart rate correlated with increasing impairment of GLS. None of the clozapine group had a clinical, electrocardiographic (ECG) or biochemical history suggestive of myocarditis, and the authors postulated a direct toxic effect of clozapine on the heart.

Tachycardia is a recognized cause of cardiomyopathy (Gupta and Figueredo, 2014; Umana et al., 2003), and sustained tachycardia is not uncommon with long-term clozapine (Cohen et al., 2001). Rostagno et al. (2012) reported that 54% of patients on long-term clozapine had a resting heart rate in excess of $100 \ \text{min}^{-1}$. Barnes and McPhillips (1999) note that elevated heart rate is a consequence of the antimuscarinic effect of antipsychotics and clozapine, with the greatest muscarinic potency, has the greatest effect on heart rate. Interestingly, Barnes and McPhillips (1999) also observed that olanzapine, with little muscarinic effect, does not change heart rate but tachycardia is a recognized adverse effect of quetiapine, despite negligible muscarinic activity. There may be a connection between this effect of quetiapine on heart rate and the published cases of cardiomyopathy.

Another cardiac effect of clozapine which may predispose the patient to cardiomyopathy is a reduction in heart rate variability, indicative of autonomic dysregulation (Cohen et al., 2001), which has also been observed in patients taking haloperidol and olanzapine in comparison with healthy controls, but effects were significantly greater with clozapine.

Low selenium concentrations in plasma and red cells have been noted in patients taking clozapine and the deficiency has been invoked as a cause of both myocarditis and cardiomyopathy (Vaddadi et al., 2003).

Thus, several mechanisms are proposed for the development of clozapine-induced cardiomyopathy, and all may apply. These are as the long-term consequence of the development of myocarditis; sustained clozapine-induced tachycardia; reduced heart rate variability; and impaired GLS. Inflammatory cytokines may contribute as may reduced plasma selenium concentrations. These possible mechanisms strengthen the case for a causal association between clozapine and cardiomyopathy.

2.5 CLINICAL AND LABORATORY FEATURES

2.5.1 Myocarditis

Clozapine-induced myocarditis typically develops in the third week after initiation of clozapine (Haas et al., 2007; Ronaldson et al., 2011b), but cases of delayed onset occurring after more than 2 months of clozapine therapy have been reported (Haas et al., 2007; Ronaldson et al., 2015a). These latter may have been precipitated by an event resulting in a rapid increase in clozapine plasma concentration such as discontinuation (usually for noncompliance) and reinitiation, smoking cessation (Brownlowe and Sola, 2008), drug–drug interaction resulting in reduced clozapine metabolism, or illness associated with inflammation (Leung et al., 2014), but the possibility that late cases may occur without a precipitating event cannot be excluded. Nevertheless, the critical period is the first 4 weeks after commencing clozapine and this is the period when patients should be monitored for this outcome and clinician suspicion should be high.

Fever with elevation of C-reactive protein (CRP) is the usual signal for the onset of myocarditis in a patient commencing clozapine (Fig. 2.1, point 2)

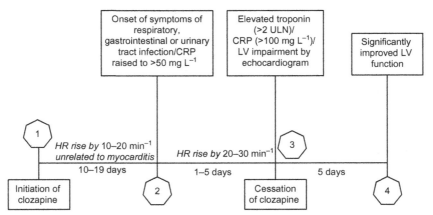

FIGURE 2.1 The typical evolution of clozapine-induced myocarditis. Abbreviations: *CRP*, C-reactive protein; *HR*, heart rate; *LV*, left ventricular; *ULN*, upper limit of normal. *Used with permission from Ronaldson, K.J., Taylor, A.J., Fitzgerald, P.B., Topliss, D.J., McNeil, J.J., 2011b. A new monitoring protocol for clozapine induced myocarditis based on an analysis of 75 cases and 94 controls. Aust. N. Z. J. Psychiatry 45 (6), 458–465.*

(Ronaldson et al., 2011b). The fever is commonly accompanied by symptoms attributable to respiratory tract infection including cough, sore throat, rhinorrhea, and myalgia, but less commonly the patient may suffer severe diarrhea and vomiting. Symptoms consistent with urinary tract infection occur occasionally.

Tachycardia is also a feature of myocarditis, but this frequently occurs with clozapine initiation without development of myocarditis (Ronaldson et al., 2011b). Monitoring heart rate during initiation may assist in the early diagnosis of myocarditis, as an increase to more than $120 \, min^{-1}$ or by $30 \, min^{-1}$ may accompany myocarditis (Fig. 2.1, points 1–3). Most patients experience a drop in blood pressure with the onset of myocarditis and monitoring blood pressure from clozapine initiation will assist the cause of any hypotension to be identified with improved specificity. Chest pain occurs in about 50% of cases of myocarditis, and for a few it develops early in the course of clozapine before other signs, symptoms, or laboratory features are apparent. Chest pain has also been described in those not developing myocarditis. Elevated respiration rate ($>20 \, min^{-1}$) is observed in some patients with the onset of myocarditis.

Signs and symptoms indicative specifically of heart failure, basal crepitations, third heart sounds, peripheral edema, and raised jugular venous pressure, are not common and development is usually coincident on the rise in troponin and/or presence of left ventricular dysfunction detectable by echocardiography (Ronaldson et al., 2011b). Myocarditis may also develop without symptoms in patients commencing clozapine and some of these cases have been fatal. Asymptomatic cases have been identified by routine monitoring and thus serious outcomes have been prevented (see Section 2.10.1) (Ronaldson et al., 2011a,b).

2.5.1.1 *Laboratory and investigative features*

In a typical case of myocarditis where the patient displays symptoms consistent with infectious illness, raised CRP may herald its onset (Fig. 2.1, point 2; Fig. 2.2a) (Ronaldson et al., 2011b, 2015b). After 1–5 days, the patient will be found to have raised troponin (Fig. 2.2b), and up to 7 or 8 days after the troponin peak and withdrawal of clozapine, a maximum eosinophil count will be recorded in about 60% of cases (Fig. 2.2c). It should be noted that not only is peripheral eosinophilia not present in all cases, when it is present its development is typically delayed, and around 30% of patients not developing myocarditis have eosinophilia within a similar time frame in relation to the initiation of clozapine (Fig. 2.2d) (Ronaldson et al., 2010, 2011b, 2015b).

Evidence to date supports the use of troponin I or T together with CRP in the monitoring and diagnosis of clozapine-induced myocarditis (Ronaldson et al. 2011b). Troponin raised to more than twice the upper limit of normal or CRP greater than $100 \, mg \, L^{-1}$ is suggestive of the presence of myocarditis and indicative of the need to withdraw clozapine immediately (Ronaldson

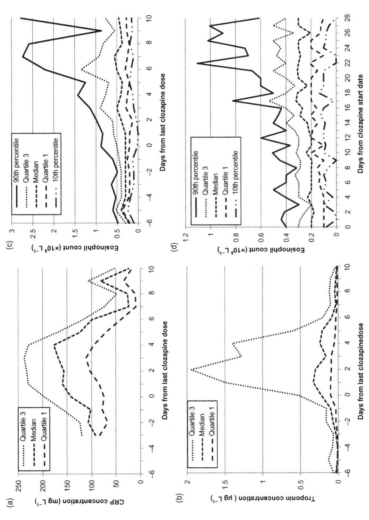

FIGURE 2.2 The evolution of (a) C-reactive protein (CRP), (b) troponin I/T, and (c) eosinophil count with time in cases, using the day of the last dose of clozapine (stop date for myocarditis) as the reference. The precipitous drop in the 90th percentile for eosinophil count on day 9 arises from the lack of data from cases with high counts on that day. Descriptive statistics (mean ± standard deviation, range) for number of results available for each day were for CRP 21 ± 14, 5–48; troponin I/T 29 ± 23, 7–83; eosinophil count 30 ± 19, 9–77. (d) The evolution of eosinophil counts (upper limit of normal 0.4–0.6 × 10⁹ L⁻¹) in control patients using the day clozapine therapy was started as the reference. Descriptive statistics for number of results available for each day mean ± standard deviation 49 ± 25, range 17–104. *Used with permission from Ronaldson, K.J., Fitzgerald, P.B., McNeil, J.J., 2015b. Evolution of troponin, C-reactive protein and eosinophil count with the onset of clozapine-induced myocarditis. Aust. N. Z. J. Psychiatry 49 (5), 486–487. doi:10.1177/0004867414566871.*

et al., 2011b). Echocardiography is used to ascertain cardiac involvement in the absence of raised troponin and to determine whether supportive treatment in the form of medication or mechanical means is required. Around 70% of cases have discernible left ventricular impairment by echocardiography (Ronaldson et al., 2011b). An early (i.e., with onset of fever or raised CRP) normal troponin level does not exclude myocarditis (Figs. 2.1 and 2.2) (Ronaldson et al., 2011b, 2015a,b). Repeated measurements are necessary for exclusion or confirmation of myocardial involvement, although not all cases have raised troponin (Caforio et al., 2013; Ronaldson et al., 2011b).

The B-type natriuretic peptide (BNP) has been used as an alternative to echocardiography in the diagnosis of heart failure, but the results of this test for a small number of cases of myocarditis are variable and it is not reliable (Annamraju et al., 2007; Caforio et al., 2013). Published results for N-terminal proBNP (NT-proBNP) are available for only two cases (Annamraju et al., 2007). Creatine kinase and creatine kinase-MB (cardiac-specific fraction) may be raised above normal in 30–40% of cases, but this is not a sufficient response for routine use in monitoring (Ronaldson et al., 2010, 2011b). Use of erythrocyte sedimentation rate to assist diagnosis of myocarditis of any cause has been recommended by the European Society of Cardiology (Caforio et al., 2013), although insufficient data specific to clozapine-induced myocarditis are currently available. Cardiac magnetic resonance imaging (CMR) is the only noninvasive technique which can give a result diagnostic of myocarditis. Nevertheless, a negative CMR result, or one that is less than definitive, does not exclude myocarditis (Ariyarajah et al., 2010; Belloni et al., 2007; Caforio et al., 2013).

A critical factor to emphasize is the variability in response observed between different parameters. A patient may have moderate or even severe left ventricular dysfunction with a LVEF of less than 30% and yet have only mildly elevated troponin; conversely a patient may have very high troponin and normal LVEF by echocardiography (Caforio et al., 2013). Similarly, the extent of late enhancement by CMR may not correlate with LVEF (Danti et al., 2009), and it is essential to ascertain cardiac function (i.e., LVEF) in cases of suspected myocarditis by echocardiography, or some more sophisticated cardiac visualization technique such as CMR.

In the presence of myocarditis, an ECG usually displays nonspecific abnormalities, including ST-T-elevation, T-wave inversion, and left bundle branch block (Caforio et al., 2013; Ronaldson et al., 2010). Endomyocardial biopsy (EMB) is still the gold standard for diagnosis of myocarditis, but it is invasive, is subject to considerable interobserver variation, and requires sampling of the affected area. A major advantage is that EMB identifies the etiology. Since myocarditis caused by clozapine responds rapidly to withdrawal of clozapine, and occurrence within 4 weeks of clozapine commencement supports this association, the imperative to confirm the cause and diagnosis using EMB is diminished (Caforio et al., 2013; Holmvang and Dec, 2012).

2.5.2   Cardiomyopathy

Cardiomyopathy with clozapine develops slowly and insidiously and may become manifest at any time after the period of clozapine initiation. The most frequent initial clinical symptom of cardiomyopathy is shortness of breath, particularly with mild to moderate exercise, which may have worsened noticeably over a period of time (Phan and Taylor, 2002; Tanner and Culling, 2003). Elevated heart rate and hypotension may also feature, and one case was thought to be having panic attacks (Sagar et al., 2008). Several studies (Chow et al., 2014a; Murch et al., 2013; Rostagno et al., 2011b) and a separately reported case identified with routine monitoring (Floreani and Bastiampillai, 2008) indicate cardiomyopathy may progress to considerable severity without overt symptoms.

The diagnostic technique usually employed for diagnosing cardiomyopathy is the measurement of LVEF, or left ventricular wall thickness for hypertrophic cardiomyopathy, by echocardiography, but other parameters such as GLS have also been used (Chow et al., 2014b). CMR can be used to accurately measure left ventricular systolic function, chamber size and wall thickness, and is especially useful if echocardiographic image quality is poor (Lakdawala et al., 2013). More particularly, delayed enhancement of the ventricular myocardium, following the administration of gadolinium-based contrast medium, occurring in a noncoronary distribution (often mid-wall location) is strongly suggestive of nonischemic cardiomyopathy. Laboratory parameters associated with inflammation, such as troponin, CRP, eosinophil count, and ESR, are not typically raised. Rostagno et al. (2011b) observed that NT-proBNP predicted LVEF (AUC 0.87) in clozapine recipients, but only three of the participants had LVEFs of less than 50%. Further studies are required to support this finding. According to Chow et al. (2014a), the diagnostic value of BNP and NT-proBNP for cardiomyopathy has not been demonstrated.

2.6   DIFFERENTIAL DIAGNOSIS

2.6.1   Myocarditis

A difficulty with the diagnosis of myocarditis is that the signs and symptoms are nonspecific, and in particular clozapine-induced myocarditis frequently presents as influenza or less frequently as a severe gastrointestinal infection, or rarely even a urinary tract infection (Ronaldson et al., 2011b, 2015a). In addition, some of the features of myocarditis, tachycardia, fever, and eosinophilia may occur benignly with initiation of clozapine (Ronaldson et al., 2010, 2011b). Thus, without suspicion of myocarditis on the part of treating physicians and an active attempt to investigate for it, a case of myocarditis is unlikely to be correctly diagnosed.

There is no evidence that family history or personal history of or risk factors for cardiovascular disease are influencing factors in the risk of myocarditis. However, the presence of such risk factors may point to an alternative cardiac or cardiovascular diagnosis (Caforio et al., 2013). Suspected myocarditis developing within 4 weeks of commencing clozapine, documented using CRP, troponin, and suitable determination of left ventricular function and responding rapidly to withdrawal of clozapine, has a high likelihood of being clozapine-induced myocarditis. Nevertheless, there are potentially confounding diagnoses (Fig. 2.3). Myocarditis may develop

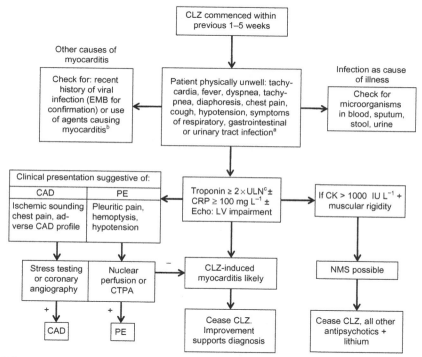

FIGURE 2.3 Differential diagnosis for suspected myocarditis in a patient who commenced clozapine titration 1−5 weeks previously.

[a]These signs and symptoms are a guide. Not all will be present and it is not possible to be prescriptive about the number that should be before commencing to investigate further.

[b]Among other agents potentially causing myocarditis are: antineoplastics (5-fluorouracil, doxorubicin, gefitinib, idarubicin, cyclophosphamide), antibiotics (ampicillin, sulfamethoxazole/trimethoprim, cefaclor, minocycline), drugs of abuse (alcohol, amphetamines, cocaine, ecstacy), and other (carbamazepine, ACE inhibitors, mesalazine, dobutamine).

[c]A normal troponin result at the time of onset of illness or initial rise in CRP does not exclude myocarditis; troponin investigation should be repeated daily until illness resolves or raised result obtained.

Abbreviations: *BP*, blood pressure; *CAD*, coronary artery disease; *CLZ*, clozapine; *CK*, creatine kinase; *CRP*, C-reactive protein; *CTPA*, computed tomographic pulmonary angiography; *Echo*, echocardiography; *EMB*, endomyocardial biopsy; *LV*, left ventricular; *NMS*, neuroleptic malignant syndrome; *PE*, pulmonary embolism.

following a viral infection and other medications besides clozapine can cause this adverse reaction (Caforio et al., 2013; Cooper, 2009; Magnani and Dec, 2006). Exposure to such a medication within a suitable time frame may indicate an alternative cause. In this situation withdrawal of both clozapine, if it has been commenced in the previous 5 weeks, and the other drug would be advised.

Since the suggested monitoring and diagnosis strategy is heavily reliant on troponin, it must be acknowledged that while troponin is very sensitive to myocarditis, it may also be raised in the presence of other conditions including myocardial infarction, hypertension, sepsis, pulmonary embolism, and marked renal insufficiency (Wu et al., 2007). Coronary angiography or stress testing will exclude or confirm coronary artery disease, but a response to withdrawal of clozapine may be sufficient to identify the nature of the illness. Many patients developing myocarditis have hypotension, and most have a drop in blood pressure with the onset of myocarditis (Ronaldson et al., 2011b). Ensuring patients with hypertension at baseline are adequately treated and monitoring blood pressure during clozapine initiation should avoid hypertension becoming a competing diagnosis. The possibility of sepsis may cause diagnostic confusion, when the patient has signs and symptoms consistent with serious infectious illness. The presence of left ventricular dysfunction on echocardiography or evidence of myocarditis by CMR will resolve this confusion, but will not be found in all cases of myocarditis. Recovery following withdrawal of clozapine and culture samples negative for pathogens will suggest that clozapine-induced myocarditis was the cause of the illness; and if initiation of clozapine occurred in the previous 2−4 weeks, there will be added support for a diagnosis of myocarditis.

Pneumonia shares many signs and symptoms with myocarditis, such as fever, dyspnea, tachycardia, and chest pain, and has been reported to occur in patients treated with clozapine, particularly during the initiation period (Kuo et al., 2013; Ronaldson et al., 2015a; Taylor et al., 2009). As a hypersensitivity reaction, myocarditis may be accompanied by pneumonia in some cases. Patients with suspected pneumonia in the early weeks of clozapine therapy should undergo evaluation for infectious disease, and also be referred to a cardiologist for investigation of cardiac involvement, associated with myocarditis.

Pulmonary embolism is a recognized adverse reaction of clozapine (Tripp, 2011) and is addressed in detail elsewhere in this book (see Chapter 3, Pulmonary Embolism). As an alternative cause of raised troponin and with some common symptoms, it is another potentially confounding event. Nuclear ventilation perfusion imaging or computed tomographic pulmonary angiography will confirm or exclude the presence of pulmonary embolism.

Serotonin syndrome and neuroleptic malignant syndrome (NMS) may also have similar features to myocarditis (see Chapter 10, Neuroleptic

Malignant Syndrome). Serotonin syndrome has not been associated with clozapine use, and certainly not with its initiation, and in the absence of concurrent escalating use of agents which increase serotonin, it is unlikely to occur (Fitzsimons et al., 2005; Raja, 2011). However, cases of NMS with clozapine, including with its initiation, have been reported. The original definition for NMS included fever, rigidity, and elevated creatine kinase as major indicative features (Levenson, 1985), but it has been proposed that clozapine causes atypical NMS where rigidity, hyperthermia, and raised creatine kinase are either absent or reduced compared with a typical case (Karagianis et al., 1999). When rigidity and elevated CK ($>1000 \, \text{IU L}^{-1}$) are not considered essential features for a diagnosis of NMS and the patient is not investigated for cardiac impairment, a case of myocarditis could be diagnosed as NMS, especially if the time to onset is within the first month after commencing clozapine (Baciewicz et al., 2002; Karagianis et al., 1999).

2.6.2 Cardiomyopathy

Cardiomyopathy occurring in a long-term user of clozapine could have other causes, particularly if the individual is obese and has diabetes mellitus, both of which are common among patients with schizophrenia, especially those taking clozapine (Fitzsimons et al., 2005; Marder et al., 2004; Raja, 2011). In addition, familial cardiomyopathy, heart failure following multiple episodes of myocardial infarction, and heart failure associated with sarcoidosis or autoimmune disease are all possible causes, as well as alcohol abuse and cocaine and methamphetamine use. Thus differential diagnosis for clozapine-induced cardiomyopathy involves taking a personal and family history of cardiovascular disease and recent history of drug abuse, documenting BMI and checking for the presence of diabetes mellitus. Familial cases of cardiomyopathy may be reported as "heart attacks" and such reports should not be accepted at face value. Clozapine should not be excluded too readily as a contributing cause even in the presence of multiple other factors.

The most common symptom of cardiomyopathy is exertional breathlessness, but cardiomyopathy develops insidiously and may be without symptoms (Chow et al., 2014a; Floreani and Bastiampillai, 2008; Hoehns et al. 2001; Rostagno et al., 2011b). Tachycardia may be present, but fever is described only in cases with time to onset less than 6 weeks and these probably involved the inflammation typical of myocarditis (Kikuchi et al., 2013; Pastor and Mehta, 2008). Troponin I or T and CRP concentrations were typically normal in published cases. Almost all published cases were diagnosed using echocardiography which showed the left ventricular dysfunction with enlarged ventricular chamber characteristic of dilated cardiomyopathy (Makhoul et al., 2008; Novo et al., 2010; Rostagno et al., 2008) and occasionally hypertrophic cardiomyopathy with wall thickening (Bobb et al., 2010; Roh et al., 2006; Tanner and Culling, 2003). Echocardiography is the diagnostic method of choice (Chow et al., 2014a). Hypertrophy can also be detected on ECG (Wexler et al., 2009). In addition, the presence cardiomyopathy has been investigated using BNP levels to distinguish breathlessness caused by heart failure and that caused by other etiologies (Wexler et al., 2009), but its specificity and sensitivity have not been adequately investigated. Very high values (normal <100 pg mL^{-1}) may indicate acutely decompensated heart failure.

Withdrawal of clozapine in cases of cardiomyopathy may not result in a discernible improvement in the short term, but over a longer period of months, improvement in, if not full recovery of, left ventricular function is to be expected (Rostagno et al., 2008; Tanner and Culling, 2003).

2.7 COMPLICATIONS AND SIGNIFICANT SEQUELAE

Clozapine-induced myocarditis may be fatal and the case fatality rate in case series varies from 0% to 75% (Ronaldson et al., 2015a). There is some suggestion from Australian data (Ronaldson et al., 2015a) that mortality is reduced and may be less than 10% if clozapine is initiated in the context of monitoring for myocarditis. The reasons are twofold. Monitoring for myocarditis identifies more cases (increased denominator) and those identified are likely to have clozapine ceased before the myocarditis becomes life-threatening (decreased numerator). Death in the acute phase of myocarditis is more likely in severe or fulminant cases in which catastrophic heart failure leads to death, although even mild and asymptomatic cases may be fatal, with arrhythmia the postulated cause of fatality (Kitulwatte et al., 2010; Ronaldson et al., 2011a).

Evidence suggests that all those who survive the acute phase of myocarditis with prompt withdrawal of clozapine recover fully, except for some with severe left ventricular impairment (Annamraju et al., 2007; Merrill et al., 2006; Ronaldson et al., 2010). One case, published in 2014, with little left ventricular impairment (LVEF 54%) was diagnosed by elevated creatine kinase and the presence of a focus of late gadolinium enhancement on CMR. The patient was found to have persisting myocardial scarring at 14 months despite echocardiography displaying a normal image (LVEF 58%) (Chow et al., 2014a). While symptomatic recovery may be complete, the long-term effects on cardiac health of developing myocarditis are unknown. An approach to long-term monitoring or medical intervention for these cases has not been formulated.

The issue of long-term sequelae if clozapine is not withdrawn in a case of myocarditis is rather different. First, in five documented mild cases, clozapine was continued with or without temporary suspension of clozapine or dose reduction and continuation appeared to present no ongoing risk to cardiac function (Ronaldson et al., 2012a). The judgment that these cases were mild was based on troponin result (range $0.08-0.8\ \mu g\ L^{-1}$; ULN $0.03-0.2\ \mu g\ L^{-1}$) and three of the cases also had normal echocardiography. Second, myocarditis, despite moderate severity, may be missed and clozapine continued. In such cases the assault which caused the injury is sustained and the expected consequence is cardiomyopathy (Kilian et al., 1999). For obvious reasons, there are no reliable data to permit a comprehensive description of these cases. A published case of cardiomyopathy may have followed an episode of myocarditis at 4 weeks (Leo et al., 1996). This patient had an LVEF of 18% at 6 months. Treatment with frusemide and enalapril, following clozapine withdrawal, led to some recovery in function to an LVEF of 33% 3 months later.

Clozapine-induced cardiomyopathy may occur in patients without a past history of myocarditis by other causal pathways including persistent tachycardia (see Section 2.4.2). Data on prognosis with cardiomyopathy caused by clozapine, with or without clozapine continuation and with or without intervention using cardiac medication are limited. Two published cases were fatal and were not diagnosed until autopsy (Hoehns et al., 2001; Reinders et al., 2004) and one case included among the eight described by Kilian et al. (1999) was fatal 2 years after diagnosis. Nevertheless, in one case described by Rostagno et al. (2008), the patient was able to recommence clozapine successfully with concurrent use of carvedilol and captopril. Moreover, this patient had continuing improvement in left ventricular function to an LVEF of more than 60% despite ongoing clozapine therapy.

2.8 RISK STRATIFICATION FOR DEATH OR PERMANENT DISABILITY

Among a total of 76 cases of clozapine-induced myocarditis, Ronaldson et al. (2011a) reviewed 10 fatal cases, diagnosed at autopsy. Three were asymptomatic. Only four had cardiac-specific investigations (troponin or creatine kinase MB) and the result was normal for one (at the time of cardiac arrest) and elevated but not alarmingly so for the other three. All three with determinations for creatine kinase had results in excess of $1000\ U\ L^{-1}$. Since only 3 of 65 surviving cases had creatine kinase results in excess of $1000\ U\ L^{-1}$ ($p = 0.0004$), this may be an indicator of risk of fatal outcome (Ronaldson et al., 2011a). Two other possible risk factors for fatality were identified by comparison with nonfatal cases: BMI greater than $30\ kg\ m^{-2}$ (60% vs 26%; $p = 0.03$) and longer duration of clozapine use before cessation for myocarditis (mean 21 vs 17 days; $p = 0.006$). Age and smoking status did not change the risk of death.

One published fatal case had an exceedingly high BNP result ($12,265\ pg\ mL^{-1}$) (Annamraju et al., 2007), but BNP is affected by factors other than degree of heart failure and the degree of BNP elevation is of little prognostic significance (Guglin et al., 2007; Law et al., 2010).

Although most nonfatal cases of myocarditis recover completely or almost completely, severe left ventricular impairment (LVEF < 30%) with myocarditis or cardiomyopathy is an indication that the patient may suffer permanent impairment or decline over a period of time to death (Kilian et al., 1999).

2.9 MANAGEMENT

2.9.1 Myocarditis

Most cases of clozapine-induced myocarditis recover on withdrawal of clozapine without further intervention. More severe cases, as determined by echocardiography or other suitable cardiac visualization technique, are treated empirically and require supportive treatment which may be treatment with an angiotensin-converting enzyme (ACE) inhibitor or an angiotensin II receptor antagonist and a β-blocker with or without mechanical ventilation (Caforio et al., 2013). Use of corticosteroids and other immunosuppressive agents has produced variable results in nonviral myocarditis (Caforio et al., 2013). Treatment with corticosteroids has been described in some published case reports of clozapine-induced myocarditis (Annamraju et al., 2007; Pieroni et al., 2004; Razminia et al., 2006). Results of an experimental study suggest that steroid treatment may prevent arrhythmias (Park et al., 2014) which are considered a primary cause of mortality with myocarditis. Patients with persistent left ventricular dysfunction, particularly if the LVEF is less than 40%, may require cardiac medication until recovery of function is complete.

A patient developing a hypersensitivity reaction, such as myocarditis, would not usually be rechallenged with the causative agent. However, rechallenge with clozapine after myocarditis has been conducted successfully in about 50% of cases (Manu et al., 2012; Ronaldson et al., 2012b). The incentive for such a risky experiment has been the improvement in mental health observed during the few weeks the patient was taking clozapine before it was ceased for myocarditis. This is often in a context in which insufficient response had been achieved with other antipsychotics agents.

2.9.1.1 Rechallenge

An analysis of cases of rechallenge considered whether certain factors may influence the success: severity of the initial event; delay from the initial event to rechallenge; and slow clozapine titration during rechallenge (Ronaldson et al., 2012b). None of these appeared to be critical factors. However, if rechallenge is considered desirable, it should be conducted with the consent of the patient and the patient's family after communication of the potential risks and benefits, and with added care in monitoring for an adverse outcome. Slow dose titration and avoidance of sodium valproate, if possible, will do no harm during rechallenge and may improve the outcome, and coprescription of an ACE inhibitor and a β-blocker may protect against myocarditis, although there are no human data to support this strategy (Abdel-Wahab et al., 2014; Wang et al., 2008).

2.9.2   Cardiomyopathy

A diagnosis of cardiomyopathy automatically leads to withdrawal of clozapine. Patients with cardiomyopathy should be prescribed an ACE inhibitor or angiotensin II receptor antagonist and a β-blocker (Wexler et al., 2009). If there is peripheral edema or other evidence of fluid overload a diuretic would be beneficial. Reduced salt intake should be advised, but may be difficult to implement in those whose diet is suboptimal. Alcohol, cocaine, and amphetamines should be avoided, as should endurance and competitive sport, even if the cardiomyopathy is mild. Smoking cessation is also recommended. In those with ongoing severe systolic dysfunction an implantable cardioverter-defibrillator will reduce the risk of sudden cardiac death (Lakdawala et al., 2013). Heart transplantation may be an option to be considered in those whose function does not improve sufficiently and who have severe symptoms of heart failure (Lakdawala et al., 2013; Wexler et al., 2009).

Case reports suggest that recovery from clozapine-induced cardiomyopathy usually occurs over several months, but that most patients have improvement, if not full recovery, in left ventricular function following withdrawal of clozapine and treatment with cardiac-supportive medication (Leo et al., 1996; Pastor and Mehta, 2008; Phan and Taylor, 2002). Even two cases with severe left ventricular impairment (LVEF 18% and 9%, respectively), treated with an ACE inhibitor and a diuretic with or without a β-blocker, had significant recovery in function to LVEF 33% and 43%, respectively, within 3 months (Leo et al., 1996; Tanner and Culling, 2003).

2.9.2.1   Rechallenge

For many patients, clozapine is the only antipsychotic which has effectively controlled symptoms and permitted a reasonable quality of life. The effect of clozapine discontinuation, described in case reports, is a rapid decline into psychosis which cannot be controlled by other treatment modalities (Bobb et al., 2010; Rostagno et al., 2011a). Although this scenario has not been adequately studied, it may be that patients developing cardiomyopathy, or at least those whose left ventricular dysfunction or hypertrophy is not too severe, may continue clozapine while they are medicated for heart failure (Rostagno et al., 2008).

2.10 PREVENTION

2.10.1 Myocarditis

The case–control study cited earlier indicated that the risk of myocarditis in patients commencing clozapine can be reduced by slow clozapine dose titration and by avoiding sodium valproate, but these precautions do not eliminate the risk altogether (Ronaldson et al., 2012d). In fact, a third of cases had no identified risk factors. An alternative strategy is to follow an effective evidence-based monitoring protocol. This cannot prevent myocarditis, but it can reduce the risk of serious outcomes in the short and long term, by catching myocarditis before it becomes either severe, and therefore life-threatening, or the insult is sustained leading to cardiomyopathy and further decline.

On the basis of an analysis of 75 cases of myocarditis and 94 control patients commencing clozapine without myocarditis, a monitoring protocol for clozapine-induced myocarditis has been developed (Fig. 2.4) (Ronaldson et al., 2011b). The inclusion of control patients permitted consideration of features associated with clozapine initiation and not necessarily attributable to the onset of myocarditis.

The following is a description of the significance of the elements of the monitoring guidelines. Most cases of myocarditis occur in the third week of clozapine therapy and almost all within the first month after initiation. Hence, monitoring for the first 4 weeks of clozapine use is a rational approach. Conducting baseline echocardiography will detect cardiac disease needing intervention in all patients commencing clozapine and also enable the diagnosis of myocarditis, if it develops, to be made with considerable specificity (Murch et al., 2013; Ronaldson et al., 2012c). Checking and recording vital signs from clozapine initiation will assist the clinician to separate the effects of clozapine initiation from the onset of myocarditis, which, for example, may develop with a further increase in heart rate and a decrease in blood pressure.

CRP and troponin I or T were found to be the most effective parameters for monitoring for the onset of myocarditis; eosinophilia occurs with and without myocarditis and may be delayed after the rise in troponin by several days (Ronaldson et al., 2010, 2011b). Thus monitoring eosinophil count is not of diagnostic value. Development of fever and a moderate rise in CRP with other symptoms suggestive of infective illness typically occur 3–5 days prior to a rise in troponin (Fig. 2.1, point 2; Fig. 2.2). It is essential to adequate monitoring to realize that a normal troponin result at the time of onset of signs and symptoms of illness or rise in CRP does not exclude myocarditis. Because of this characteristic of myocarditis, the guidelines recommend checking troponin and CRP daily until either the features of illness normalize or the presence of myocarditis is confirmed. Although troponin is a sensitive indicator of myocarditis, some cases develop without a documented rise in

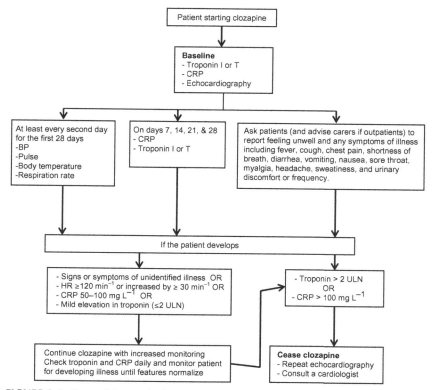

FIGURE 2.4   Protocol for monitoring patients commenced on clozapine for clozapine-induced myocarditis. Abbreviations: *BP*, blood pressure; *CRP*, C-reactive protein; *HR*, heart rate; *ULN*, upper limit of normal. *Used with permission from Ronaldson, K.J., Taylor, A.J., Fitzgerald, P.B., Topliss, D.J., McNeil, J.J., 2011b. A new monitoring protocol for clozapine induced myocarditis based on an analysis of 75 cases and 94 controls. Aust. N. Z. J. Psychiatry 45 (6), 458–465. Available from: http://dx.doi.org/10.3109/00048674.2011.572852.*

troponin (Ronaldson et al., 2011b). Almost all of these have had a CRP result in excess of 100 mg L^{-1}. Cardiac involvement in these cases has been confirmed by echocardiography. Echocardiography is also essential for assessment of left ventricular impairment. A patient may have a slight rise in troponin, but yet have moderate to severe left ventricular impairment; conversely a substantial rise in troponin is not necessarily an indicator of severe left ventricular dysfunction. Echocardiography will indicate whether the patient requires medical or mechanical intervention (Ronaldson et al., 2011b).

Myocarditis may also develop without symptoms and some fatal cases have been asymptomatic, with diagnosis at autopsy (Ronaldson et al., 2011a). Nonfatal asymptomatic cases have been identified by routine monitoring (Ronaldson et al., 2011b). Hence, checking CRP and troponin weekly for the first 4 weeks should proceed even in the absence of signs and symptoms of illness.

2.10.2 Cardiomyopathy

Monitoring for clozapine-induced cardiomyopathy using annual echocardiography has been recommended (Berk et al., 2007), but has subsequently been deemed not cost-effective (Murch et al., 2013). As for myocarditis, monitoring does not prevent cardiomyopathy, but increases the chances of early detection before the condition becomes symptomatic and severe. Ideally, a strategy involving screening long-term clozapine patients by clinical examination and biomarker testing for candidates for echocardiography would solve the problem of excessive cost. However, cardiomyopathy in the early stages is subclinical and Chow et al. (2014a) have declared that even the most promising of the biomarkers for which routine testing is available, NT-proBNP, is not an adequate measure of left ventricular function. Currently there is no cheaper alternative to replace echocardiographic surveillance.

Nevertheless, there is one possible, though unproven, preventive strategy. Those with sustained tachycardia may have a lower risk of developing cardiomyopathy if their heart rate is controlled using a β-blocker and the medication titrated to a favorable heart rate (Cohen et al., 2001; Stryjer et al., 2009), but with caution because orthostatic hypotension may develop (see Chapter 4, Orthostatic Hypotension) (Bradley and Davis, 2003). Clearly, the association of sustained tachycardia with the development of cardiomyopathy, the benefit of treatment to reduce heart rate and the development of a cost-effective monitoring scheme for cardiomyopathy in patients taking clozapine long term are matters for further investigation.

ACKNOWLEDGMENT

The author wishes to thank Dr. Andrew Taylor, Cardiologist, Alfred Hospital, Melbourne, for checking the manuscript.

REFERENCES

Abdel-Wahab, B.A., Metwally, M.E., El-khawanki, M.M., Hashim, A.M., 2014. Protective effect of captopril against clozapine-induced myocarditis in rats: role of oxidative stress, proinflammatory cytokines and DNA damage. Chem. Biol. Interact. 216, 43−52.

Alpert, M.A., Lavie, C.J., Agrawal, H., Aggarwal, K.B., Kumar, S.A., 2014. Obesity and heart failure: epidemiology, pathophysiology, clinical manifestations, and management. Transl. Res. 164 (4), 345−356.

Annamraju, S., Sheitman, B., Saik, S., Stephenson, A., 2007. Early recognition of clozapine-induced myocarditis. J. Clin. Psychopharmacol. 27 (5), 479−483.

Ansari, A., Maron, B.J., Berntson, D.G., 2003. Drug-induced toxic myocarditis. Tex. Heart. Inst. J. 30 (1), 76−79.

Ariyarajah, V., Shaikh, N., Garber, P.J., Kirkpatrick, I., McGregor, R., Jassal, D.S., 2010. Cardiovascular magnetic resonance in mild to moderate clozapine-induced myocarditis: is there a role in the absence of electrocardiographic and echocardiographic abnormalities?. J. Magn. Reson. Imaging 31 (6), 1473−1476.

Baciewicz, A.M., Chandra, R., Whelan, P., 2002. Clozapine-associated neuroleptic malignant syndrome. Ann. Intern. Med. 137 (5 Pt 1), 374.

Barnes, T.R., McPhillips, M.A., 1999. Critical analysis and comparison of the side-effect and safety profiles of the new antipsychotics. Br. J. Psychiatry 174 (Suppl. 38), 34−43.

Belloni, E., De Cobelli, F., Esposito, A., Mellone, R., Gentinetta, F., Meloni, C., et al., 2007. Myocarditis associated with clozapine studied by cardiovascular magnetic resonance. J. Cardiovasc. Magn. Reson. 9 (3), 591−593.

Berk, M., Fitzsimons, J., Lambert, T., Pantelis, C., Kulkarni, J., Castle, D., et al., 2007. Monitoring the safe use of clozapine: a consensus view from Victoria, Australia. CNS Drugs 21 (2), 117−127.

Bhatia, M.S., Gupta, R., Dhawan, J., 2009. Myocarditis after overdose of conventional antipsychotics. World J. Biol. Psychiatry 10 (4 Pt 2), 606−608. Available from: http://dx.doi.org/10.1080/15622970701678815.

Bobb, V.T., Jarskog, L.F., Coffey, B.J., 2010. Adolescent with treatment-refractory schizophrenia and clozapine-induced cardiomyopathy managed with high-dose olanzapine. J. Child Adolesc. Psychopharmacol. 20 (6), 539−543.

Bradley, J.G., Davis, K.A., 2003. Orthostatic hypotension. Am. Fam. Physician 68 (12), 2393−2398.

Brakoulias, V., Bannan, E., Cohen, P., Geary, G., 2005. Amisulpride and cardiomyopathy. Aust. N. Z. J. Psychiatry 39 (8), 738.

Brownlowe, K., Sola, C., 2008. Clozapine toxicity in smoking cessation and with ciprofloxacin. Psychosomatics 49 (2), 176.

Bush, A., Burgess, C., 2008. Fatal cardiomyopathy due to quetiapine. N. Z. Med. J. 121 (1268), 78−79. Available from: <http://www.nzma.org.nz/journal/120-1268/2909/>.

Caforio, A.L., Pankuweit, S., Arbustini, E., Basso, C., Gimeno-Blanes, J., Felix, S.B., et al., 2013. Current state of knowledge on aetiology, diagnosis, management, and therapy of myocarditis: a position statement of the European Society of Cardiology Working Group on Myocardial and Pericardial Diseases. Eur. Heart. J. 34 (33), 2636−2648. Available from: http://dx.doi.org/10.1093/eurheartj/eht210.

Chow, V., Feijo, I., Trieu, J., Starling, J., Kritharides, L., 2014a. Successful rechallenge of clozapine therapy following previous clozapine-induced myocarditis confirmed on cardiac MRI. J. Child Adolesc. Psychopharmacol. 24 (2), 99−101. Available from: http://dx.doi.org/10.1089/cap.2013.0098.

Chow, V., Yeoh, T., Ng, A.C.C., Pasqualon, T., Scott, E., Plater, J., et al., 2014b. Asymptomatic left ventricular dysfunction with long-term clozapine treatment for schizophrenia: a multi-centre cross-sectional cohort study. Open Heart 1, e000030. Available from: http://dx.doi.org/10.1136/openhrt-2013-000030.

Christoffersen, R.K., Vestergard, L.D., Hoimark, L., Vesterby, A., 2011. [Eosinophilic myocarditis and sudden unexpected death in a younger patient treated with antipsychotics]. [Danish]. Ugeskr. Laeger. 173 (44), 2799−2800.

Chung, W.H., Hung, S.I., Hong, H.S., Hsih, M.S., Yang, L.C., Ho, H.C., et al., 2004. A marker for Stevens Johnson syndrome. Nature 428, 486.

Coffey, S., Williams, M., 2011. Quetiapine-associated cardiomyopathy. N. Z. Med. J. 124 (1337), 105−107. Available from: <http://www.nzma.org.nz/journal/124-1337/4744/>.

Cohen, H., Loewenthal, U., Matar, M., Kotler, M., 2001. Association of autonomic dysfunction and clozapine. Heart rate variability and risk for sudden death in patients with schizophrenia on long-term psychotropic medication. Br. J. Psychiatry 179, 167−171.

Cohen, D., Bogers, J.P., van Dijk, D., Bakker, B., Schulte, P.F., 2012. Beyond white blood cell monitoring: screening in the initial phase of clozapine therapy. J. Clin. Psychiatry 73 (10), 1307−1312.

Cooper, L.T., 2009. Myocarditis. N. Engl. J. Med. 360 (15), 1526−1538.

Couchman, L., Morgan, P.E., Spencer, E.P., Flanagan, R.J., 2010. Plasma clozapine, norclozapine, and the clozapine:norclozapine ratio in relation to prescribed dose and other factors: data from a therapeutic drug monitoring service, 1993-2007. Ther. Drug Monit. 32 (4), 438−447.

Coulter, D.M., Bate, A., Meyboom, R.H., Lindquist, M., Edwards, I.R., 2001. Antipsychotic drugs and heart muscle disorder in international pharmacovigilance: data mining study. Br. Med. J. 322 (7296), 1207−1209.

Daly, A.K., Donaldson, P.T., Bhatnagar, P., Shen, Y., Pe'er, I., Floratos, A., et al., 2009. HLA-B*5701 genotype is a major determinant of drug-induced liver injury due to flucloxacillin. Nat. Genet. 41 (7), 816−819.

Danti, M., Sbarbati, S., Alsadi, N., et al., 2009. Cardiac magnetic resonance imaging: diagnostic value and utility in the follow-up of patients with acute myocarditis mimicking myocardial infarction. Radiol. Med. 114, 229−238.

Diaz, F.J., Santoro, V., Spina, E., Cogollo, M., Rivera, T.E., Botts, S., et al., 2008. Estimating the size of the effects of co-medications on plasma clozapine concentrations using a model that controls for clozapine doses and confounding variables. Pharmacopsychiatry 41 (3), 81−91.

Diaz, F.J., Eap, C.B., Ansermot, N., Crettol, S., Spina, E., de Leon, J., 2014. Can valproic acid be an inducer of clozapine metabolism? Pharmacopsychiatry 47 (3), 89−96.

Escaut, L., Liotier, J.Y., Albengres, E., Cheminot, N., Vittecoq, D., 1999. Abacavir rechallenge has to be avoided in case of hypersensitivity reaction. AIDS 13 (11), 1419−1420.

Fitzsimons, J., Berk, M., Lambert, T., Bourin, M., Dodd, S., 2005. A review of clozapine safety. Expert Opin. Drug Saf. 4 (4), 731−744.

Floreani, J., Bastiampillai, T., 2008. Successful re-challenge with clozapine following development of clozapine-induced cardiomyopathy. Aust. N. Z. J. Psychiatry 42 (8), 747−748.

Goldstein, J.I., Fredrik Jarskog, L., Hilliard, C., Alfirevic, A., Duncan, L., Fourches, D., et al., 2014. Clozapine-induced agranulocytosis is associated with rare HLA-DQB1 and HLA-B alleles. Nat. Commun. 5, 4757. Available from: http://dx.doi.org/10.1038/ncomms5757.

Guglin, M., Hourani, R., Pitta, S., 2007. Factors determining extreme brain natriuretic peptide elevation. Congest. Heart Fail. 13 (3), 136−141.

Gullestad, L., Ueland, T., Vinge, L.E., Finsen, A., Yndestad, A., Aukrust, P., 2012. Inflammatory cytokines in heart failure: mediators and markers. Cardiology 122 (1), 23−35.

Gupta, S., Figueredo, V.M., 2014. Tachycardia mediated cardiomyopathy: pathophysiology, mechanisms, clinical features and management. Int. J. Cardiol. 172 (1), 40−46.

Haas, S.J., Hill, R., Krum, H., Liew, D., Tonkin, A., Demos, L., et al., 2007. Clozapine-associated myocarditis: a review of 116 cases of suspected myocarditis associated with the use of clozapine in Australia during 1993-2003. Drug Saf. 30 (1), 47−57.

Hetherington, S., McGuirk, S., Powell, G., Cutrell, A., Naderer, O., Spreen, B., et al., 2001. Hypersensitivity reactions during therapy with the nucleoside reverse transcriptase inhibitor abacavir. Clin. Ther. 23 (10), 1603−1614.

Hoehns, J.D., Fouts, M.M., Kelly, M.W., Tu, K.B., 2001. Sudden cardiac death with clozapine and sertraline combination. Ann. Pharmacother. 35 (7−8), 862−866.

Holmvang, G., Dec, G.W., 2012. CMR in myocarditis: valuable tool, room for improvement. JACC Cardiovasc. Imaging 5 (5), 525−527.

Hung, S.-I., Chung, W.-H., Liou, L.-B., Chu, C.-C., Lin, M., Huang, H.-P., et al., 2005. HLA-B*5801 allele as a genetic marker for severe cutaneous adverse reactions caused by allopurinol. Proc. Natl. Acad. Sci. U.S.A. 102 (11), 4134−4139.

Karagianis, J.L., Phillips, L.C., Hogan, K.P., LeDrew, K.K., 1999. Clozapine-associated neuroleptic malignant syndrome: two new cases and a review of the literature. Ann. Pharmacother. 33 (5), 623−630.

Kelly, D.L., Wehring, H.J., Linthicum, J., Feldman, S., McMahon, R.P., Love, R.C., et al., 2009. Cardiac-related findings at autopsy in people with severe mental illness treated with clozapine or risperidone. Schizophr. Res. 107 (2−3), 134−138.

Kenchaiah, S., Evans, J.C., Levy, D., Wilson, P.W., Benjamin, E.J., Larson, M.G., et al., 2002. Obesity and the risk of heart failure. N. Engl. J. Med. 347 (5), 305−313.

Kidd, S., Chopra, P., Stone, J., Jackson, T., Gwee, K., Maynard, S., et al., 2013. Monitoring of long-term cardiac complications in patients receiving clozapine. Australas. Psychiatry 21 (1), 77−78.

Kikuchi, Y., Ataka, K., Yagisawa, K., Omori, Y., Shimizu, K., Kanbayashi, T., et al., 2013. Clozapine-induced cardiomyopathy: a first case in Japan. Schizophr. Res. 150 (2−3), 586−587.

Kilian, J.G., Kerr, K., Lawrence, C., Celermajer, D.S., 1999. Myocarditis and cardiomyopathy associated with clozapine. Lancet 354 (9193), 1841−1845.

Kitulwatte, I.D., Kim, P.J.H., Pollanen, M.S., 2010. Sudden death related myocarditis: a study of 56 cases. Forensic Sci. Med. Pathol. 6 (1), 13−19.

Kluge, M., Schuld, A., Schacht, A., Himmerich, H., Dalal, M.A., Wehmeier, P.M., et al., 2009. Effects of clozapine and olanzapine on cytokine systems are closely linked to weight gain and drug-induced fever. Psychoneuroendocrinology 34 (1), 118−128.

Kuo, C., Yang, S.Y., Liao, Y.T., Chen, W.J., Lee, W.C., Shau, W.Y., et al., 2013. Second-generation antipsychotic medications and risk of pneumonia in schizophrenia. Schizophr. Bull. 39 (3), 648−657.

Lakdawala, N.K., Winterfield, J.R., Funke, B.H., 2013. Dilated cardiomyopathy. Circ. Arrhythm. Electrophysiol. 6 (1), 228−237.

Law, C., Glover, C., Benson, K., Guglin, M., 2010. Extremely high brain natriuretic peptide does not reflect the severity of heart failure. Congest. Heart Fail. 16 (5), 221−225.

Leo, R.J., Kreeger, J.L., Kim, K.Y., 1996. Cardiomyopathy associated with clozapine. Ann. Pharmacother. 30 (6), 603−605.

Leung, J.G., Nelson, S., Takala, C.R., Goren, J.L., 2014. Infection and inflammation leading to clozapine toxicity and intensive care: a case series. Ann. Pharmacother. 48 (6), 801−805.

Levenson, J.L., 1985. Neuroleptic malignant syndrome. Am. J. Psychiatry 142, 1137−1145.

Magnani, J.W., Dec, G.W., 2006. Myocarditis: current trends in diagnosis and treatment. Circulation 113, 876−890.

Makhoul, B., Hochberg, I., Rispler, S., Azzam, Z.S., 2008. Dilated cardiomyopathy: an unusual complication of clozapine therapy. Nat. Clin. Pract. Cardiovasc. Med. 5 (9), 566−570.

Mallal, S., Phillips, E., Carosi, G., Molina, J.-M., Workman, C., Tomazic, J., et al., 2008. HLA-B*5701 screening for hypersensitivity to abacavir. N. Engl. J. Med. 358 (6), 568−579.

Manu, P., Sarpal, D., Muir, O., Kane, J.M., Correll, C.U., 2012. When can patients with potentially life-threatening adverse effects be rechallenged with clozapine? A systematic review of the published literature. Schizophr. Res. 134 (2−3), 180−186.

Marder, S.R., Essock, S.M., Miller, A.L., Buchanan, R.W., Casey, D.E., Davis, J.M., et al., 2004. Physical health monitoring of patients with schizophrenia. Am. J. Psychiatry 161 (8), 1334–1349.

Marti, V., 2005. Sudden cardiac death due to risperidone therapy in a patient with possible hypertrophic cardiomyopathy. Ann. Pharmacother. 39 (5), 973.

Merrill, D.B., Ahmari, S.E., Bradford, J.-M.E., Lieberman, J.A., 2006. Myocarditis during clozapine treatment. Am. J. Psychiatry 163 (2), 204–208.

Meth, M.J., Sperber, K.E., 2006. Phenotypic diversity in delayed drug hypersensitivity: an immunologic explanation. Mt. Sinai J. Med. 73 (5), 769–776.

Montastruc, G., Favreliere, S., Sommet, A., Pathak, A., Lapeyre-Mestre, M., Perault-Pochat, M. C., et al., 2010. Drugs and dilated cardiomyopathies: a case/noncase study in the French PharmacoVigilance Database. Br. J. Clin. Pharmacol. 69 (3), 287–294.

Murch, S., Tran, N., Liew, D., Petrakis, M., Prior, D., Castle, D., 2013. Echocardiographic monitoring for clozapine cardiac toxicity: lessons from real-world experience. Australas. Psychiatry 21 (3), 258–261.

Novo, G., Assennato, P., Augugliaro, S., Fazio, G., Ciaramitaro, G., Coppola, G., et al., 2010. Midventricular dyskinesia during clozapine treatment? J. Cardiovasc. Med. 11 (8), 619–621.

Nymark, T.B., Hovland, A., Bjornstad, H., Nielsen, E.W., 2008. A young man with acute dilated cardiomyopathy associated with methylphenidate. Vasc. Health Risk Manag. 4 (2), 477–479.

O'Connell, K.E., Thakore, J., Dev, K.K., 2014. Pro-inflammatory cytokine levels are raised in female schizophrenia patients treated with clozapine. Schizophr. Res. 156 (1), 1–8.

Park, H., Park, H., Lee, D., et al., 2014. Increased phosphorylation of Ca(2+) handling proteins as a proarrhythmic mechanism in myocarditis. Circ. J. 78, 2292–2301.

Pastor, C.A., Mehta, M., 2008. Masked clozapine-induced cardiomyopathy. J. Am. Board Fam. Med. 21 (1), 70–74.

Phan, K.L., Taylor, S.F., 2002. Clozapine-associated cardiomyopathy. Psychosomatics 43 (3), 248.

Pieroni, M., Cavallaro, R., Chimenti, C., Smeraldi, E., Frustaci, A., 2004. Clozapine-induced hypersensitivity myocarditis. Chest 126 (5), 1703–1705.

Pollmacher, T., Hinze-Selch, D., Mullington, J., 1996. Effects of clozapine on plasma cytokine and soluble cytokine receptor levels. J. Clin. Psychopharmacol. 16 (5), 403–409.

Raja, M., 2011. Clozapine safety, 35 years later. Curr. Drug Saf. 6 (3), 164–184.

Razminia, M., Salem, Y., Devaki, S., Shah, N., Khosla, S., 2006. Clozapine induced myopericarditis: early recognition improves clinical outcome. Am. J. Ther. 13 (3), 274–276.

Reinders, J., Parsonage, W., Lange, D., Potter, J.M., Plever, S., 2004. Clozapine-related myocarditis and cardiomyopathy in an Australian metropolitan psychiatric service. Aust. N. Z. J. Psychiatry 38 (11–12), 915–922.

Roesch-Ely, D., Van Einsiedel, R., Kathofer, S., Schwaninger, M., Weisbrod, M., 2002. Myocarditis with quetiapine. Am. J. Psychiatry 159 (9), 1607–1608.

Roh, S., Ahn, D.H., Nam, J.H., Yang, B.H., Lee, B.H., Kim, Y.S., 2006. Cardiomyopathy associated with clozapine. Exp. Clin. Psychopharmacol. 14 (1), 94–98.

Ronaldson, K.J., Taylor, A.J., Fitzgerald, P.B., Topliss, D.J., Elsik, M., McNeil, J.J., 2010. Diagnostic characteristics of clozapine induced myocarditis identified by an analysis of 38 cases and 47 controls. J. Clin. Psychiatry 71 (8), 976–981.

Ronaldson, K.J., Taylor, A.J., Fitzgerald, P.B., Topliss, D.J., McNeil, J.J., 2011a. Clinical course and analysis of ten fatal cases of clozapine-induced myocarditis and comparison with 66 surviving cases. Schizophr. Res. 128, 161–165.

Ronaldson, K.J., Taylor, A.J., Fitzgerald, P.B., Topliss, D.J., McNeil, J.J., 2011b. A new monitoring protocol for clozapine induced myocarditis based on an analysis of 75 cases and 94 controls. Aust. N. Z. J. Psychiatry 45 (6), 458−465.

Ronaldson, K.J., Fitzgerald, P.B., Taylor, A.J., McNeil, J.J., 2012a. Continuation of clozapine following mild myocarditis. Aust. N. Z. J. Psychiatry 46 (9), 910−911.

Ronaldson, K.J., Fitzgerald, P.B., Taylor, A.J., McNeil, J.J., 2012b. Observations from 8 cases of clozapine rechallenge after development of myocarditis. J. Clin. Psychiatry 73 (2), 252−254.

Ronaldson, K.J., Fitzgerald, P.B., Taylor, A.J., Topliss, D.J., McNeil, J.J., 2012c. Clozapine-induced myocarditis and baseline echocardiography. Aust. N. Z. J. Psychiatry 46 (10), 1006−1007.

Ronaldson, K.J., Fitzgerald, P.B., Taylor, A.J., Topliss, D.J., Wolfe, R., McNeil, J.J., 2012d. Rapid clozapine dose titration and concomitant sodium valproate increase the risk of myocarditis with clozapine: a case-control study. Schizophr. Res. 141 (2−3), 173−178.

Ronaldson, K.J., Fitzgerald, P.B., McNeil, J.J., 2015a. Clozapine-induced myocarditis, a widely overlooked adverse reaction. Acta Psychiatr. Scand. 132 (4), 231−240. Available from: http://dx.doi.org/10.1111/acps.12416.

Ronaldson, K.J., Fitzgerald, P.B., McNeil, J.J., 2015b. Evolution of troponin, C-reactive protein and eosinophil count with the onset of clozapine-induced myocarditis. Aust. N. Z. J. Psychiatry 49 (5), 486−487. Available from: http://dx.doi.org/10.1177/0004867414566871.

Rostagno, C., Di Norscia, G., Placidi, G.F., Gensini, G.F., 2008. Beta-blocker and angiotensin-converting enzyme inhibitor may limit certain cardiac adverse effects of clozapine. Gen. Hosp. Psychiatry 30 (3), 280−283.

Rostagno, C., Domenichetti, S., Gensini, G.F., 2012. Does a subclinical cardiotoxic effect of clozapine exist? Results from a follow-up pilot study. Cardiovasc. Hematol. Agents Med. Chem. 10 (2), 148−153.

Rostagno, C., Domenichetti, S., Pastorelli, F., Gensini, G.F., 2011a. Clozapine associated cardiomyopathy: a cluster of 3 cases. Intern. Emerg. Med. 6 (3), 281−283.

Rostagno, C., Domenichetti, S., Pastorelli, F., Gensini, G.F., 2011b. Usefulness of NT-pro-BNP and echocardiography in the diagnosis of subclinical clozapine-related cardiotoxicity. J. Clin. Psychopharmacol. 31 (6), 712−716.

Rostagno, C., Pastorelli, F., Domenichetti, S., Gensini, G.F., 2011c. Cardio-vascular risks associated with clozapine treatment. Curr. Psychiatry Rev. 7 (3), 170−176.

Roussel, O., Dumillard, C., Sadeg, N., Belhadj Tahar, H., 2006. [Amisulpride poisoning. A case report]. [French]. Therapie 61 (6), 534−536.

Sagar, R., Berry, N., Sadhu, R., Mishra, S., Kahn, D.A., 2008. Clozapine-induced cardiomyopathy presenting as panic attacks. J. Psychiatr. Pract. 14 (3), 182−185.

Serrano, A., Rangel, N., Carrizo, E., Uzcategui, E., Sandia, I., Zabala, A., et al., 2014. Safety of long-term clozapine administration. Frequency of cardiomyopathy and hyponatraemia: two cross-sectional, naturalistic studies. Aust. N. Z. J. Psychiatry 48 (2), 183−192.

Stevenson, L.W., Loscalzo, J., 2012. Chapter 238. Cardiomyopathy and myocarditis. In: 18th ed. Longo, D.L., Fauci, A.S., Kasper, D.L., Stephen, L.H., Jameson, J.L., Loscalzo, J. (Eds.), Harrison's Principles of Internal Medicine, vol. 2. McGraw-Hill Medical, New York, NY, pp. 1951−1970.

Stryjer, R., Timinsky, I., Reznik, I., Weizman, A., Spivak, B., 2009. Beta-adrenergic antagonists for the treatment of clozapine-induced sinus tachycardia: a retrospective study. Clin. Neuropharmacol. 32 (5), 290−292.

Tanner, M.A., Culling, W., 2003. Clozapine associated dilated cardiomyopathy. Postgrad. Med. J. 79 (933), 412—413.

Taylor, D.M., Douglas-Hall, P., Olofinjana, B., Whiskey, E., Thomas, A., 2009. Reasons for discontinuing clozapine: matched, case-control comparison with risperidone long-acting injection. Br. J. Psychiatry 194 (2), 165—167.

Therapeutic Goods Administration. Australian Government. Database of Adverse Event Notifications (DAEN). Retrieved (January 12, 2015) from: <https://www.tga.gov.au/database-adverse-event-notifications-daen>.

Tripp, A.C., 2011. Nonfatal pulmonary embolus associated with clozapine treatment: a case series. Gen. Hosp. Psychiatry 33 (1), 85.e85-86.

Umana, E., Solares, A., Alpert, M.A., 2003. Tachycardia-induced cardiomyopathy. Am. J. Med. 114, 51—55.

Vaddadi, K.S., Soosai, E., Vaddadi, G., 2003. Low blood selenium concentrations in schizophrenic patients on clozapine. Br. J. Clin. Pharmacol. 55 (3), 307—309.

Wang, J.-F., Min, J.-Y., Hampton, T.G., Amende, I., Yan, X., Malek, S., et al., 2008. Clozapine-induced myocarditis: role of catecholamines in a murine model. Eur. J. Pharmacol. 592 (1—3), 123—127.

Wassef, N., Khan, N., Shahzad, M., 2015. Quetiapine-induced myocarditis presenting as acute STEMI. BMJ Case Rep. 2015. Available from: http://dx.doi.org/10.1136/bcr-2014-207151.

Wexler, R.K., Elton, T., Pleister, A., Feldman, D., 2009. Cardiomyopathy: an overview. Am. Fam. Physician 79 (9), 778—784.

Wrigley, B.J., Lip, G.Y., Shantsila, E., 2011. The role of monocytes and inflammation in the pathophysiology of heart failure. Eur. J. Heart Fail. 13 (11), 1161—1171.

Wu, A.H., Jaffe, A.S., Apple, F.S., Jesse, R.L., Francis, G.L., Morrow, D.A., et al., 2007. National Academy of Clinical Biochemistry laboratory medicine practice guidelines: use of cardiac troponin and B-type natriuretic peptide or N-terminal proB-type natriuretic peptide for etiologies other than acute coronary syndromes and heart failure. Clin. Chem. 53 (12), 2086—2096.

Chapter 3

Pulmonary Embolism

Peter Manu[1,2], Christopher Hohman[3], James F. Barrecchia[3] and
Matisyahu Shulman[3]

[1]*Hofstra Northwell School of Medicine, Hempstead, NY, United States,* [2]*South Oaks Hospital,
Amityville, NY, United States,* [3]*Zucker Hillside Hospital, Glen Oaks, NY, United States*

3.1 EPIDEMIOLOGY

Pulmonary embolism is common (4−21/10,000 adults per year) and has a
high mortality (23−87%) if not treated (Levin et al., 2015). A majority of
patients who die from pulmonary embolism have not been diagnosed premortem, an issue related to the variability in clinical presentation, which
includes sudden death; inaccurate risk assessment; and lack of advanced
imaging technology. Together with deep vein thrombosis, the condition is
part of the clinical continuum represented by acute venous thromboembolism
(VTE). At age 45, the lifetime risk of pulmonary embolism and/or deep
venous thrombosis is 8.1% in the United States, with higher rates in patients
with obesity, sickle cell disease, and persons heterozygous for factor V
Leiden (Bell et al., 2016). The risk of VTE has been shown to increase by
up to 50% in patients treated with antipsychotic drugs (Zornberg and Jick,
2000; Hagg et al., 2008; Parker et al., 2010; Barbui et al., 2014). The drugs
most often associated with VTE are low-potency first generation antipsychotics, clozapine and olanzapine (Jönsson et al., 2012). The condition is life-
threatening, as indicated (Walker et al., 1997) by a death from pulmonary
embolism among current users of clozapine five times greater than for past
users (30 vs 6 per 100,000 person-years).

The epidemiological association between antipsychotic drugs and pulmonary thromboembolism was first studied in New Zealand and represented an
expansion of a national case−control studies of deaths produced by this condition (Parkin et al., 2003). Of the country's 122 persons aged 15−59 years who
had been recorded as fatal cases of pulmonary thromboembolism from 1990
through 1998, 75 were confirmed by thorough review of pulmonary angiography, ventilation/perfusion scans and/or duplicated expert consultations using

Life-Threatening Effects of Antipsychotic Drugs. DOI: http://dx.doi.org/10.1016/B978-0-12-803376-0.00003-4
© 2016 Elsevier Inc. All rights reserved.
59

standard criteria. Four age- and gender-matched control subjects were randomly selected from the patient panel seen in the same group practice of each fatal case of pulmonary thromboembolism. Individuals who had been given at least one prescription of psychotropics (antipsychotics, antidepressants, or other) within 3 months of the index date were considered current users. The fatal pulmonary embolism cases and control groups were compared after adjustment for weight and use of contraceptive/hormonal therapy. Sixty-two of the seventy-five fatal cases and 243 from their control group had no identifiable major risk factors, such as previous of venous thromboembolic events, prolonged immobility, major surgery, or pregnancy. Two control patients and eight fatal cases were taking antipsychotics. Of the eight cases, six were treated with thioridazine and two with haloperidol. Compared with nonusers, their adjusted odds ratio (OR) for fatal pulmonary embolism was 13.3 (95% confidence interval (CI) 2.3−76.3). Past use of antipsychotics did not carry a significantly higher risk compared with never use (OR 5.3, 95% CI 0.6−45.8). Similarly, a comparison between current users and nonusers of antidepressants indicated an OR of 4.9 (95% CI 1.1−22.5), a trend attributed by the authors to the chemical resemblance between tricyclics and phenothiazines.

The New Zealand study was followed by a report from Japan, based on the review of the medical records of 1125 individuals who had forensic autopsies performed after sudden unexpected death from Jan. 1998 to Dec. 2002 by staff pathologists in the Department of Legal Medicine at Kitasato University (Hamanaka et al., 2004). Thirty-four patients (3% of the cohort) had been treated with antipsychotic drugs for schizophrenia (32 cases), schizoaffective disorder (1 case) and mental retardation (1 case). Pulmonary embolism was identified as the cause of death in 28 patients, 8 (29%) of whom had been on antipsychotics. On logistic regression, antipsychotic drug use was associated with a significantly higher risk of dying from pulmonary embolism, as indicated by an OR of 10.49 with a 95% CI of 3.95−27.85.

The eight patients who died of pulmonary embolism during treatment with antipsychotics were all female. Their age ranged from 32 to 65 (mean 55; standard deviation 11). Seven of the eight patients had been treated with antipsychotic polytherapy, which combined conventional antipsychotics (chlorpromazine, levomepromazine, perphenazine, haloperidol, and/or bromperidol) with atypical antipsychotics (risperidone and/or zotepine). The total neuroleptic dose was substantial, an example being a patient treated with chlorpromazine 175 mg, levomepromazine 50 mg, haloperidol 18 mg, and risperidone 6 mg each day. Five patients had evidence of deep venous thrombosis at autopsy. One patient had a collagen vascular disease, which was considered a risk factor for thrombotic disease. None of the patients tested positive for anticardiolipin antibody. The body mass index was in the overweight category ($25-29.9 \text{ kg m}^{-2}$) in four cases. Age and body mass index were not independent predictors of pulmonary embolism in this cohort.

A third epidemiological analysis evaluated the risk of pulmonary embolism in the United States was assessed retrospectively in the 2006 database generated by the "Premier's Perspective," a survey of approximately 500 acute care hospitals (Allenet et al., 2012). The database provided information regarding 28,723,771 patients 18 years of age or older, of whom 450,951 had been prescribed antipsychotic drugs. There were 76,814 cases of pulmonary thromboembolism in the entire sample (0.3%) and 3764 among persons presumably treated with antipsychotics (0.83%). After adjustment for important confounders, such as age, gender, obesity, pregnancy, hormone therapy, thrombophilia, hospitalization, the OR for pulmonary thromboembolism were 1.17 (95% CI 1.13−1.21) in the population prescribed antipsychotics compared with nonusers. The ORs for conventional (1.19; 95% CI 1.13−1.25) and atypical (1.15; 95% CI 1.09−1.21) were statistically similar. Clozapine was associated with the highest risk of pulmonary thromboembolism (OR 1.46; 95% CI 1.05−2.02), followed by ziprasidone (OR 1.21; 95% CI 1.07−1.38) and chlorpromazine (OR 1.19; 95% CI 1.03−1.38). The lowest risk was noted in patients prescribed quetiapine (OR 0.97; 95% CI 0.91−1.04) and aripiprazole (OR 0.98; 95% CI 0.83−1.15). The adjusted ORs increased linearly from low-dose prescription (1.07), usual dose (1.16), tolerated dose (1.21), and high dose (1.28).

The most recent study to date used information retrieved from the Lombardy Regional Health Service, Italy regarding all individuals 18 years of age or older ($N = 144,129$) who had been prescribed treatment with antipsychotics in 2012 and 2013 (Conti et al., 2015). Cases were patients with at least one hospital admission for pulmonary embolism. Up to 20 controls, not treated with anticoagulants in the previous 12 months, matched for gender and age with each case, were extracted from the inception cohort. The exclusion criteria were a diagnosis of neoplasm, hip or lower extremity fractures, and pregnancy. Patients were classified as past users if their last prescription for antipsychotics was issued more than a year prior to the index date, recent user if they had received a prescription within 4−12 months, and current user if they had received at least one prescription in the previous 3 months. There were 269 pulmonary thromboembolic events recorded for the cohort, that is, an incidence rate of 305 cases/100,000 person-years. As a group, cases were more likely than control subjects to have a history of coronary artery disease, heart failure, stroke, and chronic liver or renal disease. Data regarding specific antipsychotics and clinical outcome of the thrombotic events were not included in the report.

A substantial majority of pulmonary thromboembolic events (84.1%) occurred in recent antipsychotic users, which translated into a doubling of the risk compared with past use (OR 2.31, 95% CI 1.16−4.59) even after adjusting for comorbid medical conditions, but not for body mass index or for level of physical activity. Recent use did not increase the risk of pulmonary thromboembolism (OR 0.96, 95% CI 0.44−2.07). Exclusive use of

TABLE 3.1 Odds Ratios of Pulmonary Embolism in Patients Treated With Antipsychotic Drugs

Authors (Year)	Odds Ratio	95% CI	N	Type of Comparison
Parkin et al. (2003)[a]	13.30	2.30−76.60	75	Users vs nonusers
Hamanaka et al. (2004)[a]	10.49	3.95−27.85	28	Users vs nonusers
Allenet et al. (2012)[b]	1.17	1.13−1.21	3764	Prescribed vs not prescribed[c]
Conti et al. (2015)[b]	2.31	1.1−4.59	232	Current vs past users

[a]Analysis of risk of death from pulmonary embolism.
[b]The study did not separate fatal and nonfatal cases.
[c]The control group consisted of members of the general population hospitalized for any cause during the period of interests, that is, not patients with a psychiatric diagnosis not prescribed antipsychotic drugs.

conventional antipsychotics was associated with a higher OR of pulmonary thromboembolism (3.52, 95% CI 1.61−7.35) than the exposure to atypical antipsychotics (OR 2.01, 95% CI 1.01−4.03). A similar incidence was calculated for cases that had recently received concomitant treatment with conventional and atypical antipsychotics (OR 4.21, 95% 1.53−11.59). The risk was greatest among individuals who had received prescriptions for two or more antipsychotics within the past 3 months (OR 5.87; 95% CI 2.48−13.89). Taken together with the previous three studies, the data strongly support an increased risk of pulmonary embolism in current users of antipsychotic drugs (Table 3.1). A caveat is the fact that in the latter two studies (Allenet et al., 2012; Conti et al., 2015) no independent investigation was conducted to validate the diagnosis of pulmonary embolism.

3.2 PATHOBIOLOGY

The way in which antipsychotic drugs increase the risk of VTE has not been elucidated. The suggested mechanism include enhanced platelet aggregation, production of antiphospholipid abnormalities, hyperprolactinemia, and venous stasis due to decreased ambulation (Jönsson et al., 2012), but data are scant and rarely independently confirmed. A key factor may prove to be the overweight and obese status of a majority of patients treated with these drugs. Virchow's triad of venous stasis, hypercoagulability, and endothelial injury (Wolberg et al., 2012) is a useful tool in understanding the development of thromboembolism and offers a sound framework for the understanding of how antipsychotic drugs may increase the risk of VTE (Fig. 3.1).

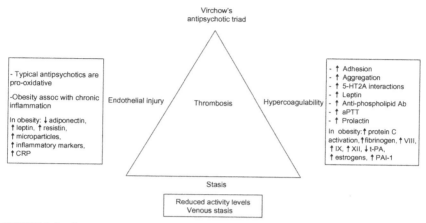

FIGURE 3.1 Components and suggested mechanisms of Virchow's triad in patients treated with antipsychotic drugs.

3.2.1 Venous Stasis as a Consequence of Obesity and Physical Inactivity

The analysis of the contribution of a stasis component of the triad to the increased risk of pulmonary embolism in patients treated with antipsychotic drugs is of the utmost importance, as it relates to obesity and low levels of physical activity. The lifestyle of the chronically psychotic patient and the antipsychotic drug treatment often lead to little physical activity and a high caloric intake (Urban et al., 2007; Ehrlich et al., 2012; Manu et al., 2015).

The presence of obesity is associated with a significant increase in the risk of pulmonary embolism. In the most recent large epidemiological survey in the United States, performed in 18 million persons over a 10-year period (1998−2008), 1.1% of obese, but only 0.6% of the nonobese were diagnosed with pulmonary embolism, for a relative risk of 2.03 (Stein et al., 2011). The relative risk was higher in the obese women than in men (2.08 vs 1.74). The highest relative risk (5.80) was observed in obese youth 11−20 years old. In contrast, the relative risk was lowest (1.41) in the cohort 61−70 years of age. Careful assessments using strain gauge outflow plethysmography, venous continuous Doppler ultrasonography, and passive venous drainage and refill testing have indicated that an increased body mass index was independently associated with the venous stasis syndrome in subjects with or without a past history of VTE (Ashrani et al., 2009). The influence of obesity on the risk of pulmonary embolism through venous stasis must be interpreted with caution, because obesity is also a prothrombotic condition, as indicated by the increased expression of plasminogen activator inhibitor-1 (PAI-1) and enhanced platelet activation (Stein et al., 2011; Samad and Ruf, 2013). The change in PAI-1 level decreases fibrinolytic activity by disrupting the conversion of plasminogen to plasmin, leading to reduced fibrin clearance, an effect compounded by adiponectin deficiency and decreased endothelial tissue-type plasminogen activator (Craft and Reed, 2010). The expression of antifibrinolytic proteins may also be enhanced by elevated levels associated with obesity (Schäfer and Konstantinides, 2014). The prothrombotic pattern is acquired, as indicated in a study of obesity-discordant monozygotic twin pairs which indicated a significant increase in the PAI-1, fibrinogen, and factors IX, XI, and XII in the obese cotwins (Kaye et al., 2012). The intrapair difference in PAI-1 and fibrinogen correlated with severity of adiposity.

Obesity is a risk factor for both VTE and atherothrombosis, an epidemiological link that is likely due to a common inflammatory mechanism for the two conditions, which is manifested by increased levels cytokines, primarily interleukin-6, interleukin 1 beta, and tumor necrosis factor-alpha, as well as by marked elevation in the titer of C-reactive protein (Piazza, 2015).

3.2.2   Hypercoagulability

3.2.2.1   Antipsychotic Drugs and Platelet Function

The effect of antipsychotic drugs on platelet function has remained a subject of debate. Axelsson et al. (2007) have observed increased platelet adhesion and aggregation after exposure to clozapine. On the other hand, clozapine (420 ng mL^{-1}), risperidone (65 ng mL^{-1}), and haloperidol (20 ng mL^{-1}) significantly reduced ADP-induced and collagen-induced platelet aggregability in vitro (Dietrich-Muszalska et al., 2010a,b).

3.2.2.2   Antiphospholipid Antibodies

Chlorpromazine use has been known to be associated with the presence of lupus-like anticoagulant, a potentially thrombogenic antiphospholipid antibody, since the 1970s (Zarrabi et al., 1979). Among 30 current users of chlorpromazine, the antibody was identified in 11 and was absent in all of the 17 patients tested who had been off this drug for more than a year (Canoso and Sise, 1982). The presence of lupus anticoagulant is significantly greater in patients with pulmonary embolism, infarction, and microthrombosis than in control subjects with arterial thrombotic events (Stojanovich et al., 2015). The interpretation of these data is difficult given the numerous antiphospholipid antibodies other than lupus anticoagulant, that is, anticardiolipin, anti-β2 Glycoprotein I, antiprothrombin, antiphosphatidyl serine, and antiphosphatidyl ethanolamine, a heterogeneous group with regard to propensity for inducing venous and arterial thrombi (Reynaud et al., 2014). It is also worth noting that although antiphospholipid antibodies have been found in up to 27% of users of antipsychotics, the frequency was similar in nonusers (Delluc et al., 2014).

3.2.2.3   Prolactin-Mediated Hypercoagulability

Most antipsychotics cause increased prolactin levels which may lead to platelet activation (Wallaschofski et al., 2003), in some instances even after a single dose (Reuwer et al., 2009). Higher prolactin is correlated with increased coagulation factors in healthy controls and risk of thrombotic events increases with increasing levels of prolactin (Stuijver et al., 2012). Prolactin is associated with increased coagulation factors VIII and vWF (Stuijver et al., 2012), as well as with biomarkers of VTE, such as D-dimer/fibrin/fibrinogen degradation products and thrombin-antithrombin complex (Ishioka et al., 2015). However, a prolactin-dependent enhancement of ADP-induced platelet activation or aggregation has not been convincingly demonstrated (Reuwer et al., 2009).

3.2.2.4   Obesity-Mediated Hypercoagulability

Obesity, another common side effect of many antipsychotic medications, is associated with a number of factors increasing risk for thrombotic events including increased levels of factors VIII, IX, XII, and fibrinogen; increased estrogen levels; and decreased levels of antithrombotic molecules (Ehrlich et al., 2012).

3.2.3   Endothelial Injury

Endothelial injury can occur via a variety of mechanisms in psychotic patients. Physical restraints may produce vascular trauma in psychotic patients. Typical antipsychotics are pro-oxidative (Jeding et al., 1995) and may play a role in oxidative injury to vessel walls. Obesity may affect the vascular endothelium through its association with chronic inflammation, increased leptin, resistin, and microparticles, decreased adiponectin (Ehrlich et al., 2012), and increased C-reactive protein (Carrizo et al., 2008).

3.3   CLINICAL AND LABORATORY FEATURES

3.3.1   Clinical Presentation

Pulmonary thromboembolism must be considered in the presence of new onset or worsening chest pain, dyspnea, and hypotension. The presence of hypoxemia, hemoptysis, and painful or asymmetric edema of lower extremities increases the probability of acute pulmonary embolism. Clinicians should also be aware that psychiatric patients with pulmonary embolism may report only fatigue, or decrease their participation in group sessions, instead of focusing on dyspnea (Tripp, 2011).

Hemodynamically unstable patients, that is, those with sustained hypotension or in shock have an all-cause mortality rate of 31.8%, while in patients with pulmonary embolism presenting with stable hemodynamic parameters, the observed mortality rate was 3.4% (Casazza et al., 2012). Survivors may develop chronic thromboembolic pulmonary hypertension, a major, but infrequent (less than 4%) complication (Agnelli and Becattini, 2010). The intrinsic risk factors for pulmonary embolism are age older than 70, previous VTE, and inherited hypercoagulable states (Lapner, 2013). There are also numerous acquired risk factors (Lapner, 2013), of which obesity and prolonged immobility are quite common in psychiatric patients (Table 3.2). The relative impact of risk factors, evaluated during a 15-year period in Olmsted County, MN, indicated that the highest risk is attributable to hospitalization for surgery (24%) or medical illness (22%), nursing home residence (22%), and malignancy (16%) (Heit et al., 2002).

The presentation of pulmonary embolism in patients treated with antipsychotic drugs is often characterized by components of the classic triad chest pain-dyspnea-hypotension. In the case of a 25-year-old patient with schizoaffective disorder treated with olanzapine 20 mg per day for 3 months, the pulmonary embolism produced sudden onset of back pain radiating to the left side of the chest. The chest pain was followed, a few hours later, by shortness of breath and hemoptysis (Borras et al., 2008). The patient was not hypoxic and had no ultrasonographic evidence of deep vein thrombosis of lower extremities. The diagnosis of pulmonary embolism was established by computerized tomographic pulmonary angiography. A coagulopathy was excluded after a thorough work-up. The patient was maintained on warfarin without complications, but with intermittent nonadherence. He was then started on risperidone (3 mg per day), but 3 weeks later he developed chest pain, dyspnea, and hemoptysis, associated with multiple peripheral pulmonary emboli demonstrated on computerized tomography. Risperidone was continued, but a third episode occurred 4 months later, while the patient

TABLE 3.2 Acquired Risk Factors for Pulmonary Embolism

Malignancy or current cancer chemotherapy
Limb paralysis, major trauma or orthopedic surgery
Obesity
Pregnancy or puerperium
Prolonged immobility
General anesthesia
Antiphospholipid antibodies
Heparin-induced thrombocytopenia
Estrogen therapy

was adequately anticoagulated. Recurrent episodes of pulmonary embolism in a patient treated with clozapine had a similar presentation with acute dyspnea (Munoli et al., 2013).

The time lag between the start of treatment with an antipsychatic drug and pulmonary embolism is quite variable. One 32-year-old patient had been on olanzapine 10 mg per day for a year prior to developing pleuritic chest pain, fever, and hemoptysis due to bilateral large vessel pulmonary emboli and right lower lobe infarction. In contrast, a 62-year-old developed a fatal saddle embolus occluding the right ventricular outflow tract only 4 days after starting olanzapine for agitation (Hill et al., 2008).

Other presentations are specific for psychiatric settings, particularly those involving recent use of physical restraints (Cecchi et al., 2012) or complicating neuroleptic malignant syndrome (Pandya et al., 2007) or catatonia (Larsen et al., 2011; Clinebell et al., 2014). An illustrative case is that of a 35-year-old physically healthy male with a diagnosis of schizophrenia, admitted for severe agitation and acute persecutory delusions (Cecchi et al., 2012). There was no history of coagulopathy or VTE, no other known risk factors except for a long history of cigarette smoking, and no evidence of traumatic injury produced during the agitated state. The patient received a dose of 4 mg of risperidone, followed by a standing regimen of haloperidol 5 mg and chlorpromazine 100 mg three times daily. He remained agitated and aggressive and was placed in restraints using padded bracelets for 6 days, from which he was released for 45 minutes on the day 2 and 60 minutes on day 5. Immediately after the restraints were removed on day 6, the patient became dizzy and collapsed to the floor. He was unconscious, cyanotic, and dyspneic upon transfer to a medical intensive care unit. A presumptive diagnosis of pulmonary embolism was made and the patient was appropriately anticoagulated with unfractionated heparin. He remained comatose and died after 5 days. The autopsy identified thrombosis in the right femoral-popliteal venous axis and emboli in the right pulmonary artery. The microscopic examination of the thrombi indicated pyknotic neutrophils, macrophages, and fibrinous ribbon deposition, suggesting that the thromboembolic event had occurred within 8 days of death. Another instructive case is that of a 27-year-old obese female admitted for catatonia and treated with risperidone, quetiapine, sertraline, and lorazepam (Tripp, 2011). The patient became hypotensive on the second hospital day, then entered cardiorespiratory arrest. The death was attributed to the bilateral pulmonary thromboemboli discovered on autopsy.

Fever, leukocytosis, inflammatory markers (high erythrocyte sedimentation rate), and ill-defined opacities on chest radiographs have been described as part of the presenting clinical picture in olanzapine-associated pulmonary embolism (Toringhibel et al., 2011) and may render difficult the differentiation from pneumonia. Fever was also the presenting complaint in a 40-year-old male with a paliperidone-associated pulmonary embolism, and occurred together with increased irritability and mild dyspnea (Şengül et al., 2014).

Changes in the antipsychotic drug therapy (dosage or type) may increase the risk of pulmonary embolism, as suggested, for example, by the clinical course of a 42-year-old female with schizoaffective disorder refractory to treatment with flupenthixol decanoate (200 mg intramuscularly once weekly) and amisulpride (400 mg twice daily) (McInerney and McDonald, 2012). Over a 12 week hospitalization her drug regimen was changed to flupenthixol decanoate 400 mg per week, amisulpride 600 mg twice daily, aripiprazole 30 mg per day plus olanzapine 10 mg per day given as needed for agitation. She had no physical complaints during the medication titration period, until she developed chest pain, which was not associated with dyspnea or hypotension. An electrocardiogram and a chest radiograph revealed no abnormalities. D-Dimer level was three times the upper limit of normal and the computerized tomographic pulmonary angiography visualized pulmonary emboli in the lower lobes. However, in other cases, the effect of the change does not appear related to the dose, as in the case of a patient who had tolerated quetiapine 600 mg per day, but developed chest pain and dyspnea after she was cross-tapered to clozapine 175 mg per day (Tripp, 2011). In at least two cases (Munoli et al., 2013; Chate et al., 2013) no recurrence was observed after switching from clozapine to haloperidol.

3.3.2 Diagnosing Pulmonary Embolism in Psychiatric Patients

3.3.2.1 Probability Assessments

The diagnostic sequence in patients suspected of pulmonary embolism starts with an estimation of the probability of the event, which is performed using clinical decision rules known as the Wells score and Revised Geneva score (Penaloza et al., 2013).

The *Wells score* assigns 3 points for clinical signs of deep venous thrombosis, such as edema and pain; 1.5 points each for previous history of deep venous thrombosis or pulmonary embolism, immobilization or surgery within the past 4 weeks, or heart rate >100 beats minute^{-1}; and 1.0 point each for the presence of hemoptysis and history of malignancy (Wells et al., 2000). The absence of an alternative diagnosis more likely than pulmonary embolism adds 3 points. A score of at least 7 indicates high probability, while moderate probability is suggested by a score of $2-6$. Patients with a score of $0-1$ are considered to have low probability for pulmonary embolism.

In the *Revised Geneva score*, 5 points are entered for heart rate >94 beats minute^{-1}; 4 points for unilateral lower extremity edema or pain on deep vein palpation; 3 points each for history of deep venous thrombosis or pulmonary embolism, unilateral lower extremity pain, and heart rate $75-94$ beats minute^{-1}; 2 points each for fracture of the lower extremity or surgery under general anesthesia within the past 4 weeks, active malignancy, and hemoptysis; and 1 point for persons older than 65 years of age

(Le Gal et al., 2006). A score greater than 10 suggests high probability. Moderate clinical probability is indicated by a score of 4−10.

Prospective assessments of the utility of the *Wells score* indicated that the categories corresponded to 1.3% for low probability, 16.2% for moderate, and 37.5% for high probability of pulmonary embolism (Wells et al., 2001). Recent data indicate that unstructured clinician *gestalt* performs at least as well as these scores for the identification of patients with low and high probability of pulmonary embolism (Penaloza et al., 2013). The *Revised Geneva score* appears to correlate with the fatality rate, which was 0% (95% CI 0−5.4) in the low probability and 14.3% (95% CI 6.3−28.2) in the high probability category (Bertoletti et al., 2013). Testing for pulmonary embolism may not be necessary if all of the following conditions are met: no previous venous thromboembolic event, no treatment with estrogens, no recent trauma or surgery, age <50 years, arterial oxygen saturation >94% on room air, heart rate <100 beats minute^{-1}, no hemoptysis, and no unilateral leg swelling (Kline et al., 2008; Freund et al., 2015). The probability of pulmonary embolism in these cases is 1%, with a 95% CI of 0.6−1.6% (Kline et al., 2008).

3.3.2.2 Laboratory Tests and Imaging Investigations

3.3.2.2.1 D-Dimer

The determination of D-dimer, a product of acute thrombi degradation by fibrinolysis, is a common first step in the investigation of patients with symptoms suggestive of pulmonary embolism. Immunoturbidimetric and enzyme-linked immunoabsorbant assays have sensitivities of at least 95%, but specificity of only approximately 40% (Lapner, 2013; Le Gal et al., 2015), so that the positive likelihood ratio is a moderate 1.64 (Le Gal et al., 2015). The specificity is influenced by the presence of clinical entities that increase the level of the D-dimer in the absence of acute thrombosis, such as pregnancy, infection, inflammation, trauma, malignancy, and postsurgical status (Lapner, 2013; Le Gal et al., 2015). D-Dimer should not be used as a primary screening test, that is, prior to a clinical assessment, because of the relatively high rate of false-positive results (Lapner, 2013). Values lower than 500 ng mL^{-1} are considered to rule out pulmonary embolism in patients with low probability of this condition (Le Gal et al., 2015). Patients with "positive" results on D-dimer testing should be referred immediately for the most precise diagnostic imaging procedure available (Le Gal et al., 2015). The D-dimer concentrations increase with age, decreasing the utility of the above threshold to rule out pulmonary embolism in patients older than 50. An age-adjusted cut-off, calculated as age (years) × 10, has been tested prospectively in a study in which patients with D-dimer value between the conventional and the age-adjusted cut-offs did not undergo further investigations and were not anticoagulated (Righini et al., 2014). Among the 331 patients observed, only 1 had a thromboembolic event diagnosed in the 3 months follow-up period.

3.3.2.2.2 Computed Tomographic Pulmonary Angiography

The identification of thrombi on computed tomography using intravenous contrast material has become the main testing modality for the diagnosis of pulmonary embolism. The test has high sensitivity and specificity, but its diagnostic accuracy, as indicated by the positive predictive value, correlates with the size of the occluded artery (Lapner, 2013), ranging from a low of 25% for isolated subsegmental thrombi to 97% for thrombosis occurring in the main pulmonary artery or its lobar branches. From a clinical standpoint, the absence of thrombi on computed tomography pulmonary angiography is considered to rule out a thromboembolic event, as only 1.3% (95% CI, 0.7—2.0%) of patients in this category have shown evidence of progressive venous thrombosis in the following 3 months (Van Belle et al., 2006). Recent data (Mos et al., 2014) have moved the risk of venous thrombosis in patients with a negative computed tomographic angiography slightly higher (2.8%; 95% CI 1.2—5.5) and indicated one fatality in 253 patients (0.4%; 95% CI 0.02—1.9). The negative predictive value of the multi detector computerized tomography is quite high (95%), and can be further improved to 97% by a ultrasonographic or tomographic evaluation of the veins of the lower extremities (Agnelli and Becattini, 2010).

3.3.2.2.3 Ventilation-Perfusion Scanning

Ventilation-perfusion scanning is used in the diagnosis of pulmonary embolism when the computerized tomographic pulmonary angiography is not available or contraindicated by the presence of renal insufficiency or history of allergic reaction to injectable contrast material. The positive predictive value of findings indicating a high probability of pulmonary arterial occlusion is in the 85—90% range (Agnelli and Becattini, 2010). The test is more valuable when the findings are normal, because with a negative predictive value of 97% it essentially rules out acute thrombosis of pulmonary arteries (Agnelli and Becattini, 2010). In a randomized study comparing patients in whom acute thrombosis was excluded, 6 of 611 (1%) patients who had a negative ventilation-perfusion scan and 2 of 561 patients ruled out by computed tomographic pulmonary angiography had clinical evidence of VTE during a 3-month follow-up period (Anderson et al., 2007). The operating characteristics of the ventilation-perfusion scanning can be improved by single-photon emission computed tomography, particularly in patients without significantly abnormal chest radiographs or severe chronic obstructive pulmonary disease (Leblanc and Paul, 2010).

3.3.2.2.4 Venous Ultrasonography

A ultrasonographic examination of the lower extremities positive for deep venous thrombosis in a hemodynamically stable patient suspected of pulmonary embolism allows the initiation of anticoagulant therapy and may obviate the need for additional imaging with computerized tomography or ventilation-perfusion scanning (Agnelli and Becattini, 2010).

3.3.2.2.5 Echocardiography

Echocardiographic evaluations indicating right ventricular dysfunction have limited utility and are indicated for hemodynamically unstable, critically ill patients investigated in settings in which computerized tomographic pulmonary angiography is not available (Agnelli and Becattini, 2010). The presence of diastolic dysfunction on the echocardiogram performed within 72 hours of the diagnosis of acute pulmonary embolism may have prognostic implications, as their OR of in-hospital mortality is 2.71 (95% CI 0.59−12.44) compared with patients with normal diastolic function (Cho et al., 2014). Patients with signs of right ventricular overload and elevated troponin or brain natriuretic peptide require careful monitoring, as they may develop hemodynamic decompensation and require systemic thrombolysis for reperfusion (Konstantinides, 2014).

3.4 PREVENTION AND MANAGEMENT

3.4.1 Intravenous Unfractionated Heparin and Oral Vitamin K Antagonists

The standard treatment of acute pulmonary embolism is rapid anticoagulation, traditionally accomplished with unfractionated heparin administered intravenously, followed by long-term use of an oral vitamin K antagonist. Thrombolytic therapy and embolectomy are reserved for cases with severe cardiopulmonary dysfunction.

3.4.2 Subcutaneous Low Molecular Weight Heparin and Oral Vitamin K Antagonists

Current practice has challenged the use of unfractionated heparin and has demonstrated the noninferiority of other anticoagulant modalities, some of which may allow shorter hospital stays and even exclusive outpatient treatment. The once daily subcutaneously administered low molecular weight heparin tinzaparine, available in Europe, was the first alternative to intravenous heparin, and was shown to have a similar rate of recurrent thromboembolism when compared with heparin 1 week (2.9% vs 3.0%) and 90 days (5.9% vs 7.1%) after the initial episode, and a similar risk of major bleeding (Simonneau et al., 1997). Likewise, enoxaparin, a low molecular weight heparin available in North America, given subcutaneously twice daily in dosages adjusted for weight (1 mg kg^{-1} per dose) was noninferior to intravenous unfractionated heparin, based on frequency of recurrent VTE after 1 week (0% vs 3.3%) and 90 days (3.4% vs 10%), without major bleeding episodes or deaths in the two groups (Findik et al., 2002). Enoxaparin monotherapy without oral anticoagulation for up to 3 months has been also used with good results (Beckman et al., 2003).

Patients with acute pulmonary embolism may not need admission to a medical unit, but could receive anticoagulant therapy in an outpatient. In an open label noninferiority trial involving cases recruited after presenting with pulmonary embolism to emergency departments in Switzerland, France, Belgium, and the United States, the patients were treated with subcutaneous enoxaparin for 5 days, followed by oral anticoagulation with vitamin K antagonist for at least 90 days (Aujesky et al., 2011). Patients randomly assigned to outpatient treatment were discharge within 24 hours from the time of diagnosis, while the inpatient group remained in the hospital for the duration of the enoxaparin treatment. All patients were considered at low risk of death from pulmonary embolism, that is, were not hypoxemic (as determined by a value of at least 60 mmHg partial oxygen pressure by arterial blood gas analysis or at least 90% oxygen saturation by pulse oximetry), had a systolic blood pressure greater than 100 mmHg, did not have chest pain requiring opioid treatment, were not considered at high risk of bleeding, had no evidence of severe impairment of renal function, and no known barriers to treatment adherence, such as psychosis, dementia, homelessness, or alcohol abuse. The primary outcome, defined as recurrent thrombophlebitis within 90 days after the onset of anticoagulation in this "low-risk" population, was similar in the outpatient and inpatient groups (0.6% vs 0%). The quality of the evidence is suboptimal given the small sample size (Yoo et al., 2014). Nonetheless, the work has been considered an adequate "proof of concept" (Howard and Salooja, 2011), but its applicability to patients treated with antipsychotic drugs, who were excluded by the design of the study, remains to be established.

3.4.3   Oral Factor Xa Inhibitor

The introduction of rivaroxaban, an oral factor Xa inhibitor, in the treatment of pulmonary embolism has represented true progress, at least in terms of patients' convenience. The main published trial recruited 4832 patients with acute, symptomatic pulmonary embolism and randomly assigned them to receive therapy with subcutaneous enoxaparin followed by oral vitamin K antagonist or oral rivaroxaban, administered a fixed dose of 15 mg twice daily for 21 days and 20 mg daily thereafter (EINSTEIN-PE Investigators et al., 2012). The treatment modalities were similar with regard to recurrent VTE (1.8% vs 2.1%, hazard ratio 1.12, 95% CI 0.75−1.68) and frequency of major bleeding events (2.2% vs 1.1%, hazard ratio 0.49, 95% CI 0.31−0.79). The use of rivaroxaban as a single-drug regimen decreased significantly the length of hospital stay after a diagnosis of pulmonary embolism (van Bellen et al., 2014).

3.4.4   Primary Prevention

VTE prophylaxis has not been prospectively studied in individuals treated with antipsychotic drugs and any recommendation must be considered an extrapolation of data and guidelines used for nonsurgical patients. An analysis of 10 trials enrolling 20,717 patients which compared heparin prophylaxis with no prophylaxis indicated a reduced risk for pulmonary embolism (relative ratio 0.69, 95% CI 0.52−0.90), translating into avoidance of four events per 1000 persons treated, without a significant change in the risk of major bleeding (Qaseem et al., 2011). However, in medical inpatients, prophylaxis does not decrease the number of fatal outcomes of pulmonary embolism (Spencer et al., 2014). Evidence from nine trials ($n = 14,435$) indicated that unfractionated heparin, administered subcutaneously 2−3 per day and one daily dose of low molecular weight heparin were equally effective for prophylaxis (Qaseem et al., 2011).

Recent guidelines published by the American College of Chest Physicians (Kahn et al., 2012) recommend the use of the Padua Prediction Score (Barbar et al., 2010) in hospital medical patients, which can be used as a template for patients receiving antipsychotic drugs (Table 3.3). Patients with a risk score greater than 4 should be considered at increased risk for VTE and prescribed prophylactic treatment if they are at low risk of

TABLE 3.3 Risk Score for Venous Thromboembolism in Psychiatric Patients

Risk Factors	Points
Factors Common in Psychiatric Patients	
Reduced mobility (voluntary, restraints, pathology)	3
Treatment with antipsychotic drugs	1
Obesity	1
Standard Risk Factors in Nonsurgical Patients	
Previous venous thromboembolism	3
Thrombophilic pathology	3
Active malignancy	3
Recent limb trauma	2
Age 70 or older	1
Major acute or chronic pathology (assign 1 point/condition)	1
Estrogen treatment	1

bleeding. In the commonest scenarios, prophylaxis will be needed by obese individuals treated with antipsychotic drugs who have impaired mobility due to deconditioning or use of physical restraints, catatonic states, or recent limb trauma produced by falls or altercations. The gradient between the risk of VTE and duration of nonsurgical immobility has not been established (Cushman, 2007), but a duration exceeding 24 hours deserves attention. A high risk of VTE should also be considered in older dementia patients with heart or respiratory failure and an acute infection leading to the use of an antipsychotic for control of behavioral disturbance. The most important risk factors for bleeding in nonsurgical inpatients are active gastroduodenal ulcer, thrombocytopenia (with platelet count less than $50,000 \, \text{mm}^{-3}$), age older than 85, and liver or renal failure (Kahn et al., 2012).

3.4.5 Secondary Prevention

The standard approach to the duration of oral anticoagulation after an episode of pulmonary embolism is based on assessing whether the thrombotic event was provoked by a temporary, reversible condition, or was either unprovoked, recurrent, or associated with an irreversible condition (Agnelli and Becattini, 2010). Patients in the first of these categories should be anticoagulated for 3 months, while the others should be considered candidates for indefinite anticoagulation, if justified after periodic reevaluations of the risk—benefit ratio (Agnelli and Becattini, 2010). The 3-month mandatory anticoagulation is considered "active treatment" for the diagnosed thromboembolic event, while the extension of treatment is considered "secondary prevention," and reduces the risk of recurrent VTE by about 90% if the vitamin K antagonist is used to maintain an international normalized ratio (INR) for the prothrombin time at around 2.5 (Kearon and Akl, 2014). Indefinite anticoagulation makes sense for patients with a pulmonary embolus diagnosed during treatment with antipsychotics if these psychotropic drugs must be continued, particularly if the patient has other risk factors for VTE, such as obesity and significantly reduced ambulation.

The low cost of vitamin K antagonists makes them attractive, but monitoring requirements to maintain the target INR may not be achieved by a population with severe mental illness. Costlier, but equally effective alternatives for extended or indefinite anticoagulation include rivaroxaban (20 mg daily), apixaban (2.5—5 mg daily), or dabigatran (150 mg twice daily) (Kearon and Akl, 2014). These drugs are safer, as they are associated with a significantly lower risk of intracranial bleeding (Kearon and Akl, 2014). Bleeding complications are more likely to occur in patients older than 65 and in those with previous bleeding episode, metastatic malignancy, hepatic or renal failure, thrombocytopenia, anemia, and concomitant treatment with antiplatelet agents (Kearon and Akl, 2014). For psychiatric patients who refuse to take oral medication, the anticoagulation can be achieved with enoxaparin or other low molecular weight heparin. Patients who refuse to be anticoagulated may benefit from treatment with low-dose aspirin (Kearon and Akl, 2014), which has been shown to reduce the risk of recurrent VTE by 35% (Piazza, 2015).

REFERENCES

Agnelli, G., Becattini, C., 2010. Acute pulmonary embolism. N. Engl. J. Med. 363, 266−274.

Allenet, B., Schmidlin, S., Genty, C., Bosson, J.L., 2012. Antipsychotic drugs and risk of pulmonary embolism. Pharmacoepidemiol. Drug Saf. 21, 42−48.

Anderson, D.R., Khan, S.R., Rodger, M.A., Kovacs, M.J., Morris, T., Hirsch, A., et al., 2007. Computed tomographic pulmonary angiography vs. ventilation-perfusion lung scanning in patients with suspected pulmonary embolism: a randomized controlled trial. JAMA 298 (23), 2743−2753.

Ashrani, A.A., Silverstein, M.D., Lahr, B.D., Petterson, T.M., Bailey, K.R., Melton 3rd, L.J., et al., 2009. Risk factors and underlying mechanisms for venous stasis syndrome: a population-based case-control study. Vasc. Med. 14 (4), 339−349.

Aujesky, D., Roy, P.M., Verschuren, F., Righini, M., Osterwalder, J., Egloff, M., et al., 2011. Outpatient versus inpatient treatment for patients with acute pulmonary embolism: an international, open-label, randomized, non-inferiority trial. Lancet 378 (9785), 41−48.

Axelsson, S., Hägg, S., Eriksson, A.C., Lindahl, T.L., Whiss, P.A., 2007. In vitro effects of antipsychotics on human platelet adhesion and aggregation and plasma coagulation. Clin. Exp. Pharmacol. Physiol. 34 (8), 775−780.

Barbar, S., Noventa, F., Rossetto, V., Ferrari, A., Brandolin, B., Perlati, M., et al., 2010. A risk assessment model for the identification of hospitalized medical patients at risk for venous thromboembolism: the Padua Prediction Score. J. Thromb. Haemost. 8 (11), 2450−2457.

Barbui, C., Conti, V., Cipriani, A., 2014. Antipsychotic drug exposure and risk of venous thromboembolism: a systematic review and meta-analysis of observational studies. Drug Saf. 37, 79−90.

Beckman, J.A., Dunn, K., Sasahara, A.A., Goldhaber, S.Z., 2003. Enoxaparin monotherapy without oral anticoagulation to treat acute symptomatic pulmonary embolism. Thromb. Haemost. 89 (6), 953−958.

Bell, E.J., Lutsey, P.L., Basu, S., Cushman, M., Heckbert, S.R., Lloyd-Jones, D.M., et al., 2016. Lifetime risk of venous thromboembolism in two cohort studies. Am. J. Med. 129 (3), 339. e19−339.e26, pii:S0002-9343(15)01018-9.

Bertoletti, L., Legal, G., Aujesky, D., Sanchez, O., Roy, P.M., Verschuren, F., et al., 2013. Prognostic value of the Geneva prediction rule in patients with pulmonary embolism. Thromb. Res. 132, 32−36.

Borras, L., Eytan, A., de Timary, P., Constant, E., Huguelet, P., Hermans, C., 2008. Pulmonary thromboembolism associated with olanzapine and risperidone. J. Emerg. Med. 35, 159−161.

Canoso, R.T., Sise, H.S., 1982. Chlorpromazine-induced lupus anticoagulant and associated immunologic abnormalities. Am. J. Hematol. 13 (2), 121−129.

Carrizo, E., Fernández, V., Quintero, J., Connell, L., Rodríguez, Z., Mosquera, M., et al., 2008. Coagulation and inflammation markers during atypical or typical antipsychotic treatment in schizophrenia patients and drug-free first-degree relatives. Schizophr. Res. 103 (1), 83−93.

Casazza, F., Becattini, C., Bongarzoni, A., Cuccia, C., Roncon, L., Favretto, G., et al., 2012. Clinical features and short term outcomes of patients with acute pulmonary embolism. The Italian Pulmonary Embolism Registry (IPER). Thromb. Res. 130, 847−852.

Cecchi, R., Lazzaro, A., Catanese, M., Mandarelli, G., Ferracuti, S., 2012. Fatal thromboembolism following physical restraint in a patient with schizophrenia. Int. J. Legal Med. 126, 477−482.

Chate, S., Patted, S., Nayak, R., Patil, N., Pandurangi, A., 2013. Pulmonary thromboembolism associated with clozapine. J. Neuropsychiatry Clin. Neurosci. 25, e3−e6.

Cho, J.H., Kaw, R., Chhabra, J., Kola, S., Mahata, I., Shahani, S., et al., 2014. Prognostic implications of diastolic dysfunction in patients with acute pulmonary embolism. BMC Res. Notes 7, 610 (September 6; epub).

Clinebell, K., Azzam, P.N., Gopalan, P., Haskett, R., 2014. Guidelines for preventing common complications of catatonia: case report and literature review. J. Clin. Psychiatry 75, 644−651.

Conti, V., Venegoni, M., Cocci, A., Fortino, I., Lora, A., Barbui, C., 2015. Antipsychotic drug exposure and risk of pulmonary embolism: a population-based, nested case-control study. BMC Psychiatry 15, 92 (epub). Available from: http://dx.doi.org/10.1186/s12888-015-0479-9.

Craft, M.K., Reed, M.J., 2010. Venous thromboembolic disease and hematologic considerations in obesity. Crit. Care Clin. 26 (4), 637−640.

Cushman, M., 2007. Epidemiology and risk factors for venous thrombosis. Semin. Hematol. 44, 62−69.

Delluc, A., Rousseau, A., Le Galudec, M., Canceil, O., Woodhams, B., Etienne, S., et al., 2014. Prevalence of antiphospholipid antibodies in psychiatric patients users and non-users of antipsychotics. Br. J. Haematol. 164 (2), 272−279.

Dietrich-Muszalska, A., Rabe-Jablonska, J., Nowak, P., Kontek, B., 2010a. The first-and second-generation antipsychotic drugs affect ADP-induced platelet aggregation. World J. Biol. Psychiatry 11 (2−2), 268−275.

Dietrich-Muszalska, A., Rabe-Jabłońska, J., Olas, B., 2010b. The effects of the second generation antipsychotics and a typical neuroleptic on collagen-induced platelet aggregation in vitro. World J. Biol. Psychiatry 11 (2−2), 293−299.

Ehrlich, S., Leopold, K., Merle, J.V., Theophil, I., Haag, W., Lautenschlager, M., et al., 2012. Trajectories of agouti-related protein and leptin levels during antipsychotic-associated weight gain in patients with schizophrenia. J. Clin. Psychopharmacol. 32 (6), 767−772.

EINSTEIN-PE Investigators, Buller, H.R., Prins, M.H., Lensin, A.W., Decousus, H., Jacobson, B.F., et al., 2012. Oral rivaroxaban for the treatment of symptomatic pulmonary embolism. N. Engl. J. Med. 366, 1287−1297.

Findik, S., Erkan, M.L., Selcuk, M.B., Albavrak, S., Atici, A.G., Doru, F., 2002. Low-molecular weight heparin versus unfractionated heparin in the treatment of patients with acute pulmonary thromboembolism. Respiration 69, 440−444.

Freund, Y., Rousseau, A., Guyot-Rousseau, F., Claessens, Y.E., Hugli, O., Sanchez, O., et al., 2015. PERC rule to exclude the diagnosis of pulmonary embolism in emergency low-risk patients: study protocol for the PROPER randomized controlled study. Trials 16 (1), 537.

Hagg, S., Bate, A., Stahl, M., Spigset, O., 2008. Association between venous thromboembolism and antipsychotics. A study of the WHO database of adverse drug reactions. Drug Saf. 31, 685−694.

Hamanaka, S., Kamijo, Y., nagai, T., Kurihara, K., Tanaka, K., Soma, K., et al., 2004. Massive pulmonary thromboembolism demonstrated at necropsy in Japanese psychiatric patients treated with neuroleptics including atypical antipsychotics. Circ. J. 68, 850−852.

Heit, J.A., Ofallon, W.M., Petterson, T.M., Lohse, C.M., Silverstein, M.D., Mohr, D.N., et al., 2002. Relative impact of risk factors for deep vein thrombosis and pulmonary embolism: a population-based study. Arch. Intern. Med. 162, 1245−1248.

Hill, M.A., MacRedmond, R., Hollywood, P., O'Neill, S., Morgan, R., 2008. Massive pulmonary emboli associated with olanzapine. Ir. Med. J. 101, 186.

Howard, L., Salooja, N., 2011. Outpatient management of pulmonary embolism. Lancet 378, 5−6.

Ishioka, M., Yasui-Furukori, N., Sugawara, N., Furukori, H., Kudo, S., Nakamura, K., 2015. Hyperprolactinemia during antipsychotics treatment increases the level of coagulation markers. Neuropsychiatr. Dis. Treat. 11, 477.

Jeding, I., Evans, P.J., Akanmu, D., Dexter, D., Spencer, J.D., Aruoma, O.I., et al., 1995. Characterization of the potential antioxidant and pro-oxidant actions of some neuroleptic drugs. Biochem. Pharmacol. 49 (3), 359−365.

Jönsson, A.K., Spigset, O., Hägg, S., 2012. Venous thromboembolism in recipients of antipsychotics: incidence, mechanisms and management. CNS Drugs 26 (8), 649−662.

Kahn,, S., Lim,, W., Dunn,, A.S., Cushman,, M., Dentali,, F., Akl,, E.A., et al., 2012. Prevention of VTE in nonsurgical patients: antithrombotic therapy and prevention of thrombosis, 9th ed: American College of Chest Physicians Evidence-Based Clinical Practice Guidelines. Chest 141 (2 Suppl.), 195S−225S.

Kaye, S.M., Pietilainene, K.H., Kotronen, A., Joutsi-Korhonen, L., Kaprio, J., Yki-Jarvinen, H., et al., 2012. Obesity-related derangements of coagulation and fibrinolysis: a study of obesity-discordant monozygotic twin pairs. Obesity 20, 88−94.

Kearon, C., Akl, E.A., 2014. Duration of anticoagulant therapy for deep vein thrombosis and pulmonary embolism. Blood 123, 1794−1801.

Kline, J.A., Courtney, D.M., Kabrhel, C., Moore, C.L., Smithline, H.A., Plewa, M.C., et al., 2008. Prospective multicenter evaluation of the pulmonary embolism rule-out criteria. J. Thromb. Haemost. 6 (5), 772−780.

Konstantinides, S., 2014. 2014 ESC Guidelines on the diagnosis and management of acute pulmonary embolism. Eur. Heart J. 35, 3145−3151.

Lapner, S.T., 2013. Diagnosis and management of pulmonary embolism. BMJ 346, f757.

Larsen, H.H., Ritchie, J.C., McNutt, M.D., Musselman, D.L., 2011. Pulmonary embolism in a patient with catatonia: an old disease, changing times. Psychosomatics 52, 387−391.

Le Gal, G., Righini, M., Roy, P.M., Sanchez, O., Aujesky, D., Bounameaux, H., et al., 2006. Prediction of pulmonary embolism in the emergency department: the revised Geneva score. Ann. Intern. Med. 144, 165−171.

Le Gal, G., Righini, M., Wells, P.S., 2015. D-dimer for pulmonary embolism. JAMA 313, 1668−1669.

Leblanc, M., Paul, N., 2010. V/Q SPECT and computed tomographic pulmonary angiography. Semin. Nucl. Med. 40, 426−441.

Levin, D., Seo, J.B., Kiely, D.G., Hatabu, H., Gefter, W., van Beek, E.J.R., et al., 2015. Triage for suspected acute pulmonary embolism: think before opening Pandora's box. Eur. J. Radiol. 84 (6), 1202−1211 (epub).

Manu, P., Dima, L., Shulman, M., Vancampfort, D., De Hert, M., Correll, C.U., 2015. Weight gain and obesity in schizophrenia: epidemiology, pathobiology, and management. Acta Psychiatr. Scand. 132 (2), 97−108 (epub).

McInerney, S.J., McDonald, C., 2012. Idiopathic pulmonary thromboembolism in the course of intensive psychiatric inpatient care: case report and treatment guidelines. BMJ Case Rep. 2012, (epub).

Mos, I.C., Douma, R.A., Erkens, P.M., Kruip, M.J., Hovens, M.M., van Houten, A.A., et al., 2014. Diagnostic outcome management study in patients with clinically suspected recurrent acute pulmonary embolism with a structured algorithm. Thromb. Res. 133, 1039−1044.

Munoli, R.N., Praharaj, S.K., Bhat, S.M., 2013. Clozapine-induced recurrent pulmonary thromboembolism. J. Neuropsychtry Clin. Neurosci. 25, 3.

Pandya, H.N., Keyes, M.J., Christenson, B.C., 2007. Electroconvulsive therapy in a schizophrenic patient with neuroleptic malignant syndrome and pulmonary embolism: a case report. Psychiatry (Edgmont) 4 (4), 21.

Parker, C., Coupland, C., Hippisley-Cox, J., 2010. Antipsychotic drugs and risk of venous thromboembolism: nested case-control study. BMJ 341, c4245.

Parkin, L., Skegg, D.C., Herbison, G.P., Paul, C., 2003. Psychotropic drugs and fatal pulmonary embolism. Pharmacoepidemiol. Drug Saf. 12, 647−652.

Penaloza, A., Verschuren, F., Meyer, G., Quentin-Georget, S., Soulie, C., Thys, F., et al., 2013. Comparison of the unstructured gestalt, the Wells score, and the revised Geneva score to estimate pretest probability for suspected pulmonary embolism. Ann. Emerg. Med. 62, 117−126.

Piazza, G., 2015. Beyond Virchow's triad: does cardiovascular inflammation explain the recurrent nature of venous thromboembolism? Vasc. Med. 20, 102−104.

Qaseem, A., Chou, R., Humphrey, L.L., Starkey, M., Shekelle, P., Clinical Guideline Committee of the American College of Physicians, 2011. Venous thromboembolism prophylaxis in hospitalized patients: a clinical practice guideline from the American College of Physicians. Ann. Intern. Med. 155, 625−632.

Reuwer, A.Q., Nieuwland, R., Fernandez, I., Goffin, V., van Tiel, C.M., Schaap, M.C., et al., 2009. Prolactin does not affect human platelet aggregation or secretion. Thromb. Haemost. 101 (6), 1119−1127.

Reynaud, Q., Lega, J.C., Mismetti, P., Chapelle, C., Wahl, D., Cathébras, P., et al., 2014. Risk of venous and arterial thrombosis according to type of antiphospholipid antibodies in adults without systemic lupus erythematosus: a systematic review and meta-analysis. Autoimmun. Rev. 13 (6), 595−608.

Righini, M., Van Es, J., Den Exter, P.L., Roy, P.M., Verschuren, F., Ghuysen, A., et al., 2014. Age-adjusted D-dimer cutoff levels to rule out pulmonary embolism: the ADJUST-PE study. JAMA 311, 1117−1124.

Samad, F., Ruf, W., 2013. Inflammation, obesity, and thrombosis. Blood 122, 3415−3422.

Schäfer, K., Konstantinides, S., 2014. Mechanisms linking leptin to arterial and venous thrombosis: potential pharmacological targets. Curr. Pharm. Des. 20 (4), 635−640.

Şengül, M.C., Kaya, K., Yilmaz, A., Şengül, C., Serinken, M., 2014. Pulmonary thromboembolism due to paliperidone: report of 2 cases. Am. J. Emerg. Med. 32 (7), 814.e1−814.e2.

Simonneau, G., Sors, H., Charbonnier, B., Page, Y., Laaban, J.P., Azarian, R., et al., 1997. A comparison of low-molecular weight heparin with unfractionated heparin for acute pulmonary embolism. The THESEE Study Group. Tinzaparine ou Heparine Standard: Evaluations dans l'Embolie Pulmonaire. N. Engl. J. Med. 337, 663−669.

Spencer, A., Cawood, T., Frampton, C., Jardine, D., 2014. Heparin-based treatment to prevent symptomatic deep venous thrombosis, pulmonary embolism or death in general medical inpatients is not supported by best evidence. Intern. Med. J. 44, 1054−1065.

Stein, P.D., Matta, F., Goldman, J., 2011. Obesity and pulmonary embolism: the mounting evidence of risk and the mortality paradox. Thromb. Res. 128, 518−523.

Stojanovich, L., Djokovic, A., Kontic, M., 2015. Antiphospholipid-mediated thrombosis: interplay between type of antibodies and localisation of lung, and cardiovascular incidences in primary antiphospholipid syndrome. Clin. Exp. Rheumatol. 33 (4), 531−536.

Stuijver, D.J., Debeij, J., van Zaane, B., Dekkers, O.M., Smit, J.W., Büller, H.R., et al., 2012. Levels of prolactin in relation to coagulation factors and risk of venous thrombosis. Results of a large population-based case-control study (MEGA-study). Thromb. Haemost. 108 (3), 499.

Toringhibel, M., Adam, T., Arghir, O.C., Gima, E., 2011. Acute massive pulmonary embolism associated with olanzapine therapy and no significant personal history in a young male—case report and literature review. Pneumologia 60, 82−84.

Tripp, A.C., 2011. Nonfatal pulmonary embolus associated with clozapine treatment: a case series. Gen. Hosp. Psychiatry 33, 85e5−85e6.

Urban, A., Masopust, J., Malý, R., Hosak, L., Kalnicka, D., 2007. Prolactin as a factor for increased platelet aggregation. Neuroendocrinol. Lett. 28 (4), 518−523.

Van Belle, A., Buller, H.R., Huisman, M.V., Kaasiager, K., Kamphuisen, P.W., Kramer, M.H., et al., 2006. Effectiveness of managing suspected pulmonary embolism using an algorithm combining clinical probability, D-Dimer testing, and computed tomography. JAMA 295, 172−179.

van Bellen, B., Bmaber, L., Correa de Cravalho, F., Prins, M., Wang, M., Lensing, A.W., 2014. Reduction in the length of stay with rivaroxaban as a single-drug regimen for the treatment of deep vein thrombosis and pulmonary embolism. Curr. Med. Res. Opin. 30, 829−837.

Walker, A.M., Lanza, L.L., Arellano, F., Rothman, K.J., 1997. Mortality in current and former users of clozapine. Epidemiology 8 (6), 671−677.

Wallaschofski, H., Eigenthaler, M., Kiefer, M., Donne, M., Hentschel, B., Gertz, H.J., et al., 2003. Hyperprolactinemia in patients on antipsychotic drugs causes ADP-stimulated platelet activation that might explain the increased risk for venous thromboembolism: pilot study. J. Clin. Psychopharmacol. 23 (5), 479−483.

Wells, P.S., Anderson, D.R., Rodger, M., Ginsberg, J.S., Kearon, C., Gent, M., et al., 2000. Derivation of a simple clinical model to characterize patients probability of pulmonary embolism: increasing the models utility with the SimpliRED D-dimer. Thromb. Haemost. 83, 416−420.

Wells, P.S., Anderson, D.R., Rodger, M., Stiell, J., Dreyer, J.F., Barnes, D., et al., 2001. Excluding pulmonary embolism at bedside without diagnostic imaging: management of patients with suspected pulmonary embolism presenting to the emergency department by using a simple clinical model and D-dimer. Ann. Intern. Med. 135, 98−107.

Wolberg, A.S., Aleman, M.M., Leiderman, K., Machlus, K.R., 2012. Procoagulant activity in hemostasis and thrombosis: Virchow's triad revisited. Anesth. Analg. 114 (2), 275−285.

Yoo, H.H., Queluz, T.H., El Dib, R., 2014. Outpatient versus inpatient treatment for acute pulmonary embolism. Cochrane Database Syst. Rev. 11, CD010019. Available from: http://dx. doi.org/10.1002/14651858.CD010019.pub2.

Zarrabi, M.H., Zucker, S., Miller, F., Derman, R.M., Romano, G.S., Hartnett, J.A., et al., 1979. Immunologic and coagulation disorders in chlorpromazine-treated patients. Ann. Intern. Med. 91 (2), 194−199.

Zornberg, G.L., Jick, H., 2000. Antipsychotic drug use and risk of first-time idiopathic venous thromboembolism: a case-control study. Lancet 356, 1219−1223.

Chapter 4

Orthostatic Hypotension

James J. Gugger[1] and Megan J. Ehret[2]

[1]*Johns Hopkins School of Medicine, Baltimore, MD, United States,*
[2]*Fort Belvoir Community Hospital, Fort Belvoir, VA, United States*

4.1 EPIDEMIOLOGY

4.1.1 Prevalence

Orthostatic or postural hypotension, defined by one or more of the following criteria within 2−5 minutes of standing: (1) at least a 20 mmHg fall in systolic blood pressure; (2) at least a 10 mmHg fall in diastolic pressure; (3) symptoms of cerebral hypoperfusion, is one of the most common cardiovascular side effects of antipsychotic drugs (Michelsen and Meyer, 2007; Drici and Priori, 2007; Casey, 1997; Consensus Statement, 1996). Slow dose titration of antipsychotics is often necessary to minimize the risk of orthostasis potentially leaving the patient at subtherapeutic doses for a prolonged period of time. Symptomatic orthostasis may even prevent escalation to a dose that is optimal for the control of psychotic symptoms. Identification of factors that increase the risk of orthostatic hypotension and proper treatment can minimize this potentially severe complication of antipsychotic treatment. Orthostatic hypotension is associated with neurodegenerative diseases, frailty in elderly patients, chronic heart disease hypertension, and diabetes. This review describes the risk factors for antipsychotic-associated orthostatic hypotension and provides a comprehensive evaluation of treatment strategies. Literature retrieval was accessed through MEDLINE (1977−2015) for publications in English using the terms: antipsychotic drug and orthostatic hypotension. Clinical trials with data on antipsychotic side effects and reference lists from literature retrieved were also included in this review. Some treatment recommendations are extrapolated from reports on the treatment of orthostatic hypotension secondary to tricyclic antidepressants, monoamine oxidase inhibitors, and autonomic failure.

Life-Threatening Effects of Antipsychotic Drugs. DOI: http://dx.doi.org/10.1016/B978-0-12-803376-0.00004-6
© 2016 Elsevier Inc. All rights reserved.

All antipsychotic agents are associated with orthostatic hypotension (Michelsen and Meyer, 2007; Drici and Priori, 2007; Casey, 1997), although the incidence and severity varies. The incidence of orthostatic hypotension in patients taking antipsychotic agents is described below; however, comparison between studies should be done with caution due to significant differences in the demographic profile of each study and differing methods of assessment for orthostasis.

The largest source of comparative data comes from The Clinical Antipsychotic Trials of Intervention Effectiveness (CATIE) trial, a large, federally-funded study, comparing the relative effectiveness and tolerability of second generation antipsychotic drugs to first generation antipsychotics (represented by the mid-potency phenothiazine, perphenazine). Table 4.1 shows rates of orthostatic hypotension in patients participating in phases 1−3 of CATIE (Lieberman et al., 2005; McEvoy et al., 2006; Stroup et al., 2006, 2007, 2009). Clozapine and quetiapine had the greatest incidence of orthostatic hypotension, as high as 24% and 27%, respectively, likely due to high affinity for the α_1-adrenoceptor. Among the more recently introduced antipsychotic agents, iloperidone appears to have the highest incidence of orthostatic hypotension (19.5% compared to 8.3% in patients taking placebo in a randomized controlled trial) (Citrome, 2009a) while the incidence of orthostasis with paliperidone, lurasidone, and asenapine is less than 2% (Product Information, 2013; Meltzer et al., 2008; Citrome, 2009b).

There is much less data on the incidence of orthostatic hypotension with older antipsychotic agents, although low-potency (i.e., agents with low potency for the dopamine (D2)-receptor) phenothiazine antipsychotics like chlorpromazine and thioridazine are generally considered the most likely to cause orthostatic hypotension (Casey, 1997). Almost no quantitative data exists for higher-potency phenothiazine antipsychotics (perphenazine, loxapine, trifluoperazine, fluphenazine, and thiothixene) (Casey, 1997; Michelsen and Meyer, 2007; Mackin, 2008; Swett et al., 1977; Bishop and Gallant, 1970; Gershon et al., 1970; Hansen et al., 1997; Simpson and Cuculic, 1976), but they are generally considered to infrequently cause orthostatic hypotension. In an iloperidone study, the incidence of orthostatic hypotension with haloperidol (used as an active control) was 15.3% versus 8.3% for placebo (Weiden et al., 2008).

Since intramuscular (IM) administration generally results in higher and more rapid elevation of plasma concentrations than oral administration (Product Information, 2014a; Curry, 1971), there is theoretically a greater risk of orthostatic hypotension with use of the IM route of administration. A large study ($n = 2011$) evaluated the safety of IM olanzapine relative to other IM antipsychotic agents (primarily haloperidol). Orthostatic hypotension occurred in 2.4% of patients receiving olanzapine versus 4.2% in those receiving any other antipsychotic agent (Chandrasena et al., 2009). Very little data exists for the other IM antipsychotics. In a trial of IM

TABLE 4.1 Percentage of Patients Reporting Orthostatic Faintness in Phases 1–3 of the CATIE Trial

CATIE Study	Aripiprazole	Clozapine	Two Agents	Fluphenazine Decanoate	Olanzapine	Perphenazine	Quetiapine	Risperidone	Ziprasidone
Phase (Lieberman et al., 2005)	–	–	–	–	9	11	11	11	13
Phase 1 (Stroup et al., 2007)	–	–	–	–	8	–	18	3	–
Phase 2 (Stroup et al., 2006)	–	–	–	–	7	–	13	6	4
Phase 2E (McEvoy et al., 2006)	–	12	–	–	5	–	27	6	–
Phase 3 (Stroup et al., 2009)	6	24	10	0	10	0	12	0	8

chlorpromazine (dosed at 1 mg kg^{-1} with a maximum dose 100 mg) for the treatment of migraine, 18% (18/100) of patients developed orthostasis (Iserson, 1983). Although the frequency was not defined, orthostasis was the most common side effect of chlorpromazine in a trial comparing the efficacy of IM chlorpromazine and IM haloperidol in 50 patients with psychotic agitation; orthostasis was not mentioned as a side effect of haloperidol (Ritter et al., 1972).

4.1.2   Genetic Vulnerability

There is a paucity of data regarding the genetic risk for the development of orthostatic hypotension and syncope from antipsychotic medications. Poor metabolizer status due to mutations in the genes coding for various cytochrome p450 enzymes may put an individual at an increased risk for the development of this adverse effect due to the accumulation of the medication. One study has demonstrated in a total of 180 patients treated with clozapine who were genotyped for the CYP1A2 − 1545C > T polymorphism (rs2470890) that those with the TT genotype had numerically (but insignificantly) more frequent (82% vs 71%) and more severe orthostatic hypotension than the wildtype in addition to other adverse effects. The researchers caution that the results are tentative and larger samples are needed to determine the effect of this polymorphism on the development of adverse effects with clozapine (Viikki et al., 2014).

4.2   PATHOBIOLOGY

Rising from a supine position causes 0.5−1 L of blood to pool in the lower extremity and splanchnic circulation resulting in a decline in venous return and ventricular filling. Stroke volume and cardiac output are depressed as a consequence. Baroreceptors, located in the aorta and carotid arteries, detect a small drop in blood pressure and activate the sympathetic nervous system. Increased adrenergic tone causes vasoconstriction resulting in increased systemic vascular resistance, an effect mediated by postsynaptic α_1-adrenoceptors on vascular smooth muscle cells, and acceleration of heart rate, which is mediated primarily by postsynaptic myocardial β_1-receptors (Westfall and Westfall, 2006a; Smith et al., 1994). This response facilitates the maintenance of blood pressure after postural changes. The vasodilatory effect of α_1-adrenoceptor blockade by antipsychotic agents attenuates the increase in systemic vascular resistance and leads to an orthostatic drop in blood pressure. The decline in blood pressure putatively results in cerebral hypoperfusion leading to the neurological symptoms of orthostasis such as dizziness or lightheadedness, cognitive impairment, asthenia, headache, and visual disturbance (Mets, 1995).

Young patients treated with a α_1-adrenoceptor antagonist often develop sinus tachycardia with minimal changes in postural blood pressure reflecting an adequate autonomic reflex. This is especially common with clozapine because it is a potent α_1-adrenoceptor antagonist with anticholinergic properties that further contribute to tachycardia (Young et al., 1998). Elderly patients treated with a α_1-adrenoceptor antagonist are more likely to develop significant postural blood pressure changes without a dramatic increase in heart rate owing to an age-dependent decline in baroreflex sensitivity (Tonkin and Wing, 1994; Laitinen et al., 2004). This likely explains the increase in falls and other adverse sequelae seen in this population.

4.3   CLINICAL AND LABORATORY FEATURES

Symptoms of orthostatic hypotension are protean and may include complaints of dizziness or lightheadedness, cognitive impairment, asthenia, headache, and visual disturbance (Mets, 1995). To complicate matters, the correlation between subjective report of postural dizziness and postural hypotension appears to be weak (Ensrud et al., 1992; Scalco et al., 2000). In addition, psychotic patients are often unable to effectively convey symptoms of cerebral hypoperfusion to clinicians due to negative symptoms, paranoia, or formal thought disorder (Kaplan, 1959). Additionally, complaints may be bizarre or seemingly unrelated to postural hypotension. For example, a report describes the manifestations of orthostatic hypotension in two chlorpromazine-treated patients as a sleep-like state (Jefferson, 1972). Sole reliance on subjective report of symptoms consistent with orthostasis may contribute to under-recognition and increase the risk of complications. It is unclear if routine monitoring of orthostatic blood pressure leads to a decrease in complications of orthostatic hypotension, but it seems prudent to monitor closely for orthostatic hypotension closely when antipsychotic agents are initiated and rapidly titrated, as in hospitalized patients. Although orthostasis may be conceptualized as an acute, dose-related side effect, there is evidence that it is also a chronic side effect. A study reported that orthostatic hypotension occurred in 77% of patients with schizophrenia who were physically healthy and on a stable dosage of an antipsychotic agent for at least 6 months (Silver et al., 1990).

A thorough evaluation of potential risk factors for orthostatic hypotension should be undertaken prior to antipsychotic initiation. In reviewing past medical history, special attention should be given to disease states that affect the autonomic nervous system and fluid status (Table 4.2). An evaluation of the patient's drug therapy regimen is necessary because concomitant drugs that affect hemodynamic tone can increase the risk of postural hypotension.

TABLE 4.2 Disease States Associated With Autonomic Dysfunction and Dehydration

Autonomic Dysfunction (Consensus Statement, 1996; Bradley and Davis, 2003; Figueroa et al., 2010; Freeman, 2008; Goldstein et al., 2002; Jordan, 2005; Jordan et al., 2000)	Dehydration (Figueroa et al., 2010; LaWall, 1980; Pirke, 1996)
Diabetes mellitus	Anorexia
Alcohol dependence	Vomiting
Parkinson's disease	Diarrhea
Multiple system atrophy	Catatonia
Pure autonomic failure	Febrile illness

4.3.1 Autonomic Failure

In autonomic failure, postganglionic fibers of the sympathetic nervous system do not release adequate amounts of norepinephrine thereby diminishing the response to orthostatic stress (Kaufmann, 2002). Patients with underlying or unrecognized disorders of the autonomic nervous system may develop severe orthostatic changes following the addition of an antipsychotic drug with high affinity for α_1-adrenoceptors. Autonomic dysfunction may occur as a consequence of diabetic neuropathy or alcoholic neuropathy (Silver et al., 1990). Autonomic failure is a common manifestation of the so-called synucleinopathies: movement disorders, which include Parkinson's disease, Lewy body dementia, and multiple system atrophy. Low-potency antipsychotics such as quetiapine and clozapine are frequently used to control psychotic symptoms in patients with Parkinson's disease (Friedman and Factor, 2000), because of the low incidence of extrapyramidal symptoms, but this combination comes with a high incidence of orthostatic hypotension which may be severe from the additive effects of drug and disease state. Antipsychotic drugs should be carefully titrated in patients with longstanding alcohol dependence, poorly controlled diabetes, movement disorders, and other disease states associated with autonomic failure.

4.3.2 Dehydration

Patients with low circulating plasma volume are under a state of adrenergic hyperactivity in order to maintain adequate cardiac output. This compensated state can be compromised by addition of an α_1-adrenoceptor blocker. An example is the case of a 45-year-old patient who presented to the emergency room with an acute exacerbation of schizophrenia (LaWall, 1980). She received 200 mg of chlorpromazine for agitation and developed syncope within about 30 minutes. She had a rapid pulse, profound hypotension, and stupor. The author postulates that the cumulative effect of the α_1-adrenoceptor blocking properties of chlorpromazine and the patient's presentation in a volume-depleted state resulted in severe orthostatic hypotension and syncope. It is important for the clinician in the emergency room to be aware of this drug-disease state interaction because patients presenting to the emergency room have often not eaten or had adequate fluid intake prior to arrival resulting in a state of hypovolemia. Since patients often receive high initial dosages of antipsychotic medications, often via the IM route, in the emergency room, special attention to fluid balance should be given to patients who are malnourished, catatonic, and to those who have a recent history of vomiting or diarrhea. IM antipsychotic medications with low affinity for the α_1-adrenoceptor, such as haloperidol, ziprasidone, or aripiprazole, may be safer for dehydrated patients than chlorpromazine or olanzapine.

4.3.3 Drug–Drug Interactions

An evaluation of the patient's pharmacotherapeutic regimen prior to treatment initiation is necessary because drug–drug interactions (e.g., antihypertensives and antipsychotics) can cause or exacerbate orthostasis. Most interactions are pharmacodynamic rather than pharmacokinetic in that the interacting agent alters hemodynamic tone in a way that exaggerates postural blood pressure changes (Table 4.3). Concurrent therapy with one of these agents may increase the risk or magnitude of postural hypotension. Medications with the greatest risk for postural hypotension include β-blockers, diuretics, calcium channel blockers, and α_2-adrenoceptor agonists (Thomas et al., 1965; Bradley and Davis, 2003; Aronow, 2009). All antihypertensive drugs may predispose older patients to symptomatic orthostasis (Aronow, 2009).

4.3.3.1 Use of β-Adrenoceptor Antagonists (β-blockers)

β-Blockers are often prescribed for the treatment of antipsychotic-induced akathisia so it is important to be aware of this pharmacodynamic interaction. β-Blockers antagonize myocardial β_1-receptors thereby decreasing heart rate and cardiac contractility, which can lower cardiac output (Westfall and Westfall, 2006b). If a patient is taking an antipsychotic that has high affinity for the α_1-adrenoceptor, β-blockade will attenuate the compensatory rise in cardiac contractility and heart rate triggered by α_1-adrenoceptor blockade. Impaired sympathetic reflexes may reduce the patient's ability to tolerate postural changes resulting in syncope or near-syncope.

There are reports of syncope after treatment with haloperidol and propranolol with positive rechallenge (Alexander et al., 1984) and severe

TABLE 4.3 Nonantipsychotic Medications That Cause Orthostatic Hypotension

Mechanism	Drugs and Drug Classes
Negative chronotropic and inotropic effects	β-Blockers (propranolol, metoprolol, atenolol) (Westfall and Westfall, 2006a), nondihydropyridine calcium channel blockers (diltiazem, verapamil) (Weber, 2002)
Reduction in systemic vascular resistance	α_1-Adrenoceptor blockers including agents prescribed for benign prostatic hyperplasia (prazosin, terazosin, doxazosin) (Westfall and Westfall, 2006a), tricyclic antidepressants (Kranzler and Cardoni, 1988; Maskall and Lam, 1993; Forster, 1989), and trazodone (Poon and Braun, 2005); arteriolar vasodilators (e.g., hydralazine, minoxidil) (Campese, 1981); dihydropyridine calcium channel blockers (e.g., amlodipine, nifedipine) (Weber, 2002; Campese, 1981); angiotensin-converting enzyme inhibitors (lisinopril, enalapril), angiotensin II receptor antagonists (losartan, valsartan) (Wong et al., 2004); opioids (Thomas et al., 1965; Crawford et al., 1996; Chambers, 1988); phosphodiesterase-5 inhibitors (e.g., sildenafil) (Prisant, 2006); ethanol (Chaudhuri et al., 1994; Narkiewicz et al., 2000)
Reduction in preload	Nitrate antianginals (isosorbide mononitrate, nitroglycerin) (Fung, 2004)
Reduction in sympathetic outflow	α_2-Adrenoceptor agonists (e.g., clonidine, guanfacine) (MacMillan et al., 1996), benzodiazepine, especially when given parenterally (Lindqvist et al., 1996; van den Berg et al., 1996), dopamine agonists (e.g., pramipexole, ropinirole), and levodopa (Durrieu et al., 1991; Haapaniemi et al., 2000)
Intravascular volume contraction	Diuretics (e.g., furosemide, hydrochlorothiazide) (Poon and Braun, 2005)
Depletion of norepinephrine from adrenergic terminals	Monoamine oxidase inhibitors (Haapaniemi et al., 2000; Turkka et al., 1997; Churchyard et al., 1997)

postural hypotension with the combination of chlorpromazine and propranolol (Vestal et al., 1979). Although there is a minor pharmacokinetic drug interaction between chlorpromazine and propranolol, the most probable explanation for postural hypotension is the pharmacodynamic interaction between an α_1-adrenoceptor blocker (chlorpromazine) and β-blocker. A study of hypertensive patients without a psychiatric disorder showed that the combination of prazosin, a high potency α_1-adrenoceptor antagonist, with a β-blocker resulted in an exaggerated orthostatic reaction after a single dose of prazosin compared to patients taking prazosin alone (Seideman et al., 1982) and the authors recommended starting α_1-adrenoceptor blocking agents at a lower dose in patients taking β-blockers. It is rational to extend this recommendation to patients on β-blocker therapy who are subsequently started on an antipsychotic agent. It would be prudent to start antipsychotic agents at a lower dose, make conservative dose adjustments, and carefully monitor patients on concurrent β-blocker therapy.

Young patients often experience reflex tachycardia without postural hypotension when taking antipsychotic drugs, especially clozapine (Young et al., 1998). Several authors recommend low dose propranolol to treat neuroleptic-induced reflex tachycardia (Young et al., 1998; Freitas et al., 2000; Raj et al., 2009). It is important to note, however, that sinus tachycardia is a compensatory response to the hemodynamic effects of antipsychotics (Bradley and Davis, 2003) and hence important in the maintenance of cardiac output and blood pressure. Addition of a β-blocker will further impair the baroreflex of the sympathetic nervous system.

4.3.3.2   Use of α_2-Adrenoceptor Agonists

α_2-Agonists (e.g., clonidine, guanfacine, methyldopa) stimulate presynaptic α_2-adrenoceptors in the brainstem resulting in reduced sympathetic outflow and consequently vasodilation and decreases in heart rate (Westfall and Westfall, 2006b). Again, patients who are taking antipsychotics with a high level of α_1-adrenoceptor blockade may not be able to tolerate postural changes due to impaired sympathetic reflexes conferred by α_2-agonist treatment. Fruncillo reported two patients who developed severe hypotension, which was responsive to fluids, after administration of clonidine and a typical antipsychotic (chlorpromazine in one patient and haloperidol in the other) (Fruncillo et al., 1985).

4.3.3.3   Use of α_1-Adrenoceptor Antagonists

Prazosin is an effective treatment for nightmares in patients with posttraumatic stress disorder and doxazosin, terazosin, alfuzosin, tamsulosin, and silodosin are commonly used for the symptomatic treatment of benign prostatic hyperplasia (BPH). Concomitant use of two agents with potent α_1-adrenoceptor antagonist effects (e.g., prazosin and clozapine) may increase orthostatic stress, although there are no case reports published that document such an interaction.

The α_{1A}-adrenoceptor mediates smooth muscle tone in the bladder neck and prostate as well vascular smooth muscle contraction, the α_{1B}-adrenoceptor also regulates vascular smooth muscle contraction, and the α_{1D}-adrenoceptor controls bladder contraction and sacral spinal cord innervation. Doxazosin, terazosin, and alfuzosin have similar affinity for all three subtypes of the

α_1-adrenoceptor. Tamsulosin and silodosin are selective for the α_{1A}-adrenoceptor with low affinity for the α_{1B}-adrenoreceptor, which confer a lower, albeit still present risk of orthostasis (Schwinn and Roehrborn, 2008; Cantrell et al., 2010). When concomitant treatment with an antipsychotic and anti-BPH agent is indicated, it seems logical to prescribe tamsulosin or silodosin for BPH to mitigate the potential for increased risk of orthostasis from additive effects on the α_1-adrenoceptor.

4.3.3.4   Use of Angiotensin-Converting Enzyme Inhibitors

Combining an antipsychotic with an angiotensin-converting enzyme inhibitor may cause severe orthostatic hypotension. Addition of clozapine to enalapril and diltiazem resulted in syncope in one patient. Subsequent rechallenge and titration of clozapine to 800 mg per day was facilitated by enalapril dosage reduction (Aronowitz et al., 1994). In another case, addition of captopril to chlorpromazine resulted in orthostatic hypotension and syncope. The reaction did not reoccur when each agent was given individually (White, 1986).

4.3.4   Complications and Significant Sequelae

The most well-known complication of orthostatic hypotension is syncope, which can result in fractures and intracranial hemorrhage, but orthostatic hypotension is also linked to transient ischemic attacks, ischemic stroke, myocardial infarction, and death (Rosati, 1964; Rutan et al., 1992; Masaki et al., 1998; Eigenbrodt et al., 2000; Rose et al., 2006).

4.3.5   Risk Stratification for Death or Permanent Disability

A recent meta-analysis of prospective observational studies reported on the association between prevalent orthostatic hypotension and incident major adverse cardiac and cerebrovascular events and death. A significantly increased risk of all-cause death was found (risk ratio (RR) 1.50, 95% confidence interval (CI): 1.24−1.81), as well as incident coronary heart disease (RR 1.41, 95% CI: 1.22−1.63), heart failure (RR: 2.25, 95% CI: 1.52−3.33), and stroke (RR: 1.64, 95% CI: 1.13−2.37) (Ricci et al., 2015) and in a large-scale trial examining the link between antipsychotic drugs and sudden cardiac death, autonomic dysfunction was mentioned as a possible etiologic factor (Ray et al., 2009). It remains unclear how orthostasis increases the risk of ischemic complications and mortality, but it may be related to decompensation of preexisting arteriosclerosis by hypoperfusion.

Given the association between orthostatic hypotension and vascular complications such as myocardial infarction and stroke, it may be advisable to avoid antipsychotic drugs with a high incidence of orthostatic hypotension in patients with risk factors for cardiovascular disease. Selection of antipsychotic therapy in this patient population is further complicated by the risk of metabolic syndrome and QT interval prolongation associated with antipsychotic agents. Unfortunately, no agent is devoid of all of these side effects. Given the multitude of untoward cardiovascular effects, antipsychotic agents should be prescribed to patients with risk factors for cardiovascular disease only when there is a compelling indication.

4.4   PREVENTION AND MANAGEMENT

4.4.1   Antipsychotic Selection

In patients with a compelling indication for antipsychotic therapy and a predisposition toward orthostatic hypotension (e.g., elderly patients, patients who are dehydrated, have autonomic dysfunction, or on concomitant medications that affect hemodynamic tone), careful selection of an antipsychotic agent and a prolonged dosage titration is necessary. Avoidance of a potent α_1-adrenoceptor antagonist such as chlorpromazine, clozapine, quetiapine, and iloperidone is ideal, but may not be feasible. For example, in the treatment of psychosis in Parkinson's disease, low-potency antipsychotic agents like quetiapine or clozapine are necessary to mitigate the risk of worsening parkinsonism. In this case, the lowest initial dosage possible (12.5 mg per day for clozapine or quetiapine) and a prolonged titration period are necessary to minimize the risk of orthostasis and worsening parkinsonism.

4.4.2   Antipsychotic Reinitiation

When patients discontinue their medication, clinicians often reinitiate medication at the previous dose or rapidly escalate the dose. This approach may be dangerous for clozapine due to the risk of seizures and severe orthostasis. There is a black box warning for clozapine stating that rapid escalation of clozapine can cause severe orthostatic hypotension resulting in cardiac or respiratory arrest. If therapy is interrupted for 2 days or more, clozapine should be reinitiated at the starting dose, 12.5–25 mg per day (Product Information Clozapine, 2014b). The safety of rapidly reestablishing therapeutic dosing of other antipsychotic agents can be gleaned from studies evaluating protocols for rapid initial dose escalation. Quetiapine can be initiated at a dose of 100 mg twice daily with subsequent dosage increases of 200 mg per day (Smith et al., 2005; Boidi and Ferro, 2007). Olanzapine (Karagianis et al., 2001; Baker et al., 2003) and risperidone (Feifel et al., 2000) may also be safely initiated with as much as 40 and 6 mg per day, respectively, in divided doses.

4.4.3   Antipsychotic Dosing Frequency

Antipsychotics with twice daily dosing in the official labeling (e.g., quetiapine, ziprasidone, asenapine, iloperidone) are frequently dosed once daily to enhance adherence. However, changes in dosing frequency result in changes in the pharmacokinetic profile, which may increase the risk of orthostasis. In a pilot study evaluating the relative safety of once daily and twice daily quetiapine dosage regimens, patients ($n = 21$) were first initiated on quetiapine and titrated to 400 or 600 mg per day over 4 weeks and were then randomized to once or twice daily dosing regimens for 4 weeks. Both dosing groups were then crossed-over for another 4 weeks. Symptomatic orthostatic hypotension occurred in 4/21 (19%) patients during the titration phase and 2 (10%) of these patients experienced a recurrence of symptomatic orthostatic hypotension during the cross-over phase (Chengappa et al., 2003). This potentially indicates that changes in the dosing frequency (without changing the total daily dose) could increase the risk of symptomatic orthostatic hypotension. Changing the dosing frequency from twice daily dosing to once daily dosing results in higher peak plasma concentrations and greater peak-trough variability.

When patients develop orthostatic hypotension on once daily dosing regimens of quetiapine and clozapine, giving multiple doses throughout the day, and hence lowering peak plasma concentrations and peak-trough variability, is often effective in ameliorating symptomatic orthostatic hypotension. The risk of orthostasis may also be minimized by use of an extended release formulation. Quetiapine extended release has a prolonged drug release phase resulting in lower peak plasma concentrations and less peak-trough variability when compared to the immediate release formulation of quetiapine (Figueroa et al., 2009).

When antipsychotic agents are given in multiple daily doses throughout the day, clinicians may be able to titrate the dosage more aggressively. Support for this strategy comes from the evaluation of protocols for rapid initial dose escalation of atypical antipsychotic drugs. In these studies, rapid titration of quetiapine, up to 800 mg per day in 4 days (Pae et al., 2007; Boidi and Ferro, 2007; Smith et al., 2005; Baker et al., 2003), olanzapine, up to 40 mg in the first 24 hours (Baker et al., 2003; Karagianis et al., 2001), and risperidone, up to 6 mg in the first 24 hours (Feifel et al., 2000) was possible with the use of multiple daily dosing regimens.

4.4.4   Nonpharmacological Therapy

All patients should be advised to avoid sudden postural changes especially when rising from bed in the morning and informed that physical activity, consumption of alcoholic beverages, carbohydrate-rich meals, and heat exposure may worsen orthostasis. Abdominal binders fitted to exert gentle pressure compress venous beds in the abdomen and reduce symptoms of orthostatic hypotension. The binder should be put on in the morning before rising from bed and removed at bedtime to avoid supine hypertension during sleep and if abdominal compression is insufficient, further benefit is possible with the addition of leg compression (Figueroa et al., 2010).

4.4.5 Volume Expansion

An increase in fluid intake to 1.25—2.5 L per day (5—8 glasses of water) is advisable for all patients who are not fluid-restricted (Freeman, 2008). Bolus doses of water rapidly alleviate symptoms of orthostatic hypotension in patients with autonomic failure purportedly by increasing adrenergic drive to vascular beds (Jordan, 2005). Among patients (not chosen for psychiatric status) with severe autonomic failure (multiple system atrophy), consumption of 480 mL of tap water resulted in a mean maximum increase in systolic blood pressure of 33 ± 5 mmHg within 30—35 minutes, and was sustained for more than 60 minutes (Jordan et al., 2000). Anecdotal evidence suggests aggressive hydration is also an effective measure to partially reverse orthostasis as a consequence of the α_1-adrenoceptor blocking actions of antipsychotic agents (LaWall, 1980).

A combination of aggressive hydration with an increase in salt consumption to 10 g of sodium per day is recommended for patients with orthostatic hypotension (Freeman, 2008). In a report describing patients who developed symptomatic orthostasis during titration of psychiatric medication (trazodone, desipramine, and phenelzine), sodium chloride supplementation at dosages of 1—2 g per day minimized orthostatic blood pressure changes and facilitated dose titration (Kranzler and Cardoni, 1988). Sodium chloride 1 g tablets (Munjack, 1984) are the most reasonable option if consumption of salty foods or soups is undesirable. Patients on a salt-restricted diet such as those at risk for volume overload with hypertension and those (e.g., congestive heart failure, renal, or liver failure) should not be considered candidates for increases in fluid and salt intake (Bradley and Davis, 2003; Figueroa et al., 2010).

4.4.6 Pharmacological Therapy

Pharmacological therapy is reserved for patients with orthostasis and symptoms of cerebral hypoperfusion, a compelling indication for antipsychotic treatment, and an insufficient response to nonpharmacologic measures and antipsychotic dose optimization. Pharmacologic approaches include expansion of intravascular volume with fludrocortisone or desmopressin as well as enhancement of adrenergic tone with sympathomimetic agents.

4.4.6.1 Fludrocortisone

Fludrocortisone is a synthetic mineralocorticosteroid used to treat adrenocortical deficiency and also used off-label to treat orthostatic hypotension due to pure autonomic failure. Historically, fludrocortisone was used to manage the hypotensive effects of monoamine oxidase inhibitors (Aronow, 2009; Westfall and Westfall, 2006b). Testani (1994) reported the successful treatment of symptomatic orthostatic hypotension secondary to clozapine in two patients who failed initial nonpharmacologic measures. The first patient was a 30-year-old man with paranoid schizophrenia. He experienced a mild reduction in psychotic symptoms after a 6-month trial of clozapine 325 mg per day. Repeated attempts to increase the dose to 350 mg per day resulted in symptomatic orthostatic hypotension, which was not amenable to waist-high support stockings and an increase in salt and fluid intake. Fludrocortisone 0.1 mg per day was initiated and titrated to 0.3 mg per day over 2 weeks. This dose prevented orthostatic blood pressure changes and facilitated clozapine titration to 500 mg per day over 5 months. After 6 months, the patient developed mild supine hypertension, which resolved with reduction of the fludrocortisone to 0.05 mg per day; whereas a trial discontinuation of fludrocortisone resulted in reemergence of symptomatic orthostasis. The second patient was a 33-year-old man with undifferentiated schizophrenia who developed symptomatic orthostatic hypotension after 12 weeks of clozapine treatment. Orthostatic hypotension persisted despite an increase in salt and fluid intake. Initiation of fludrocortisone 0.1 mg per day resulted in partial improvement and titration to 0.2 mg per day resulted in alleviation of orthostasis (Testani, 1994).

Based on this report, it appears that fludrocortisone is a reasonable treatment for patients who develop symptomatic orthostasis from antipsychotic medication and do not respond to fluids and other nonpharmacologic measures. Fludrocortisone should be initiated at a dose of 0.1 mg per day with a target dosage of 0.3−0.4 mg per day (Freeman, 2008). At least 4−5 days are necessary before a therapeutic improvement (Kaufmann, 2002), so dosage changes should occur at weekly intervals. Although fludrocortisone has mild glucocorticoid activity (Schimmer and Parker, 2006), exacerbation of psychopathology has not been reported in the literature. Higher doses may result in edema, fluid overload and congestive heart failure, diabetes mellitus, hypomagnesemia, hypokalemia, and supine hypertension. Routine monitoring of electrolytes and supine blood pressure is essential for patients on fludrocortisone. Monitoring of blood sugar should be intensified in patients with diabetes mellitus. When the patient is able to tolerate a therapeutic dose of an antipsychotic agent without symptomatic orthostasis, gradual down-titration of fludrocortisone is reasonable. Trial discontinuation is an especially reasonable strategy in patients with metabolic syndrome, as fludrocortisone has the potential to exacerbate hypertension and diabetes mellitus. Patients should be monitored for reemergence of significant changes in postural blood pressure and symptoms of cerebral hypoperfusion during the tapering period.

4.4.6.2 Desmopressin

Desmopressin is a vasopressin analog used for the treatment of central diabetes insipidus. It effectively reduces morning symptoms of orthostasis in patients with autonomic failure when given intranasally (5−40 μg per day) or orally (100–800 μg per day) (Mathias et al., 1986; Freeman, 2008; Stumpf and Mitrzyk, 1994). Unfortunately, there is no support for the efficacy of desmopressin for antipsychotic-induced orthostasis. Additionally, the safety concerns accumulated from experience using desmopressin in patients with schizophrenia as a treatment for clozapine-induced urinary incontinence make it less desirable. It is associated with severe hyponatremia and seizures specifically in patients with unregulated water intake (Sarma et al., 2005). Given the absence of literature support for the treatment of antipsychotic-induced orthostasis and the potential for severe side effects, desmopressin should not be used as a first-line treatment. Patients should not be considered candidates for this medication if they have a history of psychogenic polydipsia or cannot comply with water regulation and routine monitoring of serum sodium.

4.4.6.3 Sympathomimetic Agents

Sympathomimetic agents are recommended when symptomatic orthostasis persists despite adequate volume expansion (Kaufmann, 2002; Freeman, 2008). Agents that increase adrenergic tone, reported to be useful for the treatment of orthostatic hypotension due to autonomic failure, include midodrine, pseudoephedrine, phenylephrine, psychostimulants, caffeine, yohimbine, and pyridostigmine (Freeman, 2008). Of these, only a single case report exists describing the use of a sympathomimetic (midodrine) for the treatment of psychotropic-induced orthostatic hypotension.

Midodrine is an α_1-adrenoceptor agonist approved by the US Food and Drug Administration for the treatment of orthostatic hypotension. Although there is no literature supporting the use of midodrine for patients with antipsychotic-induced orthostatic hypotension, a case report demonstrated its efficacy for orthostatic hypotension secondary to nortriptyline (Maskall and Lam, 1993). The recommended initial dosage is 2.5 mg two to three times per day; with a maximum dose of 10 mg three times daily. Side effects include supine hypertension, paresthesias, pupil dilation, piloerection, and pruritus. There are several reports of dystonic reactions following the initiation of midodrine in patients with Parkinson's disease taking antipsychotics (Castrioto et al., 2008; Takahashi, 2000), so patients should be monitored closely for extrapyramidal symptoms.

4.4.7 Prevention

The relationship between α_1-adrenoceptor blockade and orthostatic hypotension is well established. Unfortunately, the orthostatic hypotensive properties of antipsychotic agents continue to be underrecognized by clinicians. Antipsychotic-treated patients are often unable to convey symptoms of cerebral hypoperfusion to clinicians because of negative symptoms, paranoia, or formal thought disorder making routine orthostatic blood pressure monitoring important, especially when antipsychotic agents are initiated and rapidly titrated. Identification of patient factors that predispose patients to orthostatic hypotension such as dehydration, autonomic dysfunction, and drug interactions prior to initiation of antipsychotic treatment will likely minimize the occurrence of symptomatic orthostasis. Patient education, cautious dosing, and nonpharmacologic approaches including increased fluid intake and abdominal binders are usually sufficient treatments. For patients that experience symptomatic orthostatic hypotension despite these measures, a trial of a pharmacological treatment such as fludrocortisone may be considered. Once symptomatic orthostatic hypotension has resolved, the clinician may continue to titrate the antipsychotic medication to a therapeutic dose. Slow tapering of the antiorthostasis medication may be considered when the patient is stable with close monitoring for recurrence of orthostatic hypotension.

REFERENCES

Alexander Jr., H.E., McCarty, K., Giffen, M.B., 1984. Hypotension and cardiopulmonary arrest associated with concurrent haloperidol and propranolol therapy. JAMA 252, 87−88.

Aronow, W.S., 2009. Treating hypertension in older adults: safety considerations. Drug Saf. 32, 111−118.

Aronowitz, J.S., Chakos, M.H., Safferman, A.Z., Lieberman, J.A., 1994. Syncope associated with the combination of clozapine and enalapril. J. Clin. Psychopharmacol. 14, 429−430.

Baker, R.W., Kinon, B.J., Maguire, G.A., Liu, H., Hill, A.L., 2003. Effectiveness of rapid initial dose escalation of up to forty milligrams per day of oral olanzapine in acute agitation. J. Clin. Psychopharmacol. 23, 342−348. Available from: http://dx.doi.org/10.1097/01. jcp.0000085406.08426.a8.

Bishop, M.P., Gallant, D.M., 1970. Loxapine: a controlled evaluation in chronic schizophrenic patients. Curr. Ther. Res. Clin. Exp. 12, 594−597.

Boidi, G., Ferro, M., 2007. Rapid dose initiation of quetiapine for the treatment of acute schizophrenia and schizoaffective disorder: a randomised, multicentre, parallel-group, open study. Hum. Psychopharmacol. 22, 299−306. Available from: http://dx.doi.org/10.1002/hup.844.

Bradley, J.G., Davis, K.A., 2003. Orthostatic hypotension. Am. Fam. Physician 68, 2393−2398.

Campese, V.M., 1981. Minoxidil: a review of its pharmacological properties and therapeutic use. Drugs 22, 257−278.

Cantrell, M.A., Bream-Rouwenhorst, H.R., Hemerson, P., Magera Jr., J.S., 2010. Silodosin for benign prostatic hyperplasia. Ann. Pharmacother. 44, 302−310. Available from: http://dx. doi.org/10.1345/aph.1M320.

Casey, D.E., 1997. The relationship of pharmacology to side effects. J. Clin. Psychiatry 58 (Suppl. 10), 55−62.

Consensus statement on the definition of orthostatic hypotension, pure autonomic failure, and multiple system atrophy. The Consensus Committee of the American Autonomic Society and the American Academy of Neurology. 1996 Neurology 46, 1470.

Castrioto, A., Tambasco, N., Rossi, A., Calabresi, P., 2008. Acute dystonia induced by the combination of midodrine and perphenazine. J. Neurol. 255, 767−768.

Chambers, J.A., 1988. The haemodynamic effects of morphine. Arch. Emerg. Med. 5, 124−125.

Chandrasena, R., Dvorakova, D., Lee, S.I., et al., 2009. Intramuscular olanzapine vs. intramuscular short-acting antipsychotics: safety, tolerability and the switch to oral antipsychotic medication in patients with schizophrenia or acute mania. Int. J. Clin. Pract. 63, 1249–1258. Available from: http://dx.doi.org/10.1111/j.1742-1241.2009.02116.x.

Chaudhuri, K.R., Maule, S., Thomaides, T., Pavitt, D., Mathias, C.J., 1994. Alcohol ingestion lowers supine blood pressure, causes splanchnic vasodilatation and worsens postural hypotension in primary autonomic failure. J. Neurol. 241, 145–152.

Chengappa, K.N., Parepally, H., Brar, J.S., Mullen, J., Shilling, A., Goldstein, J.M., 2003. A random-assignment, double-blind, clinical trial of once- vs twice-daily administration of quetiapine fumarate in patients with schizophrenia or schizoaffective disorder: a pilot study. Can. J. Psychiatry 48, 187–194.

Churchyard, A., Mathias, C.J., Boonkongchuen, P., Lees, A.J., 1997. Autonomic effects of selegiline: possible cardiovascular toxicity in Parkinson's disease. J. Neurol. Neurosurg. Psychiatry 63, 228–234.

Citrome, L., 2009a. Iloperidone for schizophrenia: a review of the efficacy and safety profile for this newly commercialised second-generation antipsychotic. Int. J. Clin. Pract. 63, 1237–1248.

Citrome, L., 2009b. Asenapine for schizophrenia and bipolar disorder: a review of the efficacy and safety profile for this newly approved sublingually absorbed second-generation antipsychotic. Int. J. Clin. Pract. 63, 1762–1784.

Crawford, M.E., Moiniche, S., Orbaek, J., Bjerrum, H., Kehlet, H., 1996. Orthostatic hypotension during postoperative continuous thoracic epidural bupivacaine-morphine in patients undergoing abdominal surgery. Anesth. Analg. 83, 1028–1032.

Curry, S.H., 1971. Chlorpromazine: concentrations in plasma, excretion in urine and duration of effect. Proc. R. Soc. Med. 64, 285–289.

Drici, M.D., Priori, S., 2007. Cardiovascular risks of atypical antipsychotic drug treatment. Pharmacoepidemiol. Drug Saf. 16, 882–890. Available from: http://dx.doi.org/10.1002/pds.1424.

Durrieu, G., Senard, J.M., Tran, M.A., Rascol, A., Montastruc, J.L., 1991. Effects of levodopa and bromocriptine on blood pressure and plasma catecholamines in parkinsonians. Clin. Neuropharmacol. 14, 84–90.

Eigenbrodt, M.L., Rose, K.M., Couper, D.J., Arnett, D.K., Smith, R., Jones, D., 2000. Orthostatic hypotension as a risk factor for stroke: the atherosclerosis risk in communities (ARIC) study, 1987-1996. Stroke 31, 2307–2313.

Ensrud, K.E., Nevitt, M.C., Yunis, C., Hulley, S.B., Grimm, R.H., Cummings, S.R., 1992. Postural hypotension and postural dizziness in elderly women. The study of osteoporotic fractures. The Study of Osteoporotic Fractures Research Group. Arch. Intern. Med. 152, 1058–1064.

Feifel, D., Moutier, C.Y., Perry, W., 2000. Safety and tolerability of a rapidly escalating dose-loading regimen for risperidone. J. Clin. Psychiatry 61, 909–911.

Figueroa, C., Brecher, M., Hamer-Maansson, J.E., Winter, H., 2009. Pharmacokinetic profiles of extended release quetiapine fumarate compared with quetiapine immediate release. Prog. Neuropsychopharmacol. Biol. Psychiatry 33, 199–204.

Figueroa, J.J., Basford, J.R., Low, P.A., 2010. Preventing and treating orthostatic hypotension: as easy as A, B, C. Cleve. Clin. J. Med. 77, 298–306. Available from: http://dx.doi.org/10.3949/ccjm.77a.09118.

Forster, H.S., 1989. Naproxen reversal of nortriptyline-induced orthostatic hypotension. J. Clin. Psychiatry 50, 356.

Freeman, R., 2008. Current pharmacologic treatment for orthostatic hypotension. Clin. Auton. Res. 18 (Suppl. 1), 14−18. Available from: http://dx.doi.org/10.1007/s10286-007-1003-1.

Freitas, J., Santos, R., Azevedo, E., Costa, O., Carvalho, M., de Freitas, A.F., 2000. Clinical improvement in patients with orthostatic intolerance after treatment with bisoprolol and fludrocortisone. Clin. Auton. Res. 10, 293−299.

Friedman, J.H., Factor, S.A., 2000. Atypical antipsychotics in the treatment of drug-induced psychosis in Parkinson's disease. Mov. Disord. 15, 201−211.

Fruncillo, R.J., Gibbons, W.J., Vlasses, P.H., Ferguson, R.K., 1985. Severe hypotension associated with concurrent clonidine and antipsychotic medication. Am. J. Psychiatry 142, 274.

Fung, H.L., 2004. Biochemical mechanism of nitroglycerin action and tolerance: is this old mystery solved? Annu. Rev. Pharmacol. Toxicol. 44, 67−85.

Gershon, S., Hekimian, L.J., Burdock, E.I., Kim, S.S., 1970. Antipsychotic properties of loxapine succinate. Curr. Ther. Res. Clin. Exp. 12, 280−285.

Goldstein, D.S., Robertson, D., Esler, M., Straus, S.E., Eisenhofer, G., 2002. Dysautonomias: clinical disorders of the autonomic nervous system. Ann. Intern. Med. 137, 753−763.

Haapaniemi, T.H., Kallio, M.A., Korpelainen, J.T., et al., 2000. Levodopa, bromocriptine and selegiline modify cardiovascular responses in Parkinson's disease. J. Neurol. 247, 868−874.

Hansen, T.E., Casey, D.E., Hoffman, W.F., 1997. Neuroleptic intolerance. Schizophr. Bull. 23, 567−582.

Iserson, K.V., 1983. Parenteral chlorpromazine treatment of migraine. Ann. Emerg. Med. 12, 756−758.

Jefferson, J.W., 1972. Atypical manifestations of postural hypotension. Arch. Gen. Psychiatry 27, 250−251.

Jordan, J., 2005. Effect of water drinking on sympathetic nervous activity and blood pressure. Curr. Hypertens. Rep. 7, 17−20.

Jordan, J., Shannon, J.R., Black, B.K., et al., 2000. The pressor response to water drinking in humans: a sympathetic reflex? Circulation 101, 504−509.

Kaplan, N.M., 1959. Hypotension as a complication of promazine therapy. AMA Arch. Intern. Med. 103, 219−223.

Karagianis, J.L., Dawe, I.C., Thakur, A., Begin, S., Raskin, J., Roychowdhury, S.M., 2001. Rapid tranquilization with olanzapine in acute psychosis: a case series. J. Clin. Psychiatry 62 (Suppl. 2), 12−16.

Kaufmann, H., 2002. Treatment of patients with orthostatic hypotension and syncope. Clin. Neuropharmacol. 25, 133−141.

Kranzler, H.R., Cardoni, A., 1988. Sodium chloride treatment of antidepressant-induced orthostatic hypotension. J. Clin. Psychiatry 49, 366−368.

Laitinen, T., Niskanen, L., Geelen, G., Lansimies, E., Hartikainen, J., 2004. Age dependency of cardiovascular autonomic responses to head-up tilt in healthy subjects. J. Appl. Physiol. 96, 2333−2340.

LaWall, J.S., 1980. Treatment of psychotropic-caused orthostatic hypotension. Psychosomatics 21, 693−694.

Lieberman, J.A., Stroup, T.S., McEvoy, J.P., et al., 2005. Effectiveness of antipsychotic drugs in patients with chronic schizophrenia. N. Engl. J. Med. 353, 1209−1223.

Lindqvist, A., Jalonen, J., Laitinen, L.A., Seppala, T., Stromberg, C., 1996. The effects of midazolam and ephedrine on post-exercise autonomic chronotropic control of the heart in normal subjects. Clin. Auton. Res. 6, 343−349.

Mackin, P., 2008. Cardiac side effects of psychiatric drugs. Hum. Psychopharmacol. 23 (Suppl. 1), 3−14. Available from: http://dx.doi.org/10.1002/hup.915.

MacMillan, L.B., Hein, L., Smith, M.S., Piascik, M.T., Limbird, L.E., 1996. Central hypotensive effects of the alpha2a-adrenergic receptor subtype. Science 273, 801−803.

Masaki, K.H., Schatz, I.J., Burchfiel, C.M., et al., 1998. Orthostatic hypotension predicts mortality in elderly men: the Honolulu Heart Program. Circulation 98, 2290−2295.

Maskall, D.D., Lam, R.W., 1993. Midodrine for TCA-induced orthostatic hypotension. J. Psychiatry Neurosci. 18, 276−277.

Mathias, C.J., Fosbraey, P., da Costa, D.F., Thornley, A., Bannister, R., 1986. The effect of desmopressin on nocturnal polyuria, overnight weight loss, and morning postural hypotension in patients with autonomic failure. Br. Med. J. (Clin. Res. Ed.) 293, 353−354.

McEvoy, J.P., Lieberman, J.A., Stroup, T.S., et al., 2006. Effectiveness of clozapine versus olanzapine, quetiapine, and risperidone in patients with chronic schizophrenia who did not respond to prior atypical antipsychotic treatment. Am. J. Psychiatry 163, 600−610.

Meltzer, H.Y., Bobo, W.V., Nuamah, I.F., et al., 2008. Efficacy and tolerability of oral paliperidone extended-release tablets in the treatment of acute schizophrenia: pooled data from three 6-week placebo-controlled studies. J. Clin. Psych. 69, 817−829.

Mets, T.F., 1995. Drug-induced orthostatic hypotension in older patients. Drugs Aging 6, 219−228.

Michelsen, J.W., Meyer, J.M., 2007. Cardiovascular effects of antipsychotics. Expert Rev. Neurother. 7, 829−839. Available from: http://dx.doi.org/10.1586/14737175.7.7.829.

Munjack, D.J., 1984. The treatment of phenelzine-induced hypotension with salt tablets: case report. J. Clin. Psychiatry 45, 89−90.

Narkiewicz, K., Cooley, R.L., Somers, V.K., 2000. Alcohol potentiates orthostatic hypotension: implications for alcohol-related syncope. Circulation 101, 398−402.

Pae, C.U., Kim, J.J., Lee, C.U., et al., 2007. Rapid versus conventional initiation of quetiapine in the treatment of schizophrenia: a randomized, parallel-group trial. J. Clin. Psychiatry 68, 399−405.

Pirke, K.M., 1996. Central and peripheral noradrenalin regulation in eating disorders. Psychiatry Res. 62, 43−49.

Poon, I.O., Braun, U., 2005. High prevalence of orthostatic hypotension and its correlation with potentially causative medications among elderly veterans. J. Clin. Pharm. Ther. 30, 173−178. Available from: http://dx.doi.org/10.1111/j.1365-2710.2005.00629.x.

Prisant, L.M., 2006. Phosphodiesterase-5 inhibitors and their hemodynamic effects. Curr. Hypertens. Rep. 8, 345−351.

Product Information, July 2013. Latuda (lurasidone hydrochloride).

Product Information, December 2014a. Zyprexa (olanzapine).

Product Information, December 2014b. Clozapine.

Raj, S.R., Black, B.K., Biaggioni, I., et al., 2009. Propranolol decreases tachycardia and improves symptoms in the postural tachycardia syndrome: less is more. Circulation 120, 725−734.

Ray, W.A., Chung, C.P., Murray, K.T., Hall, K., Stein, C.M., 2009. Atypical antipsychotic drugs and the risk of sudden cardiac death. N. Engl. J. Med. 360, 225−235.

Ricci, F., Fedorowski, A., Radico, F., Romanello, M., Tatascfiore, A., Di Nicola, M., et al., 2015. Cardiovascular morbidity and mortality related to orthostatic hypotension: a meta-analysis of prospective observational studies. Eur. Heart 36, 1609−1617.

Ritter, R.M., Davidson, D.E., Robinson, T.A., 1972. Comparison of injectable haloperidol and chlorpromazine. Am. J. Psychiatry 129, 78−81.

Rosati, D., 1964. Hypotensive side effects of phenothiazine and their management. Dis. Nerv. Syst. 25, 366−369.

Rose, K.M., Eigenbrodt, M.L., Biga, R.L., et al., 2006. Orthostatic hypotension predicts mortality in middle-aged adults: the atherosclerosis risk in communities (ARIC) study. Circulation 114, 630−636.

Rutan, G.H., Hermanson, B., Bild, D.E., Kittner, S.J., LaBaw, F., Tell, G.S., 1992. Orthostatic hypotension in older adults. The Cardiovascular Health Study. CHS Collaborative Research Group. Hypertension 19, 508−519.

Sarma, S., Ward, W., O'Brien, J., Frost, A.D., 2005. Severe hyponatraemia associated with desmopressin nasal spray to treat clozapine-induced nocturnal enuresis. Aust. N. Z. J. Psychiatry 39, 949.

Scalco, M.Z., de Almeida, O.P., Hachul, D.T., Castel, S., Serro-Azul, J., Wajngarten, M., 2000. Comparison of risk of orthostatic hypotension in elderly depressed hypertensive women treated with nortriptyline and thiazides versus elderly depressed normotensive women treated with nortriptyline. Am. J. Cardiol. 85, 1156, 1158, A9.

Schimmer, B.P., Parker, K.L., 2006. Adrenocorticotropic hormone; adrenocortical steroids and their synthetic analogs; inhibitors of the synthesis and actions of adrenocortical hormones. In: Brunton, L.L., Lazo, J.S., Parker, K.L. (Eds.), Goodman & Gilman's The Pharmacological Basis of Therapeutics, 11th ed. The McGraw-Hill Companies, Inc., New York, NY, pp. 1587−1612.

Schwinn, D.A., Roehrborn, C.G., 2008. Alpha1-adrenoceptor subtypes and lower urinary tract symptoms. Int. J. Urol. 15, 193−199.

Seideman, P., Grahnen, A., Haglund, K., Lindstrom, B., Von Bahr, C., 1982. Prazosin first dose phenomenon during combined treatment with a beta-adrenoceptor blocker in hypertensive patients. Br. J. Clin. Pharmacol. 13, 865−870.

Silver, H., Kogan, H., Zlotogorski, D., 1990. Postural hypotension in chronically medicated schizophrenics. J. Clin. Psychiatry 51, 459−462.

Simpson, G.M., Cuculic, Z., 1976. A double-blind comparison of loxapine succinate and trifluoperazine in newly admitted schizophrenic patients. J. Clin. Pharmacol. 16, 60−65.

Smith, J.J., Porth, C.M., Erickson, M., 1994. Hemodynamic response to the upright posture. J. Clin. Pharmacol. 34, 375−386.

Smith, M.A., McCoy, R., Hamer-Maansson, J., Brecher, M., 2005. Rapid dose escalation with quetiapine: a pilot study. J. Clin. Psychopharmacol. 25, 331−335.

Stroup, T.S., Lieberman, J.A., McEvoy, J.P., et al., 2006. Effectiveness of olanzapine, quetiapine, risperidone, and ziprasidone in patients with chronic schizophrenia following discontinuation of a previous atypical antipsychotic. Am. J. Psychiatry 163, 611−622.

Stroup, T.S., Lieberman, J.A., McEvoy, J.P., et al., 2007. Effectiveness of olanzapine, quetiapine, and risperidone in patients with chronic schizophrenia after discontinuing perphenazine: a CATIE study. Am. J. Psychiatry 164, 415−427.

Stroup, T.S., Lieberman, J.A., McEvoy, J.P., et al., 2009. Results of phase 3 of the CATIE schizophrenia trial. Schizophr. Res. 107, 1−12.

Stumpf, J.L., Mitrzyk, B., 1994. Management of orthostatic hypotension. Am. J. Hosp. Pharm. 51, 648, 660; quiz 697−698.

Swett Jr., C., Cole, J.O., Hartz, S.C., Shapiro, S., Slone, D., 1977. Hypotension due to chlorpromazine. Relation to cigarette smoking, blood pressure, and dosage. Arch. Gen. Psychiatry 34, 661−663.

Takahashi, H., 2000. Acute dystonia induced by adding midodrine, a selective alpha 1 agonist, to risperidone in a patient with catatonic schizophrenia. J. Neuropsychiatry Clin. Neurosci. 12, 285−286.

Testani Jr., M., 1994. Clozapine-induced orthostatic hypotension treated with fludrocortisone. J. Clin. Psychiatry 55, 497–498.

Thomas, M., Malmcrona, R., Fillmore, S., Shillingford, J., 1965. Haemodynamic effects of morphine in patients with acute myocardial infarction. Br. Heart J. 27, 863–875.

Tonkin, A.L., Wing, L.M., 1994. Effects of age and isolated systolic hypertension on cardiovascular reflexes. J. Hypertens. 12, 1083–1088.

Turkka, J., Suominen, K., Tolonen, U., Sotaniemi, K., Myllyla, V.V., 1997. Selegiline diminishes cardiovascular autonomic responses in Parkinson's disease. Neurology 48, 662–667.

van den Berg, F., Tulen, J.H., Boomsma, F., Noten, J.B., Moleman, P., Pepplinkhuizen, L., 1996. Effects of alprazolam and lorazepam on catecholaminergic and cardiovascular activity during supine rest, mental load and orthostatic challenge. Psychopharmacology (Berl.) 128, 21–30.

Vestal, R.E., Kornhauser, D.M., Hollifield, J.W., Shand, D.G., 1979. Inhibition of propranolol metabolism by chlorpromazine. Clin. Pharmacol. Ther. 25, 19–24.

Viikki, M., Kampman, O., Seppala, N., Mononen, N., Lehtimaki, T., Leinonen, E., 2014. CYP1A2 polymorphism -1545C > T (rs2470890) is associated with increased side effects to clozapine. BMC Psychiatry 14, 50.

Weber, M.A., 2002. Calcium channel antagonists in the treatment of hypertension. Am. J. Cardiovasc. Drugs 2, 415–431.

Weiden, P.J., Cutler, A.J., Polymeropoulos, M.H., Wolfgang, C.D., 2008. Safety profile of iloperidone: a pooled analysis of 6-week acute-phase pivotal trials. J. Clin. Psychopharmacol. 28, S12–S19.

Westfall, T.C., Westfall, D.P., 2006a. Neurotransmission: the autonomic and somatic motor nervous systems. In: Brunton, L.L., Lazo, J.S., Parker, K.L. (Eds.), Goodman & Gilman's The Pharmacological Basis of Therapeutics, 11th ed. The McGraw-Hill Companies, Inc., New York, NY, pp. 137–182.

Westfall, T.C., Westfall, D.P., 2006b. Adrenergic agonists and antagonists. In: Brunton, L.L., Lazo, J.S., Parker, K.L. (Eds.), Goodman & Gilman's The Pharmacological Basis of Therapeutics, 11th ed. The McGraw-Hill Companies, Inc., New York, NY, pp. 237–296.

White, W.B., 1986. Hypotension with postural syncope secondary to the combination of chlorpromazine and captopril. Arch. Intern. Med. 146, 1833–1834.

Wong, J., Patel, R.A., Kowey, P.R., 2004. The clinical use of angiotensin-converting enzyme inhibitors. Prog. Cardiovasc. Dis. 47, 116–130.

Young, C.R., Bowers Jr., M.B., Mazure, C.M., 1998. Management of the adverse effects of clozapine. Schizophr. Bull. 24, 381–390.

Part II

Hematological Complications of Treatment With Antipsychotic Drugs

Chapter 5

Severe Neutropenia and Agranulocytosis

John Lally[1] and Robert J. Flanagan[2]
[1]*King's College London, London, United Kingdom,*
[2]*King's College Hospital, London, United Kingdom*

5.1 EPIDEMIOLOGY

Many hematological disorders may be encountered in psychiatric practice. These include deficiencies in various blood constituents—leukopenia, neutropenia, agranulocytosis, thrombocytopenia, anemia—and leukocytosis, thrombocytosis, eosinophilia, and altered platelet function. In the main, the mechanisms underlying these disorders are poorly understood (Chigaev et al., 2011). Reviews of the subject are available (Duggal and Singh, 2005; Hall et al., 2003; Oyesanmi et al., 1999; Mintzer et al., 2009; Shander et al., 2011; Stübner et al., 2004).

Leukopenia is a low leukocyte count (white blood cell count, WCC). When it occurs in association with antipsychotic medication it is often due to neutropenia. Neutropenia can be defined as a neutrophil count of $<1.5\,\text{nL}^{-1}$ (Table 5.1). As neutrophils make up the majority of circulating leukocytes, neutropenia is suggested by a WCC of $<3\,\text{nL}^{-1}$. Agranulocytosis literally means an absence of circulating granular leukocytes (neutrophils, basophils, and eosinophils) (Box 5.1). In practice it is defined as a neutrophil count $<0.5\,\text{nL}^{-1}$, and is suggested by a WCC of $<1\,\text{nL}^{-1}$. To an extent these definitions are arbitrary and hence may differ slightly between centers/studies. In many cases the red cells and platelets are unaffected in neutropenia and, therefore, hematocrit and platelet counts are often normal.

Cytokines such as granulocyte-colony stimulating factor (G-CSF) and granulocyte macrophage-colony stimulating factor (GM-CSF) increase the release of granulocytes from the bone marrow storage pool into the circulation and inhibit neutrophil apoptosis. These cytokines are available as therapeutic agents (filgrastim, lenograstim) and can produce a two- to three-fold increase in the

Life-Threatening Effects of Antipsychotic Drugs. DOI: http://dx.doi.org/10.1016/B978-0-12-803376-0.00005-8
© 2016 Elsevier Inc. All rights reserved.

TABLE 5.1 Cellular Blood Components

Cell Type	Parameter	Subdivision	Adult Normal Range[a]
Erythrocytes	Hemoglobin	Male	$140-180$ g L^{-1}
		Female	$120-160$ g L^{-1}
	Packed cell volume (hematocrit)	Male	$0.40-0.50$
		Female	$0.36-0.46$
	Corrected reticulocyte count	–	$0.5-1.5\%$
Platelets	Number of cells	–	$130-400$ nL^{-1}
Leukocytes	Number of cells (white blood cell count)	–	$4.3-10.8$ nL^{-1}
	Differential cell count	Granulocyte neutrophils[b]	$2.5-7.5$ nL^{-1}
		Lymphocytes	$1.3-4.0$ nL^{-1}
		Monocytes	$0.2-1.0$ nL^{-1}

[a] $nL^{-1} = 10^3 \, \mu L^{-1} = 10^9 \, L^{-1} = 10^3 \, mm^{-3}$.
[b] "Bands" (immature neutrophils, myeloblasts) $0-4\%$, basophils $0-2\%$, eosinophils $0-7\%$.

BOX 5.1 Definitions

- Leukopenia: low white blood cell count (WCC)
- Neutropenia: neutrophil count of <1.5 nL^{-1} (suggested by WCC < 3 nL^{-1})
- Agranulocytosis: lack of circulating granular leukocytes (neutrophils, basophils, eosinophils)
  - Neutrophil count < 0.5 nL^{-1} (suggested by WCC < 1.0 nL^{-1})
  - Annual incidence (all causes) $3-12$ per million population
- Eosinophilia: eosinophil count > 0.50 nL^{-1}
- Thrombocytopenia: platelet count < 100 nL^{-1}
- Pancytopenia (anemia, neutropenia, thrombocytopenia)
  - WCC < 0.5 nL^{-1}, platelet count < 20 nL^{-1}, corrected reticulocyte count (immature erythrocyte count corrected for hematocrit) $<1\%$, hemoglobin < 100 g L^{-1}

number of leukocytes in the blood within $4-5$ hours of administration. The marginated pool, an intravascular reservoir of leukocytes in the pulmonary circulation, can also be released into the systemic circulation. Adrenaline promotes such release, hence the neutrophilic response to stress and exercise.

Out of a total of 90×10^9 granulocytes in the average man, 20% are precursors of the bone marrow pool, 75% are in the bone marrow storage pool, 3% are in the marginated pool, and 2% are in the circulating pool. Under normal conditions, some 120×10^9 granulocytes are produced daily. Inflammation increases granulocyte production. Granulocytes live for some 9 days in the bone marrow, 3–6 hours in blood, and 1–4 days in tissues. It must be borne in mind, therefore, that measurements in peripheral blood represent a small proportion of total body neutrophils.

People from certain ethnic groups, such as Yemenite Jews and Jordanians, and some people with tanned or dark skin (25–50% of Africans, for example), may normally have a neutrophil granulocyte count in the range $1.0–1.5 \text{ nL}^{-1}$, but overall show no actual deficit in neutrophils and come to no serious harm as regards incidence of infections, response to infection, etc. These individuals are said to demonstrate benign ethnic neutropenia (BEN; Haddy et al., 1999; Rajagopal, 2005; Box 5.2). A genetic polymorphism contributing to BEN in those of African descent has been identified (Reich et al., 2009).

Neutropenia may be due to either decreased production, or peripheral destruction of neutrophils (Box 5.3). Many exogenous agents can cause neutropenia. Mechanisms may involve toxic effects in the bone marrow; be related to formation of antibodies against hematopoietic precursors or mature neutrophils; or, more rarely, involve peripheral destruction of neutrophils. Agranulocytosis from any cause is rare with an annual incidence of 3–12 cases/million population (Andrès et al., 2008). The main clinical manifestations of agranulocytosis are secondary to infection and may include a fever with no clear focus, fatigue, malaise, chills, weakness, cough, sore throat, oral mucosal infection, pharyngitis, gingivitis, abscess, pneumonia, septicemia, and septic shock.

Thrombocytopenia is usually defined as a platelet count $<100 \text{ nL}^{-1}$. However, spontaneous bleeding does not become evident until the count falls below 20 nL^{-1}. Platelet counts in the range $20–50 \text{ nL}^{-1}$ can aggravate post-traumatic bleeding.

Aplastic anemia is a life-threatening disorder in which there is bone marrow failure associated with pancytopenia (anemia, neutropenia, and

---

BOX 5.2 Benign Ethnic Neutropenia

- "Occurrence of neutropenia, defined by normative data in white populations, in individuals or other ethnic groups who are otherwise healthy and who do not have repeated or severe infections" (Rajagopal, 2005)
  - BEN in 25–50% Africans and some other ethnic groups in the Middle East (including Yemenite Jews, Jordanians)
  - Only in groups that have tanned or dark skin

BOX 5.3 Some Causes of Neutropenia/Agranulocytosis

- Defective/decreased production (either leukocytes or neutrophils alone)

- Removal from the circulation

- Congenital causes
- Benign familial neutropenia
  - Benign chronic neutropenia in children
  - Chronic idiopathic neutropenia
- Dietary
  - Vitamin deficiency (cyanocobalamin, B_{12}; folate, B_9)
  - Copper deficiency
  - Malnutrition
- Myelodysplastic syndromes
- Tumors and other diseases that infiltrate bone marrow
- Aplastic anemia
- Drugs (Table 5.2)
- Destruction in enlarged spleen (hypersplenism)
- Immune destruction disease
  - Autoimmune neutropenia
  - Isoimmune neutropenia
- Neutropenia associated with metabolic disorders
- Infection
  - Bacterial (typhoid, tuberculosis)
  - Viral (EBV, hepatitis, HIV, rubella)
  - Protozoal (malaria)
- Drugs (Table 5.2)

TABLE 5.2 Some Drugs Associated With Blood Dyscrasia

Drug Group	Examples
Analgesic/antiinflammatory/antipyretic/antirheumatoid	Aminopyrine, azapropazone, diclofenac, dipyrone, glafenine, gold, ibuprofen, indometacin, naproxen, niflumic acid, oxyphenbutazone, paracetamol, penicillamine, pentazocine, phenylbutazone, piroxicam, pirprofen, propyphenazone, salicylates, sulfasalazine, sulindac
Antiarrythmic	Ajmaline, amiodarone, aprindine, procainamide, tocainide
Antiasthmatic	Theophylline
Anticoagulant	Heparin

(Continued)

TABLE 5.2 (Continued)

Drug Group	Examples
Antidepressant	Amitriptyline, amoxapine, clomipramine, desipramine, imipramine, mianserin, mirtazapine, phenelzine, trazodone
Antiepileptic	Carbamazepine, gabapentin, lamotrigine, phenytoin, pregabalin, valproate
Antihistamine	Alimemazine, cinnarizine, mebhydrolin, promethazine
Antihypertensive	ACE-inhibitors (captopril, enalapril, lisinopril, ramipril), calcium channel antagonists (amlodipine, nifedipine), hydralazine, ibopamine, methyldopa
Antimicrobial/antiinfective	Cephalosporins (cephalexin, cepahazolin, cefuroxime, cefitaxime, cephradine), ciprofloxacin, clindamycin, chloramphenicol, cotrimoxazole, dapsone, doxycycline, fusidic acid, gentamycin, levamisole, metronidazole, nalidixic acid, nitrofurantoin, norfloxacin, penicillins, pyrimethamine, ribavirin, rifampin, sulfonamides, sulfamethizole, tetracyclines
Antineoplastic	All
Antiparkinsonian	Carbidopa/levodopa
Antiplatelet	Ticlopidine
Antipsychotic	Clozapine, haloperidol, olanzapine, phenothiazines (chlorpromazine, fluphenazine, methotrimeprazine, perazine, thioridazine), quetiapine, remoxipride, risperidone, ziprasidone, zuclopentixol
Antithyroid	Carbimazole, methylthiouracil, propylthiouracil, thiamazole (methimazole)
Antiulcer	Omeprazole, pirenzepine
Anxiolytic/sedative	Barbiturates, benzodiazepines (chlordiazepoxide, clonazepam, diazepam, lorazepam), zopiclone
Carbonic anhydrase inhibitor	Acetazolamide, methazolamide
Diuretic	Chlorthalidone, hydrochlorothiazide, spironolactone
H_2-antagonist	Cimetidine, omeprazole, ranitidine
Hypoglycemic	Glibenclamide, tolbutamide
Mood stabilizer	Lithium
Uricosuric	Allopurinol

thrombocytopenia) (WCC $< 0.5\,\mathrm{nL}^{-1}$, platelet count $< 20\,\mathrm{nL}^{-1}$, corrected reticulocyte count (immature erythrocyte count corrected for hematocrit) $< 1\%$, hemoglobin $< 100\,\mathrm{g\,L}^{-1}$). The hematocrit falls less quickly than the other parameters because the erythrocyte half-life in blood is some 120 days. Unlike agranulocytosis, which is mainly drug induced, in most cases the cause of aplastic anemia remains unknown (Young et al., 2008).

Primary bone marrow disorders should be suspected in patients who present with marked leukocytosis or concurrent abnormalities in red blood cell or platelet counts in the absence of infection. The most common such bone marrow disorders can be grouped into acute leukemias, chronic leukemias, and myeloproliferative disorders. Medications commonly associated with leukocytosis include corticosteroids, lithium, and β-agonists. A WCC $> 100\,\mathrm{nL}^{-1}$ represents a clinical emergency because of the risk of cerebral infarction and hemorrhage.

Increased eosinophil or basophil counts may result from infection, allergic reaction, and other causes, and can lead to leukocytosis in some patients. Eosinophilia is the occurrence of abnormally large numbers of eosinophils in the blood (eosinophil counts $> 0.50\,\mathrm{nL}^{-1}$). In the United Kingdom it is most commonly caused by conditions such as asthma or hay fever. Worldwide the most common cause is parasitic infections. Symptoms are related to the underlying cause. Eosinophilia can be caused by drugs and on rare occasions can indicate developing tissue damage, in the heart for example.

5.1.1 Drug-Induced Dyscrasias

Although many drugs may cause a blood dyscrasia (Box 5.4; Table 5.2), such disorders account for a minority of adverse drug reactions (one or two cases with serious hematological toxicity per year per 100,000 patients). The ability of new drugs to cause a rare dyscrasia often does not become apparent until the drug is used more widely after licensing, hence such reactions may only be identified during postmarketing studies or after widespread use of the compound (King and Wager, 1998).

BOX 5.4 Drug-Induced Dyscrasia: Mechanisms
- Almost all classes of drugs can cause blood dyscrasia
- Mechanisms include:
  - Direct toxic effects on bone marrow
  - Formation of antibodies against hematopoietic precursors
  - Peripheral destruction of cells

Leukopenia was first recognized as a side effect of psychotropic medication when it was observed in association with chlorpromazine in the 1950s. Now almost all the major classes of psychotropic medications have been associated with blood dyscrasia (Stübner et al., 2004; Levin and DeVane, 1992). Often one drug may be associated with several different types of dyscrasia (Oyesanmi et al., 1999; Tables 5.3−5.5).

5.1.2   Epidemiology of Clozapine-Induced Neutropenia and Agranulocytosis

The cumulative incidence of clozapine-induced neutropenia is 2.7%, with the peak risk occurring at 6−18 weeks with an incidence of 1.27% (Munro et al., 1999). Data from a retrospective naturalistic study identified clozapine-induced neutropenia in 15 of 320 (4.7%) clozapine-treated patients (Davis et al., 2014). The cumulative incidence of clozapine-induced agranulocytosis is 0.8% at 1 year and 0.91% at 18 months (Alvir et al., 1993), that is, after

TABLE 5.3 Hematological Toxicity of Some Antipsychotic Drugs

Class	Drug	Effect
First generation	Chlorpromazine	Agranulocytosis, anemia (aplastic, hemolytic), eosinophilia, neutropenia, thrombocytopenia
	Fluphenazine	Agranulocytosis, eosinophilia, pancytopenia, leukocytosis, neutropenia, thrombocytopenia
	Haloperidol	Agranulocytosis, leukocytosis, neutropenia, lymphomonocytosis, minimal changes in erythrocyte counts
	Prochlorperazine	Agranulocytosis, neutropenia, thrombocytopenia
	Promazine	Agranulocytosis, neutropenia, thrombocytopenia
	Thioridazine	Agranulocytosis, neutropenia, thrombocytopenia
Second generation	Clozapine	Agranulocytosis, anemia, eosinophilia, leukocytosis, neutropenia, lymphopenia, thrombocytopenia, thrombocytosis
	Olanzapine	Agranulocytosis, neutropenia, leukocytosis, thrombocytopenia
	Quetiapine	Agranulocytosis, neutropenia, thrombotic thrombocytopenic purpura
	Risperidone	Agranulocytosis, anemia, leukocytosis, neutropenia, thrombocytopenia
	Ziprasidone	Agranulocytosis, neutropenia

TABLE 5.4 Hematological Toxicity of Some Antidepressants and Benzodiazepines

Class	Drug	Effect
Tricyclic antidepressant	Amitriptyline/ nortriptyline	Agranulocytosis, eosinophilia, neutropenia, thrombocytopenia
	Imipramine/ desipramine	Agranulocytosis, eosinophilia, neutropenia, thrombocytopenia
	Clomipramine	Agranulocytosis, neutropenia, pancytopenia, thrombocytopenia
Monoamine oxidase inhibitor	Tranylcypromine	Agranulocytosis, anemia, neutropenia, thrombocytopenia
Selective serotonin reuptake inhibitor	Citalopram	Anemia, impaired platelet aggregation, leukocytosis, neutropenia
	Fluoxetine	Disseminated intravascular coagulation, impaired platelet aggregation
	Fluvoxamine	Impaired platelet aggregation
	Paroxetine	Impaired platelet aggregation
	Sertraline	Anemia, impaired platelet aggregation, thrombocytopenia
Other antidepressant	Mirtazapine	Agranulocytosis, anemia, neutropenia, pancytopenia, thrombocytopenia
	Nefazodone	Anemia, neutropenia
	Trazodone	Anemia, leukocytosis, neutropenia
	Venlafaxine	Anemia, leukocytosis, neutropenia
Benzodiazepine	Chlordiazepoxide	Agranulocytosis, anemia, impaired platelet aggregation, thrombocytopenia
	Clonazepam	Anemia, eosinophilia, neutropenia, thrombocytopenia
	Diazepam	Agranulocytosis, anemia, pancytopenia, impaired platelet aggregation, thrombocytopenia
	Lorazepam	Neutropenia

1 year the risk is similar to that with chlorpromazine (chlorpromazine agranulocytosis risk up to 0.13% (King and Wager, 1998)). Data from a UK clozapine monitoring service indicated similar results, with a cumulative incidence of clozapine-associated agranulocytosis of 0.8% over a 4.5-year study period, with the incidence of both neutropenia and agranulocytosis highest at 6–18

TABLE 5.5 Hematological Toxicity of Some Mood-Stabilizing Agents

Drug	Effect
Carbamazepine	Agranulocytosis, anemia, eosinophilia, leukocytosis, leukopenia, pure erythrocyte aplasia, thrombocytopenia
Gabapentin	Leukopenia
Lamotrigine	Anemia, pancytopenia, pure erythrocyte aplasia, thrombocytopenia
Lithium	Leukocytosis, leukemia, thrombocytosis
Valproate	Anemia, neutropenia, pure erythrocyte aplasia, thrombocytopenia

weeks after commencing clozapine (Atkin et al., 1996). The risk of agranulocytosis is increased in women [risk ratio (RR) of 1.60; 95% confidence interval (CI) 0.99–2.58 with adjustment for age] and increases with age (RR 1.06; 95% CI 1.04–1.07 with adjustment for sex) (Alvir et al., 1993).

Case fatality with nonchemotherapeutic drug-induced agranulocytosis has been declining due to improved treatment options. A systematic review of case reports found mortality to be 6% without the use of G-CSF or GM-CSF, and 5% with (Andersohn et al., 2007). The mortality rate from clozapine-induced agranulocytosis is now estimated at 0.01–0.03% and the case fatality rate is estimated to be 2.2–4.2% (Cohen et al., 2012). Davis et al. (2014) identified a case fatality rate of 0.94% (mortality rate from clozapine-induced agranulocytosis 1.5/1000 treatment-years). A reason for the reduced case fatality with clozapine-induced agranulocytosis compared to that with other drugs may be the early recognition of the condition from the regular hematological monitoring required in many countries. In addition, there may be a difference in the speed of onset of agranulocytosis with different drugs.

Observations from epidemiological studies suggest that there may be different risk factors for clozapine-induced neutropenia than for agranulocytosis, further raising the possibility of slightly different etiological mechanisms. Thus, in adults, the risk of agranulocytosis increases with age (Munro et al., 1999; Atkin et al., 1996; Alvir et al., 1993), but the risk of neutropenia decreases with age. Agranulocytosis is more common in older Caucasian women and in those with a coexisting illness or abnormal blood count than in other patient groups (Alvir et al., 1993; Munro et al., 1999; Hall et al., 2003). A low baseline leukocyte count may be associated with future neutropenia, but not with agranulocytosis (Gillman, 2000). It has been suggested that a leukocyte count of 15% or more above the previous value might predict the occurrence of agranulocytosis within the next 75 days as an increase in the count is sometimes seen before a precipitous fall (Alvir et al., 1995), but this has not been confirmed.

In the United Kingdom and Ireland, neutropenia, but not agranulocytosis, is more common in dark-skinned people and there is more than twice the frequency of agranulocytosis in Asians compared to Caucasians (Munro et al., 1999). Some human leukocyte antigen (HLA) alleles, for example, HLA-B38 phenotype in Ashkenazi Jews, may be associated with clozapine-induced agranulocytosis (Meged et al., 1999; Valevski et al., 1998).

There is evidence that adherence to clozapine is improved as a result of the regular contact with clinic staff that blood monitoring requires (Patel et al., 2005). Nevertheless, there continues to be debate surrounding (1) the mechanism of clozapine-induced hematological toxicity, (2) criteria whereby clozapine may be prescribed against a background of inherent variability in healthy WBC between ethnic groups (Kelly et al., 2007; Rajagopal, 2005), (3) criteria for clozapine rechallenge in the event that clozapine treatment was suspended because the WCC fell below a critical count, and (4) options for continuing clozapine in the event of worrying falls in WCC, including measures to boost the WCC either with, or without, continued clozapine administration (Berk et al., 2007).

In the British Isles clozapine can only be prescribed if the patient, prescribing psychiatrist, and dispensing pharmacist are registered with a clozapine monitoring service (Clozaril Patient Monitoring Service (CPMS, Novartis); Denzapine Monitoring Service (DMS, Merz Pharma); or Zaponex Treatment Access System (ZTAS, Ivax/Genthon)). Dispensing of clozapine is dependent on a satisfactory full blood count (FBC) result before treatment is started. Assuming normal counts are maintained, the FBC must be monitored weekly for the first 18 weeks of clozapine treatment, fortnightly to the end of the first year of treatment, and 4-weekly thereafter. In the United States, the requirement is for weekly monitoring for 6 months, and fortnightly monitoring up until 1 year, and 4-weekly thereafter (Nielsen et al., 2016). In the Netherlands for mentally competent and adequately informed patients, quarterly monitoring after the first 6 months of clozapine treatment is permitted (Cohen and Monden, 2013). On the other hand, more frequent monitoring may be indicated at any stage if the FBC results are abnormal or the onset of features that could indicate a developing infection are seen.

There are no clear criteria for predicting the onset of neutropenia/agranulocytosis (Box 5.5). A transient neutropenia, that is, a fall and then a return of the neutrophil count to normal values at constant clozapine dose, was reported in 22% of 68 Caucasians given clozapine for the first time (Hummer et al., 1994). Transient (2−5 days) neutropenia and weekly benign variations of the neutrophil count, not necessitating the discontinuation of clozapine treatment, have also been reported in 5 Asian patients (Ahn et al., 2004). It is unclear why some patients treated with clozapine develop a transient neutropenia and experience no further adverse events, while others progress to agranulocytosis if clozapine dosage is maintained. In this so-called benign neutropenia, successful compensation by cytokines such as

BOX 5.5 Clozapine and Agranulocytosis

- In adults, risk of agranulocytosis increases with age, but risk of neutropenia decreases
- Agranulocytosis more common in women
- More than 2× frequency in Asians compared to Caucasians
- Neutropenia, but not agranulocytosis more common in black people
- Low baseline WCC may be associated with future neutropenia, but not agranulocytosis
- WCC spike of 15% or more above previous value may predict agranulocytosis within the next 75 days

G-CSF may stimulate granulopoiesis. It has been suggested that if cytokine compensation is inadequate, progressive neutropenia may then develop (Hummer et al., 1994).

5.2   PATHOBIOLOGY

Neutropenia and agranulocytosis are the most important drug-related blood dyscrasia clinically since, as compared to other blood dyscrasia, they carry an increased mortality risk (Andersohn et al., 2007). Agranulocytosis requires urgent management (Box 5.6). Regular assessment and prompt treatment can be life-saving.

With almost all drugs in common usage that can give rise to neutropenia/agranulocytosis the risk is obviously considered acceptable, even with

BOX 5.6 Drug-Induced Agranulocytosis

- Agranulocytosis most important drug-related dyscrasia
- Idiosyncratic (i.e., genetic basis), but often dose-related component
- Range of mechanisms proposed (immune/allergic, toxic metabolites, pharmacologic): likely combination of mechanisms
- More frequent in the elderly
  - More diseases/more drugs for longer than younger patients
- More frequent in females (may be effect of age)
- Consequences fever, chills, sore throat, pneumonia, septicemia, septic shock
- Generally reversible on withdrawal of causative agent
- Mortality from drug-induced agranulocytosis 5-10% in Western countries
  - Manifestations 2° to infection
- Aggressive treatment (broad-spectrum antimicrobials IV, bone marrow stimulants) may be required

chemotherapeutic agents, given the benefits derived from continued availability of the drug. Timely withdrawal of the offending agent, if appropriate, is usually successful in preventing a fatal outcome (Andersohn et al., 2007). High-risk nonchemotherapeutic drugs include antithyroid drugs (e.g., propylthiouracil), calcium dobesilate, carbamazepine, clozapine, deferiprone (L1), diclofenac, dipyrone, β-lactam antibiotics, spironolactone, sulfamethoxazole−trimethoprim, sulfasalazine, ticlopidine, and vancomycin (Curtis, 2014; Garbe, 2007; Pontikoglou and Papadaki, 2010). There may of course be risks from hitherto unsuspected sources such as the use of illicit cocaine adulterated with tetramisole, which may have confused putative identification of offending agents in recent years (Buchanan et al., 2010).

The mechanism by which neutropenia arises varies between compounds. Some drugs cause bone marrow suppression and some cause increased peripheral destruction of white cells. Most, but by no means all, drug-induced agranulocytosis is dose-related. Among psychoactive drugs, antipsychotics, including not only clozapine (approximate risk of neutropenia 1 in 30 patients), but also chlorpromazine (risk of neutropenia with phenothiazines 1 in 10,000 patients), barbiturates, and benzodiazepines are the most common causes of neutropenia and agranulocytosis. It is not widely appreciated that olanzapine has the third highest incidence of neutropenia among both first- and second-generation antipsychotics (Duggal and Singh, 2005). Other drugs that are well-recognized causes of neutropenia include antiepileptics/mood stabilizers (notably carbamazepine, risk of neutropenia approximately 1 in 200 patients). Agranulocytosis associated with antidepressant use is rare, but since early features such as fatigue and malaise are also signs of depression, it can easily be overlooked (Demler and Trigoboff, 2011; Oyesanmi et al., 1999).

Drug-induced neutropenia usually becomes manifest after 1 or 2 weeks of exposure, the degree of neutropenia that develops depending upon the dose and the duration of exposure. This being said, acute ingestion of chlorpromazine in a 5-year-old child caused neutropenia with a nadir at 45 hours postingestion (Burckart et al., 1981). Recovery of the leukocyte count usually occurs within 3−4 weeks of stopping chronic treatment. A rebound leukocytosis may occur. If the neutropenia is mild and the drug is thought essential for the patient, sometimes treatment is continued with close monitoring. If the absolute neutrophil count is above $0.5-0.7 \text{ nL}^{-1}$ or so and there is no active infection, the drug may sometimes be continued if needed in consultation with a hematologist. A bone marrow biopsy that shows cellular bone marrow is suggestive of peripheral destruction of white cells, and this may be less critical clinically. Conversely, if a bone marrow aspiration shows a hypoplastic marrow, then it indicates that the neutropenic phase may be prolonged (>1 week duration), which may necessitate the use of hematopoietic growth factors to promote granulopoiesis.

Agranulocytosis, which can be life-threatening, usually appears 3−4 weeks after the initiation of therapy, and is more frequent and tends to be more serious in the elderly. This could be because such patients tend to have multiple pathology, hence are given more drugs for longer periods and also have less bone marrow reserve than younger patients (Andrès et al., 2004). It is also more frequent in females. Before the use of antibiotics the mortality associated with agranulocytosis was some 80%. With prompt recognition and appropriate management, the mortality from drug-induced agranulocytosis is now of the order of 5−10% (Andersohn et al., 2007; Pontikoglou and Papadaki, 2010). Features associated with increased mortality include age >65 years, comorbid medical conditions, such as renal failure or septicemia, and a neutrophil count below 0.1 nL^{-1} (Andrès et al., 2011).

5.2.1 Mechanism of Clozapine-Induced Neutropenia/Agranulocytosis

As with drug-induced neutropenia/agranulocytosis in general, the mechanism by which clozapine exerts toxic effects on the bone marrow and on circulating neutrophils is thought to have a large idiosyncratic (genetic) component. However, reports of the sudden development of agranulocytosis after several years of exposure to clozapine with no detectable adverse hematological effects (Patel et al., 2002; Lahdelma and Appelberg, 2012; Sedky et al., 2005) do suggest that extragenetic factors could play a part in such patients. Clozapine-associated agranulocytosis does not appear to be a dose-related phenomenon (Alvir et al., 1993). Although smoking cessation leads to an increase in the effective clozapine dose there are no reports of neutropenia or agranulocytosis being precipitated by a change in smoking habit. There appears to be no difference in the plasma clozapine and norclozapine (N-desmethylclozapine) concentrations in patients who either do, or do not develop agranulocytosis (Hasegawa et al., 1994; Centorrino et al., 1995).

An inverse relationship between clozapine dose and the occurrence of clozapine-associated neutropenia and agranulocytosis has been reported, but it was not clear if this analysis was adjusted for the duration of clozapine treatment at the time of the index neutropenia or agranulocytosis (Munro et al., 1999). This is relevant as the clozapine dose is titrated over the first 2 or so weeks of treatment and dose increases occur thereafter until a clinical response is attained. It is possible that the inverse dose relationship is reflective of the early time to onset of the index neutropenia or agranulocytosis during the first 6−18 weeks of clozapine treatment.

Activation of clozapine, norclozapine, and/or a further metabolite, clozapine N-oxide, to electrophilic nitrenium ions may be the initial step in the events leading to neutropenia and in turn to agranulocytosis (Pirmohamed and Park, 1997; Pereira and Dean, 2006; Box 5.7).

Oxidation of clozapine by neutrophil-generated hypochlorous acid (HOCl) via the NADPH oxidase/myeloperoxidase system has been demonstrated (Dettling et al., 2000; Gardner et al., 2005; Hsuanyu and Dunford, 1999;

BOX 5.7 Clozapine and Neutropenia/Agranulocytosis

- Initial step may be metabolism to electrophilic nitrenium ion, normally detoxified by reduced glutathione
- May bind to neutrophils to cause cell death *or* could cause oxidative stress-induced neutrophil apoptosis
- If produced in liver, need some mechanism whereby affects bone marrow
- Predisposing genetic variants in the HLA region indicate immune involvement (Goldstein et al., 2014)
- Some HLA alleles (e.g., HLA-B38 phenotype in Ashkenazi Jews) may be associated with clozapine-induced agranulocytosis
- Antineutrophil antibodies may be involved—component of immune response (problem worse on rechallenge in susceptible patients)
- Different risk factors for agranulocytosis and neutropenia

Mosyagin et al., 2004). These ions are normally detoxified by reduced glutathione. However, the ions either may also bind to neutrophils to cause cell death, or could cause oxidative stress-induced neutrophil apoptosis (Husain et al., 2006). It is possible that the target in agranulocytosis could be stromal cells, neutrophil precursors in the bone marrow (Pereira and Dean, 2006), in addition to mature peripheral neutrophils, while the main target in neutropenia may only be the peripheral blood neutrophils (Duggal and Singh, 2005). Antineutrophil antibodies, possibly generated by reaction of nitrenium ions with neutrophil proteins resulting in hapten formation, may also be involved in the etiology of clozapine-induced neutropenia. The likelihood that this phenomenon is an immune-mediated reaction perhaps mediated via T lymphocytes is indicated by the fact that the reaction occurs more quickly and is more severe on rechallenge in patients who have previously developed clozapine-induced neutropenia (Dunk et al., 2006). Fehsel et al. (2005) have suggested that oxidative mitochondrial stress may cause neutrophil apoptosis in clozapine-treated patients. Apoptosis is induced in weeks 4−12 after starting clozapine, corresponding to the period when agranulocytosis is most likely to occur. Large numbers of apoptotic neutrophils were found in clozapine-treated patients who developed agranulocytosis. Therefore, drugs that are likely to induce oxidative stress in leukocytes, and thus to decrease antioxidant defences that would be necessary to prevent clozapine-induced prooxidant deleterious effects in mitochondria, should be withdrawn before starting clozapine. Examples of such drugs include nucleotide reverse transcriptome inhibitors, for example, zidovudine (AZT), diclofenac, chlorpromazine, doxorubicin (Deavall et al., 2012), and sodium valproate (Fehsel et al., 2005). Changes in the ability of platelets to aggregate in schizophrenia may also be due to oxidative stress (Dietrich-Muszalska and Olas, 2009).

Clozapine, olanzapine, and chlorpromazine are said to accumulate in mitochondria, endoplasmic reticulum, and lysosomes. These are also the antipsychotics most likely to cause neutrophil immaturity, neutropenia, and agranulocytosis (Delieu et al., 2009). Some patients started on clozapine show a benign leukocytosis, which may persist for years (Sopko and Caley, 2010), before the usual fall in WCC becomes manifest. Animal models have shown that clozapine causes an enhanced release of leukocytes from the marginated pool and the bone marrow, as well as a shortened neutrophil plasma half-life and that the subsequent fall in the WCC is due to reduced ability to produce new neutrophils (Iverson et al., 2010).

5.2.1.1 Genetic Vulnerability

It is not known why relatively few clozapine-treated patients develop neutropenia and even fewer develop agranulocytosis, although obviously genetic factors are important (Opgen-Rhein and Dettling, 2008). By analogy with paclitaxel (Sissung et al., 2006), variation in the expression of ABCB1 (P-glycoprotein, PGP; multiple-drug resistance, MDR1) may be one such factor—clozapine has been identified as a substrate for ABCB1 (Jaquenoud Sirot et al., 2009) and may interfere in the function of ABCC4 (MRP4) (Capannolo et al., 2015). Whether diet (many patients started on clozapine have a notoriously poor diet) or prior exposure to other antipsychotic drugs (almost all such patients will have been tried on other antipsychotics) influences the development of neutropenia/agranulocytosis during clozapine treatment is likewise unknown.

The most reliable genetic evidence as regards clozapine-induced agranulocytosis suggests dysfunction in the HLA system, which is comprised of genes that are important in immune system modulation. This work was prompted by the observed association between Jewish ethnicity and the incidence of carbamazepine-induced agranulocytosis. Genetic studies focused on the HLA complex to distinguish these populations, and indicated that 83% of these patients carried the HLA-B38 biomarker. These findings were even more robust when a haplotype composed of three alleles (HLA-B38, DR4, and DQw3), known to occur frequently in Ashkenazi Jews, was used (Lieberman et al., 1990). More recently, an association between variation in the HLA−DQB1 haplotype and progression to clozapine-induced agranulocytosis has been reported (5.1% risk of developing agranulocytosis if the haplotype is present, Athanasiou et al., 2011). This finding led to the launch of commercial test with a sensitivity of 22% and a specificity of 98% for detecting the haplotype. However, the test gives a 1% (0.05×0.22) chance of identifying patients at risk of developing clozapine-induced agranulocytosis, which is not very different from the risk for all patients given clozapine (0.8%) (Chowdhury et al., 2011; Verbelen et al., 2015).

Recent work has further suggested that clozapine-induced agranulocytosis is associated with several genetic variants involved in the HLA−DQB1 locus (a single amino acid at HLA−DQB1 (126Q) and an amino acid change in the extracellular binding pocket of HLA-B (158T)) (Goldstein et al., 2014). Be this as it may, no reliable genetic test to indicate patients at especial risk from clozapine-induced agranulocytosis currently exists (Verbelen et al., 2015).

5.3 CLINICAL AND LABORATORY FEATURES

Idiosyncratic, drug-induced agranulocytosis is a rare event, with an annual incidence of 2.4−15.4 cases per million (Andrès et al., 2008). The first clinical sign of developing neutropenia/agranulocytosis is likely to be the development of pyrexia associated with infection. Thus investigation of pyrexia in a patient taking a drug which is a recognized cause of neutropenia/agranulocytosis should include measurement of total and differential leukocyte count. Patients, nurses, and other carers should be advised to report pyrexia promptly. Drug-induced neutropenia/agranulocytosis is uncommon and there is at present no way available to detect its occurrence before the decline in blood neutrophils becomes apparent. A high index of suspicion is therefore important including the recognition that drugs may be the cause of the problem (Bhatt and Saleem, 2004; Hall et al., 2003; Oyesanmi et al., 1999; Box 5.3).

It is good practice to measure the leukocyte count and the differential count before starting treatment with a drug that may cause neutropenia so that there is a baseline value in case problems occur later, and leukocyte and neutrophil counts should be monitored during treatment if feasible (Box 5.8). The use of more than one drug known to cause neutropenia at any one time should be avoided if at all possible. Hence, physicians should be wary of coprescription of clozapine, carbamazepine, valproate, proton pump inhibitors, such as omeprazole, and other drugs known to cause neutropenia or agranulocytosis (Lahdelma and Appelberg, 2012; Demler and Trigoboff, 2011; Imbarlina et al., 2004; Philipps et al., 2012; Sedky

---

BOX 5.8 Recognition and Management of Drug-Induced Agranulocytosis

- Recognize that drugs can cause neutropenia/agranulocytosis
  - Patients may lack presenting features (e.g., abscess in the elderly); fever may be only sign of infection
- Ensure normal WCC and differential count before starting treatment
- Monitor WCC and neutrophils during treatment if feasible
  - Monotherapy if possible
- Withdraw drug early if count drops and safe to do so
- Manage any diagnosed condition (e.g., sepsis) aggressively

and Lippmann, 2006). For example, there is a report of patient who developed neutropenia on clozapine and valproate that resolved on withdrawal of valproate (Pantelis and Adesanya, 2001). Patients and carers must be warned to report any new onset of fever/infection to their nurse or physician, since not only may this be the first sign of developing agranulocytosis, but also other conditions such as myocarditis and thermoregulatory disturbances can present in this way (Ronaldson et al., 2010; Kerwin et al., 2004; Fitzsimons et al., 2005).

The most important aspect of managing drug-induced neutropenia/agranulocytosis is early detection and prompt withdrawal of the offending drug if the leukocyte count drops significantly and it is safe to discontinue the drug. In most cases discontinuation will lead to a return to normal neutrophil values. However, since a marked neutropenia may result in life-threatening infection, intravenous empiric broad-spectrum antibacterial and antifungal therapy may be required after blood, urine, and any other relevant samples have been cultured. A fever in a neutropenic patient that should prompt antibiotic use has been defined as a single oral temperature measurement of $\geq 38.5°C$ or a temperature of $\geq 38.0°C$ for ≥ 1 hour. Such empiric treatment is usually continued until the neutropenia and signs of infection have resolved. If a rebound in the neutrophil count is delayed, or if a marked neutropenia with concomitant fever occurs, neutrophil release may be stimulated using G-CSF or GM-CSF (Bhatt and Saleem, 2004; Berliner et al., 2004). Other measures such as reverse barrier nursing may be required. All cases of agranulocytosis should be discussed with a hematologist.

5.3.1   Clozapine-Induced Neutropenia/Agranulocytosis

Clozapine is recognized as a potential cause of neutropenia, which may progress to agranulocytosis (Box 5.9). The mandatory hematological monitoring that is undertaken with clozapine means that more is known about the blood dyscrasia related to this drug than about blood dyscrasia that occur in association with most other drugs. It should be emphasized that (1) neutropenia and agranulocytosis induced by clozapine may have different etiological mechanisms and (2) clozapine can have a range of other effects on blood components including anemia, eosinophilia, leukocytosis, lymphopenia, thrombocytopenia, and thrombocytosis (Herceg et al., 2010). In a 15-year naturalistic retrospective study of clozapine use, hematological side-effects accounted for 45% of all side-effect related clozapine discontinuations and 13% of all discontinuations were related to hematological indices (Davis et al., 2014), highlighting the heavy patient burden associated with these adverse effects. White males in the 40−49 year age range appear to be at higher risk of neutropenia (Demler et al., 2016).

BOX 5.9 Clozapine and Blood Dyscrasia

- Clozapine well known to cause blood dyscrasia
  - Risk of neutropenia 1 in 30 patients
  - Risk of agranulocytosis 1 in 120 patients (1 in 1200 after 1 year)
- Increased risk of eosinophilia (eosinophil count > 0.5 nL^{-1}), especially in women (23%, men 7%)
  - Typically occurs at between 3 and 5 weeks: resolves spontaneously
  - If WCC < 3.5 nL^{-1} monitor for possible agranulocytosis or myocarditis
- May also cause anemia, lymphopenia, leukocytosis, thrombocytopenia
- Genetic factors important, but likely to be dose-related and immunological components as well
  - Risk of neutropenia/agranulocytosis highest at 6−18 weeks
- Likely that neutropenia due to toxic effect on mature neutrophils, while agranulocytosis due to bone marrow toxicity
  - Reversible on stopping (2−3 weeks)
- Proactive hematological monitoring very successful in preventing deaths from agranulocytosis
  - Risk of death estimated at 1 in 10,000 patients (2012)
- Can stimulate neutrophil production (lithium, G-CSF, GM-CSF), but may mask agranulocytosis

---

5.4   PREVENTION AND MANAGEMENT

Reports of agranulocytosis associated with clozapine led to its withdrawal in the 1970s in a number of countries and continue to limit its use (Fitzsimons et al., 2005). The reintroduction of clozapine in the 1980s was accompanied by the requirement for regular FBC monitoring, and if the total leukocyte and/or neutrophil counts indicate the development of neutropenia or agranulocytosis, clear criteria exist for drug withdrawal (Table 5.6) and patient management (Box 5.10). This strategy has largely prevented deaths from this serious adverse reaction—nowadays the reported mortality rate from clozapine-induced agranulocytosis is 0.01−0.03% (Cohen et al., 2012) and the risk of death from clozapine-induced agranulocytosis is estimated at 4 per 100,000 patients per year (Balda et al., 2015).

Blood leukocyte counts must be performed daily in patients in whom clozapine-associated neutropenia is suspected until the condition resolves. Efforts to develop laboratory screening tests designed to differentiate benign and life-threatening neutropenia, including monitoring of endogenous G-CSF concentrations and the use of a hydrocortisone test (Jauss et al., 2000; Murry and Laurent, 2001; Pollmächer et al., 1997), have not come to fruition.

With clozapine-induced agranulocytosis, the mean duration of the fall in WCC was 29 ± 13 days, meaning that for 50% of patients ($N = 68$) the

TABLE 5.6 Blood Dyscrasia: Definitions and Relationship to Clozapine Use in the British Isles

Dyscrasia	Explanation	No of Cells (nL^{-1})		
		Normal Range (BEN)[a]	Caution in Dispensing (BEN)[a]	Advise Stop Clozapine Then Confirm Result[b]
Leukopenia	Deficiency in white blood cells	3.5−11 (3−11)	3−3.5 (2.5−3)	<3.0
Neutropenia	Deficiency in neutrophil granulocytes	2−8 (1.5−7)	1.5−2 (1.0−1.5)	<1.5
Agranulocytosis	Severe deficiency of granular leukocytes (neutrophils, basophils, and eosinophils)	−	−	<0.5
Thrombocytopenia	Deficiency in platelets	130−400	−	<50

[a]*BEN, benign ethnic neutropenia—prescription allowed after hematology review.*
[b]*Prior to Jan. 2003, the limits for leukopenia, neutropenia, and thrombocytopenia were compulsory rather than advisory, necessitating immediate, indefinite cessation of clozapine.*

WCC began to decline ≥ 4 weeks before agranulocytosis developed. In only 6 patients was the fall in WCC of ≤ 2 weeks duration, but 16 had no WCC below 3.5 nL^{-1} within 8 days of the diagnosis of agranulocytosis (Alvir et al., 1995). The time to onset of clozapine-induced agranulocytosis (2−4 months, 96% in the first 6 months of treatment; Alvir et al., 1993) is generally longer than the 2−4 weeks more commonly seen with other drugs (median time to onset of agranulocytosis postinitiation of chlorpromazine 45 days, e.g., Andersohn et al., 2007). Balda et al. (2015) reported that most (83%) of agranulocytoses occurred in the first 3 months of clozapine treatment in the cohort studied. As with most other drug-induced blood dyscrasia, clozapine-induced neutropenia and agranulocytosis are normally fully reversible on withdrawal of the drug, the leukocyte count returning to pretreatment values within 2−3 weeks (Fig. 5.1). Unfortunately, even weekly FBC monitoring does not always identify a developing neutropenia

---

BOX 5.10 Management of Clozapine-Induced Neutropenia/Agranulocytosis

- Stop clozapine immediately if WCC < 3 (<2.5 BEN) and/or neutrophil count < 1.5 (<1.0 BEN) nL^{-1}
- Assess patient's physical state for evidence of (systemic) infection. Symptoms may be minimal
  - Fever (body temperature >38.5°C or >38°C sustained for >1 h)
- Assess for other medications that may be causing/contributing to neutropenia
  - Ask about cocaine use
- Investigations:
  - FBC with differential count
  - Renal and liver function tests; CRP
  - Blood and urine cultures
  - Other investigations as guided by symptoms (e.g., chest X-ray, sputum culture, stool culture)
- Evaluate for autoimmune disease (SLE, RA)
- Evaluate for nutritional deficiency (Vitamin B$_{12}$, folate)
- If evidence of infection (e.g., fever) or if agranulocytosis (neutrophil count < 0.5 nL^{-1})[1] then:
  - Admission to acute hospital necessary
  - No single empirical therapy regimen recommended except for broad-spectrum intravenous antibiotics
  - Liaise with local microbiology department and modify treatment based on nature of infection/sepsis and local patterns of antibiotic resistance
- If prolonged neutropenia and failure to respond to broad-spectrum antibiotics after 3−7 days of appropriate treatment, prompt use of antifungal therapy is indicated
- Consider the use of G-CSF if clinically unstable and agranulocytosis present
- If apyrexial and neutrophil count ≥ 0.5 nL^{-1} at 48 h low-risk and no cause for neutropenia found consider changing to oral antibiotics
- If still pyrexial at 48 h
  - If clinically stable continue with initial antibacterial therapy
  - If clinically unstable antibacterial therapy should be rotated or cover broadened based on clinical assessment

---

1. If both present, then febrile neutropenia.

and give sufficient warning so as to prevent progression to agranulocytosis because, as with other drug-induced neutropenias, the onset can be rapid. If a high temperature or other sign of infection is observed, an FBC should be performed urgently (Box 5.11). Clozapine should be withdrawn as a precautionary measure if the core temperature is >38.5°C until the FBC results are available. The guidance on missed doses is that if clozapine can be restarted in under 48 hours, then dosage may be continued as before. If the period missed

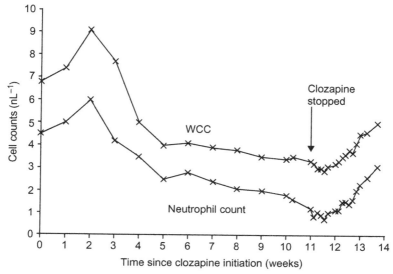

FIGURE 5.1 Plot of WCC and neutrophil counts in a 26-year-old male patient prescribed clozapine (see Box 5.12 for further details).

BOX 5.11 Clozapine: Cautions

- Individual risk factors for neutropenia/agranulocytosis (increasing age, female, etc.) are an inadequate basis on which to make decisions in individual patients
- Need to maintain vigilance especially in first 6–18 weeks
- Do not coprescribe drugs such as carbamazepine that may have similar hematological toxicity
- Warn patients/carers to report to nurse/physician any new onset of fever/infection (or constipation—Chapter 6, Gastrointestinal Hypomotility and Dysphagia)
- Do immediate FBC if high temperature or other signs of infection
- Withdraw clozapine if core temperature > 38.5°C until FBC known
- If clozapine discontinued:
  - <48 h—continue at usual dose
  - >48 h—retitrate
  - >72 h—weekly FBC, 6 weeks

---

is longer than 48 hours, then dose titration should be undertaken as in a clozapine-naïve subject. If the period without clozapine is between 3 days and 4 weeks, then FBC should be monitored weekly for at least 6 weeks on restarting.

BOX 5.12 Clozapine Rechallenge After Neutropenia

- Caucasian male, 26 years, nonsmoker, diagnosis of treatment resistant schizophrenia. Sodium valproate introduced to augment olanzapine. No history of neutropenia. Olanzapine discontinued and clozapine introduced, but developing neutropenia in the absence of infection necessitated clozapine withdrawal at week 11 (Fig. 5.1)
- The patient had shown a good early response to clozapine and for the first time in 2 years was less distressed by psychotic symptoms, most notably there was a diminution in auditory hallucinations and he was able to begin to integrate better with peers and staff. Clozapine dosage before withdrawal was 400 mg per day (plasma clozapine and norclozapine concentrations 0.40 and 0.28 mg L^{-1}, respectively)
- Subsequent to clozapine discontinuation, the neutrophil nadir was 0.7 nL^{-1} and the duration of neutropenia 8 days. The patient was managed conservatively. However, a rebound psychosis occurred, with an intensification of psychotic symptoms at 3 weeks postclozapine and associated behavioral disturbance
- Trials of many antipsychotics failed to alleviate symptoms and he remained in hospital over the next 12 months. Due to the unremitting nature of his symptoms and his marked functional impairment clozapine rechallenge was initiated after a careful risk:benefit analysis, discussions with the patient and his family, and with a hematologist
- Sodium valproate was discontinued prior to clozapine rechallenge. Lithium carbonate was commenced 4 weeks prior to and continued after clozapine initiation. Lithium dosage was titrated to 800 mg per day (serum lithium concentrations 0.6−0.7 mmol L^{-1})
- At week 5 clozapine dosage was 500 mg per day (plasma clozapine and norclozapine 0.45 and 0.31 mg L^{-1}, respectively), but neutropenia occurred and clozapine was discontinued (Fig. 5.4). The next day a neutrophil nadir 0.45 nL^{-1} was recorded and lenograstim 263 µg was given subcutaneously (patient body weight 100 kg)
- The neutrophil count normalized over the next 5 days, but a second neutropenia occurred (neutrophil nadir 0.8 nL^{-1}). The patient was pyrexial (38.1°C), but there was no hemodynamic instability, no evidence of systemic infection, and no focus of infection was identified. Nevertheless, oral antibiotics were prescribed. A second dose of lenograstim (263 µg) led to sustained normalization of the WCC and neutrophil counts. Further clozapine rechallenge was not attempted

5.4.1 Clozapine and White Blood Count Monitoring

If clozapine treatment has been continued for 1 year, the risk of clozapine-induced agranulocytosis is similar to the incidence of this disorder with drugs such as chlorpromazine that are prescribed without monitoring.

Monitoring for neutropenia/agranulocytosis is not mandatory in some countries, China for example (Wang and Li, 2012). Despite these considerations, continued (monthly) WCC monitoring is stipulated in the clozapine product licence in Europe. If patients decide that they no longer wish to be monitored in this way, it can be argued that cessation of monitoring with continued prescription of the drug (and all necessary precautions short of active monitoring) is preferable to stopping the drug since overall mortality is decreased substantially in patients treated with clozapine (Tiihonen et al., 2009; Hayes et al., 2015). Alternatively, the use of capillary (fingerprick) sampling may help persuade a patient to continue to comply with monitoring requirements. The difference between capillary and venous blood samples is mainly in the red cell content. The fingerprick sample must be sent to a laboratory that is capable of providing an accurate full WCC and neutrophil count from the sample or analyzed in an appropriate point-of-care testing device (Bogers et al., 2015).

Once clozapine is being given, blood samples for FBC monitoring are normally taken without regard to the time since the last dose of drug or the time of day. However, there may be a pronounced circadian rhythm in the leukocyte count (Porter and Mohamed, 2006; Esposito et al., 2006). In one such patient the leukocyte results were $2.9-4.2 \, \text{nL}^{-1}$ in the morning and $3.6-7.1 \, \text{nL}^{-1}$ in the afternoon, with granulocytes $0.8-1.4 \, \text{nL}^{-1}$ and $2.9-5.5 \, \text{nL}^{-1}$, respectively (Ahokas and Elonen, 1999). Circadian variations in the number of circulating neutrophils have also been described in several non-Jewish Caucasians (Esposito et al., 2004, 2005a). Clozapine may thus be withdrawn unnecessarily unless account is taken of this phenomenon. The need to measure the WCC in the afternoon if there is concern as to a fall in WCC during clozapine treatment has been emphasized (Esposito et al., 2005b; Esposito, 2007; Porter and Mohamed, 2006). There is also a suggestion that mild/moderate exercise may help raise the WCC (Phillips et al., 2000).

Neutropenia in a patient treated with clozapine could be due to causes other than clozapine (Chaves et al., 2008; Stoner et al., 2008; Igrutinović et al., 2008; Buchanan et al., 2010). The risk of inducing blood dyscrasia by initiating treatment with drugs such as β-lactam antibiotics, metronidazole, or lamotrigine, for example, in patients already being treated with clozapine should not be neglected (Andersohn et al., 2007; Urban et al., 2015). The UK CPMS (Novartis) request an extra FBC measurement when an antibiotic course has been completed, although this is not usually necessary for patients who have weekly blood tests. Any patient treated with antibiotics should be reviewed regularly to ensure there is no deterioration in condition, but this is even more pertinent in patients also receiving clozapine. Clinical staff should be vigilant in looking for signs of infection other than those present initially. If an antibiotic that is associated with a high risk of dyscrasia such as metronidazole is indicated, then closer monitoring involving additional FBC

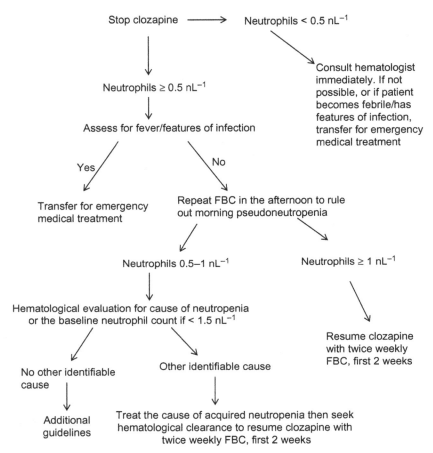

FIGURE 5.2   Use of clozapine in patients with BEN and a decreasing neutrophil count.

measurements will be required. This being said, short courses of antibiotics are unlikely to cause problems, but a 2-week course will require an FBC measurement at the end of weeks 1 and 2.

In the United Kingdom and in some other countries, such as Australia, allowance for BEN when deciding if clozapine treatment can be commenced or continued has been made for some time (Whiskey et al., 2011; Table 5.6; Figs. 5.2 and 5.3). In the United States, monitoring standards have been adapted recently to allow patients with BEN who were previously ineligible for clozapine to be able to receive it (Food and Drug Administration, 2015). Finally, the optimal management of treatment-refractory schizophrenia with clozapine and concurrent malignancy requiring myelosuppressive chemotherapy remains unclear (Barreto et al., 2015; Monga et al., 2015; Usta et al., 2014).

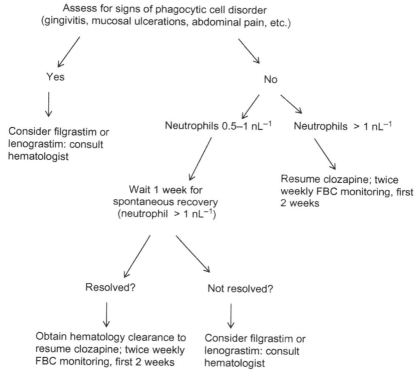

FIGURE 5.3 Use of clozapine in patients with BEN who develop neutropenia (neutrophil count $>0.5 \text{ nL}^{-1}$) and have no evidence of infection.

5.4.1.1 Clozapine Rechallenge

Further treatment with clozapine is contraindicated in a patient who has previously experienced leukopenia or neutropenia during clozapine therapy. However, this presents a dilemma if it is thought that the leukopenia or neutropenia may not have been induced by clozapine (Box 5.12). Furthermore, in some patients the risks of withholding treatment may be greater than the risk of rechallenge, and although overall rechallenge patients are 22 times more likely to develop agranulocytosis than clozapine-naïve subjects, the risk may be justified on occasion (Silvestrini et al., 2000). Bogers (2007) has suggested that bone marrow biopsy would distinguish between benign and malignant granulocytopenia. However, such a procedure is highly invasive and would not be undertaken lightly in clozapine-treated patients.

There are no clear criteria for clozapine rechallenge in the event that clozapine treatment is suspended because of developing neutropenia (Berk et al., 2007), notwithstanding the fact that several examples of successful rechallenge have been reported (Cabral et al., 2007; Bray, 2008; Wu et al., 2008;

Meyer et al., 2015). Dunk et al. (2006) reported outcome data for 53 patients (United Kingdom/Ireland) who were rechallenged with clozapine following leukopenia or neutropenia. Thirty-three (62%) patients were successfully rechallenged, including 1 who had developed agranulocytosis, and 29 were still receiving clozapine at the end of the study. Among those who developed a repeat blood dyscrasia, the event was more severe in 17, lasted longer in 12, and occurred more quickly on rechallenge in 17 than in the first instance. Rechallenge resulted in no deaths, although 9 patients developed agranulocytosis. No alternative possible cause of the blood dyscrasia was identified in 42% of those successfully versus 70% of those unsuccessfully rechallenged. Interestingly, the mean number of weeks of clozapine treatment before the initial blood dyscrasia was greater among those unsuccessfully than successfully rechallenged (82; range 1–470 vs 37; range 2–568 weeks).

In a recent systematic review, clozapine rechallenge was successful in 78/112 patients (70%) after neutropenia, and in 3/15 patients (20%) after agranulocytosis. In patients not rechallenged successfully, neutropenia recurred with a mean of 4.3 (range 0.9–156) weeks. Of 34 patients who failed rechallenge after neutropenia, 15 (44%) developed agranulocytosis during reexposure (Manu et al., 2012). In a further series (19 patients), rechallenge was successful in 15 (79%) (Meyer et al., 2015). Rechallenge after leukopenia, neutropenia, or agranulocytosis on clozapine is a risky enterprise. Careful patient selection is important (Box 5.13). If successful, rechallenge may enable long-term clozapine treatment. For the patient for whom clozapine is a last resort and the only antipsychotic providing

---

BOX 5.13 Clozapine Rechallenge: Summary

- Clozapine contraindicated if patient has had agranulocytosis from clozapine
- Rechallenge if prior leukopenia/neutropenia "off-label": patient selection paramount importance
- Only rechallenge if thought to be nonclozapine cause of dyscrasia (e.g., concurrent infection, valproate)
- Seek advice from hematologist
- If dyscrasia
  - occurred quickly (<18 weeks since clozapine introduced),
  - was severe (agranulocytosis, i.e., neutrophil count < 0.5 nL^{-1}), and
  - was prolonged (>10 days duration) need strong evidence for nonclozapine cause before rechallenge
- If rechallenge attempted suggest FBC taken:
  - Twice weekly, first 12 weeks
  - Weekly, weeks 12–52
  - Fortnightly or monthly, year 2 according to further risk assessment in consultation with hematologist

significantly, even dramatically, improved quality of life, a cautious rechallenge may be justified. If rechallenge is contemplated, the patient, their family, and carers should be apprised of the risks and potential benefit and fully informed consent of patient and family obtained. The patient should be without infection before clozapine is recommenced and the need for any current medication with known association with blood dyscrasia should be evaluated. Twice weekly monitoring of blood count is recommended for the first 3 months to ensure early identification of a fall in neutrophils.

Rechallenge should only be contemplated either if it is thought that clozapine was not the cause of the dyscrasia, that is, there are thought to be alternative explanations apart from clozapine for the first neutropenia/agranulocytosis, such as concurrent medication or infection, or if other treatment options are severely limited or nonexistent. If the dyscrasia (1) occurred quickly (<18 weeks after the initial trial of clozapine), (2) was severe, that is, progressed to agranulocytosis, (3) was prolonged (>10 days duration), or (4) the drop in neutrophils was inconsistent with previous counts and was not merely a transient neutropenia in a patient with a pattern of repeated low WBC counts, then in general strong evidence for a noncloza-pine cause of the problem is required before rechallenge is considered.

5.4.1.2 *Pharmacological Interventions*

5.4.1.2.1 **Lithium**

Lithium causes a leukocytosis, possibly via modulation of granulopoiesis through stem cell stimulation or enhanced production of G-CSF, and also a thrombocytosis. The leukocytosis is a true proliferative response (Blier et al., 1998; Ozdemir et al., 1994; Oyesanmi et al., 1999), with a twofold increase in neutrophil counts seen in lithium treated patients (Ballin et al., 1998) and with a mean increase in the neutrophil count of $2 \, nL^{-1}$ in patients treated with clozapine after the addition of lithium (Small et al., 2003). It is reversible on withdrawing lithium. Lithium-induced dyscrasia have been exploited as in the use of lithium together with cytotoxic agents while treating malignancies and have been studied in the minimization of the hematopoietic toxicity of azidothymidine (AZT). Lithium has also been coprescribed with clozapine in patients with suspected clozapine-induced neutropenia (Boshes et al., 2001), and during clozapine rechallenge with the aim of preventing a second dyscrasia (Whiskey and Taylor, 2007; Box 5.14). However, lithium might not prevent the onset of agranulocytosis with clozapine (Whiskey and Taylor, 2007; Box 5.12, Fig. 5.4) or indeed with chlorpromazine (Yen et al., 1997). The combination of lithium and clozapine may occasionally be associated with reversible neurological adverse effects, usually characterized by ataxia, coarse tremor, and myoclonus (Blake et al., 1992). Further, an increase in the incidence of neuroleptic

BOX 5.14 Clozapine: Use of Lithium and GM-CSF/G-CSF

- Lithium sometimes coprescribed during clozapine treatment/rechallenge: causes reversible leukocytosis
  - Toxic drug: dose used similar to that used as maintenance therapy in bipolar affective disorder (need to maintain serum Li > 0.4 mmol L^{-1})
  - May prevent neutropenia, but does this reduce infection risk (myeloperoxidase inhibitor)?
  - May mask the onset of agranulocytosis, leading to more severe dyscrasia
  - May mask onset of anemia
- If using lithium, start 1−2 weeks beforehand, and add clozapine if WCC has returned to normal range
  - Monitor weekly, 18 weeks and normally thereafter
- GM-CSF & G-CSF (filgrastim, lenograstim) used to treat agranulocytosis after stopping clozapine
  - Patients given G-CSF may have significantly shorter neutrophil recovery time than controls
  - G-CSF to support clozapine therapy may be considered for patients with BEN or who have experienced benign neutropenia or exhibit chronic idiopathic neutropenia (not restricted to those with ethnicity required for BEN)
- G-CSF (e.g., lenograstim 105−263 µg or filgrastim 300 µg) can be prescribed when neutrophil count drops into defined range (e.g., 1.0−1.5 nL^{-1} or 1.5−2 nL^{-1})
- G-CSF support not recommended to support rechallenge after clozapine-induced agranulocytosis

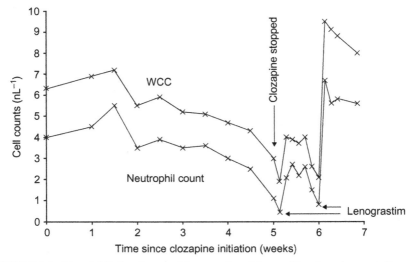

FIGURE 5.4 Plot of WCC and neutrophil counts in a 26-year-old male patient rechallenged with clozapine after developing neutropenia at 11 weeks (see Box 5.12).

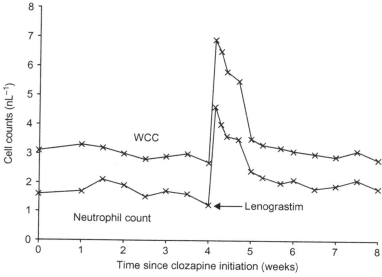

FIGURE 5.5   Plot of neutrophil count against time on clozapine in a patient who had been discontinued from clozapine because of neutropenia. BEN was diagnosed, and after clozapine rechallenge a single dose of lenograstim (105 μg) was used to avoid a second discontinuation. The clozapine dose at 3 weeks was 450 mg per day (plasma clozapine and norclozapine 0.53 and 0.29 mg L^{-1}, respectively). The previous clozapine maintenance dose was 400−500 mg per day.

malignant syndrome when lithium and clozapine are coprescribed has also been reported (Pope et al., 1986) (Fig. 5.5).

Lithium is an inhibitor of myeloperoxidase (Anderson et al., 1982; Gomez-Estrada et al., 1984; Turkozkan et al., 1993), which may explain its protective effect on clozapine-induced neutropenia, at least in part. On the other hand, inhibition of myeloperoxidase may lead to decreased resistance to infection despite an "adequate" neutrophil count.

Lithium has been used to facilitate clozapine initiation in the presence of preexisting neutropenia (Hodgson and Mendis, 2010; Suraweera et al., 2014). In the United States, lithium has been used to increase the WCC, thereby permitting less frequent WCC monitoring in patients with BEN (Papetti et al., 2004; Brunoni et al., 2008; Eseonu and Carlson, 2010; Nykiel et al., 2010; Pinninti et al., 2010). On the other hand, prescribing clozapine to a patient already prescribed lithium results predictably in a leukocytosis (Palominao et al., 2010). Tseng and Hwang (2009) described a patient who developed rhabdomyolysis during treatment with clozapine (500 mg per day) and lithium (1200 mg per day), lithium being used for the control of mania rather than to stimulate neutrophil production. The condition resolved on reducing the clozapine dose to 400 mg per day, together with rehydration.

These considerations notwithstanding, a survey of 25 patients who were rechallenged with clozapine with lithium coprescription has been reported (Kanaan and Kerwin, 2006). Lithium was given shortly before or with clozapine in 12 patients, and after clozapine (median 57 weeks after) in 13. One patient (4%) had a second episode of neutropenia or agranulocytosis (pre-2002 criteria, Table 5.6) after 4 weeks on clozapine, a very low reappearance rate. However, this one patient did show some evidence of masking of the neutropenia by lithium. At follow-up, 17 of 24 patients were still taking clozapine, but not lithium. However, 1 patient had a further episode of neutropenia 4 years after stopping lithium. In a further survey, of 35 patients coprescribed lithium, all but 2 successfully tolerated clozapine rechallenge (Manu et al., 2012). In a recent case series, 15 patients (79%) were successfully rechallenged with clozapine, with 4 of the 5 BEN patients and 8 of the remaining 10 patients receiving lithium. This provides further evidence that lithium has utility in avoiding treatment discontinuation. It is noteworthy, however, that the 4 patients who were unsuccessfully rechallenged were all prescribed lithium, indicating that lithium is not protective against clozapine-induced neutropenia (Meyer et al., 2015). Moreover, lithium does not increase neutrophil counts in all patients and attention should be paid to the possibility that other blood dyscrasia may be masked by giving lithium (Focosi et al., 2009).

In summary, lithium may be useful in increasing the WCC in patients with low baseline counts who would benefit from treatment with clozapine, or in those who develop neutropenia while treated with clozapine. If lithium is to be used prior to clozapine initiation or rechallenge, this should be started 1−2 weeks before clozapine administration, with a minimum serum lithium concentration of 0.4 mmol L^{-1} required to stimulate granulocyte production (Blier et al., 1998; Rothstein et al., 1978). Clozapine should be commenced if and only if the leukocyte count is within the normal range. FBC should be monitored weekly for 18 weeks after rechallenge, and weekly monitoring for up to 1 year should be considered. Lithium may not protect against agranulocytosis, possibly because it has a different etiology to clozapine-induced neutropenia. If the leukocyte count continues to fall despite lithium treatment, consideration should be given to discontinuing clozapine. Particular vigilance is required in patients known to be at high risk of agranulocytosis, notably older adults and those of Asian origin, during the period of highest risk, that is, the first 18 weeks of clozapine treatment.

5.4.1.2.2 G-CSF and GM-CSF

Both G-CSF and GM-CSF stimulate proliferation and differentiation of committed myeloid progenitor cells in the bone marrow (Lieschke and Burgess, 1992). In clozapine-induced agranulocytosis these drugs are usually given in doses of $4-10 \, \mu g \, kg^{-1}$. In supporting clozapine rechallenge, G-CSF has been used prophylactically before a decline in neutrophil counts has occurred that would merit a discontinuation of clozapine treatment (i.e., neutrophil count $<1.5\,nL^{-1}$) or as a continuous treatment to prevent decline in neutrophil counts for people with persistently low neutrophil counts or BEN to prevent clozapine discontinuation (Spencer et al., 2012; Meyer et al., 2015; Joffe et al., 2009; Conus et al., 2001; Rajagopal et al., 2007; Khan et al., 2013; Mathewson and Lindenmayer, 2007). In these cases, filgrastim 300 μg or lenograstim 105 or 263 μg administered subcutaneously has been used.

In one of these cases (Conus et al., 2001), further severe episodes of neutropenia developed after 10, 35, and 48 weeks of clozapine rechallenge. Each episode was treated with a single subcutaneous dose of GM-CSF, permitting clozapine continuation up to a dose of 450 mg per day at week 40. G-CSF has also been administered prophylactically. In one report (Joffe et al., 2009) two patients, who both commenced filgrastim at a dose of more than 0.3 mg per week simultaneously with clozapine rechallenge, were able to continue clozapine despite the onset of granulocytopenia/agranulocytosis, but a patient given a lower dose of filgrastim (<0.3 mg per week) developed agranulocytosis and sepsis. Manu et al. (2012) surveyed 11 cases of rechallenge after neutropenia. Seven patients given weekly doses of G-CSF successfully continued clozapine. Majczenko and Stewart (2008) describe an unsuccessful rechallenge, during which neutrophil counts fell to zero and the patient became febrile despite withholding of clozapine doses and 2 doses of filgrastim (480 μg per day). Although filgrastim was given for a total of 13 consecutive days, the patient's neutrophil count did not rise above zero for 8 days.

Giving clozapine and cytokines together is not without risks. The cytokine could mask a developing agranulocytosis and potentially result in a precipitous drop in neutrophils when the bone marrow becomes exhausted. In addition, there are no treatment options remaining if cytokines have already been used with clozapine and agranulocytosis occurs.

5.4.2   Neutropenic Risk in Clozapine-Treated Children and Adolescents

Clozapine is the drug of choice in very-early-onset schizophrenia in patients who do not respond to other antipsychotics, but, as discussed earlier, a major concern is the incidence of neutropenia/agranulocytosis (Gogtay and Rapoport, 2008). Neutropenia caused by valproate in combination with quetiapine is reported to be more common and severe in children as compared to adults (Rahman et al., 2009), but the evidence for enhanced hematological toxicity of clozapine in children is scant. In a study of 172 patients (mean age at clozapine initiation 15.0 ± 2.1 years), neutropenia (neutrophil count $<1.5\,nL^{-1}$) developed in 23 (13%) patients and agranulocytosis (neutrophil count $<0.5\,nL^{-1}$) in 1 (0.6%) patient (Gerbino-Rosen et al., 2005). Eleven (48%) of 24 patients who developed neutropenia were rechallenged successfully with clozapine. Eight (5%) patients eventually discontinued clozapine (1 because of agranulocytosis, 7 because of neutropenia). Given the relatively small number of patients, the incidence of agranulocytosis did not appear higher than that reported in adults. Similarly, in 26 patients in Korea (mean age 14.3 ± 2.1 years) treated with clozapine for more than 1 year, although 9 (27%) developed neutropenia (neutrophil count <1.5 nL^{-1}), no patient developed agranulocytosis, and all were either maintained (n = 7) on clozapine, or successfully rechallenged (n = 2) with the drug without resort to adjunctive lithium or other measures (Kim et al., 2008).

Successful use of adjunctive lithium has been reported in children who developed neutropenia when treated with clozapine (Sporn et al., 2003; Mattai et al., 2009) or with clozapine in conjunction with aripiprazole (Gagliano and Masi, 2009). However, as in adults lithium does not always raise the neutrophil count. In a 15-year-old boy who did not show a hematological response to lithium, given as a mood stabilizer before clozapine treatment was contemplated, the excessive margination of neutrophils was thought to be a possible explanation for the widely variable, but always low neutrophil count. Blood sampling was at a standardized time of day. Clozapine treatment was successfully implemented in the event, without recourse to either lithium, or G-CSF (Ragonnet et al., 2010). Concomitant treatment with lithium may have further benefit in children as it is can act as a mood-stabilizer (decreased aggression, decreased risk of suicide) (Müller-Oerlinghausen and Lewitzka, 2010), but younger children generally suffer more side-effects than older children and regular serum lithium monitoring is mandatory as with adults (Taylor et al., 2015).

5.4.3 Neutropenia/Agranulocytosis With Antipsychotics Other Than Clozapine

Agranulocytosis associated with other antipsychotics has a much lower incidence compared to that found with clozapine. As noted above, continued vigilance as to the possible occurrence of neutropenia/agranulocytosis with chlorpromazine is required (Stephan et al., 2009; Yen et al., 1997). An incidence of 0.05% has been identified for olanzapine, and 0.01% for risperidone (Stübner et al., 2004). Quetiapine, which is structurally-related to both clozapine and to olanzapine, can also cause neutropenia/agranulocytosis, but does so only rarely despite being prescribed at a higher weight for weight basis than olanzapine (Coşar et al., 2011; Cowan and Oakley, 2007; Croarkin and Rayner, 2001; Tang and Chung, 2014). This is in line with in vitro data (Pessina et al., 2006). Risperidone and ziprasidone, although structurally seemingly unrelated to clozapine, have also been associated with these problems (Montgomery, 2006; Sluys et al., 2004). In one case risperidone was implicated in the prolongation of clozapine-associated agranulocytosis (Manfredi et al., 2013). There are three case reports describing the development of neutropenia in patients treated with aripiprazole in combination with other second-generation antipsychotics (Lander and Bastiamphillai, 2011; Lim et al., 2013; Plesnicar and Plesnicar, 2008).

Oxidative metabolism of olanzapine also gives rise to a nitrenium ion and this may be the mechanism behind reports of olanzapine-induced leukopenia and neutropenia. However, as olanzapine is considerably more potent than clozapine, therapeutic doses of olanzapine are typically more than 10-fold less than those for clozapine, meaning a lower exposure to nitrenium ions formed from olanzapine (Benedetti et al., 1999; Cordes et al., 2004; Duggal et al., 2004; Stergiou et al., 2005; Stip et al., 2007; Thinn et al., 2007). This lower exposure is insufficient to offset the threefold greater myelotoxicity of olanzapine found in an in vitro study of granulocyte-macrophage progenitors (the actual results (IC90, mg L^{-1}) were: chlorpromazine (10.02 ± 0.69), olanzapine (13.43 ± 1.23), clozapine (44.71 ± 4.42), and quetiapine (137.24 ± 15.36)) (Pessina et al., 2006).

As noted above, it is thought that formation of a nitrenium cation is the initial step in the hematological toxicity of both clozapine and olanzapine (Sikora et al., 2007; Jagadheesan and Mehrtens, 2007), although one report has suggested that unactivated clozapine and to an extent norclozapine may themselves exert toxic effects on bone marrow stroma cells (Lahdelma et al., 2010). The major pathways of olanzapine metabolism include N-glucuronidation mediated by UDP-glucuronosyltransferase (UGT) 1A4 and N-demethylation, the latter catalyzed by cytochrome P450 (CYP) 1A2. CYP1A2 is subject to reversible and/or irreversible inhibition by a number of drugs and other substances, and is induced by cigarette smoking (Zhou et al., 2010). Minor pathways of olanzapine metabolism include N-oxidation and 2-hydroxylation, catalyzed by CYP2D6. Direct N-glucuronidation does not occur with clozapine, and N-desmethylolanzapine does not accumulate in plasma to the same extent as norclozapine, both factors that may help limit exposure to potentially toxic olanzapine species as compared with the situation with clozapine.

There are reports of prolongation of clozapine-induced neutropenia with olanzapine (Sayin and Cosar, 2006; Coşar et al., 2011), including that of a patient who had been treated with olanzapine (30 mg per day) with no ill effect before developing neutropenia when switched to clozapine. On withdrawal of clozapine he was again given olanzapine, but this time developed neutropenia during the third week of treatment. The WCC rose to normal on withdrawal of olanzapine (Thangadurai et al., 2006). On rare occasions patients are encountered who develop neutropenia on a range of different antipsychotics (Coşar et al., 2011). In one, challenge with fluphenazine, olanzapine, flupentixol, haloperidol, and paliperidone led to nadir neutrophil counts of 0.2 nL^{-1} with flupentixol, 0.4 nL^{-1} with paliperidone, and 0.5 nL^{-1} with olanzapine (Vila-Rodriguez et al., 2013). The patient was eventually maintained on paliperidone at the lowest effective dose (period of follow-up not given). Continued antipsychotic prescription was felt merited given the benign clinical picture associated with the neutropenia and the lack of an identified HLA genotype associated with autoimmune agranulocytosis. Neutropenia (nadir $1.1 \, nL^{-1}$) brought on by quetiapine (up to 600 mg per day) accompanied by thrombocytopenia (nadir $146 \, nL^{-1}$) has been described (Shankar, 2007). In a further patient, neutropenia (nadir $1.4 \, nL^{-1}$) became apparent on day 7 of quetiapine treatment (400 mg per day), but recovered to $2.5 \, nL^{-1}$ 5 days after stopping the drug (Yalcin et al., 2008). Subsequent treatment with amisulpride (400 mg per day for 2 days) was accompanied by a neutrophil count of $1.8 \, nL^{-1}$ and amisulpride was stopped as well—this seems unlikely to be an effect of this latter drug since exposure was very brief. Subsequent treatment with aripiprazole (20 mg per day) was accompanied by an increased neutrophil count (to $3.3 \, nL^{-1}$) after 5 weeks. A favorable response to aripiprazole was also obtained in three patients in whom clozapine had to be discontinued due to developing neutropenia (Hughes and Morcos, 2008).

There are few reports of blood dyscrasia clearly associated with either amisulpride or sulpiride (Coşar et al., 2011), with no cases of agranulocytosis reported. Alone among commonly-used antipsychotics, amisulpride and sulpiride are largely excreted unchanged. If metabolic activation of the drug is the first step in the sequence of events leading to neutropenia, prescription of amisulpride or sulpiride may be alternatives for those with a history of blood dyscrasia. Some support for this hypothesis also comes from an evaluation of peripheral blood smears of patients taking a range of antipsychotics. Of the drugs studied (flupentixol, fluphenazine, haloperidol, thioridazine, trifluoperazine, olanzapine, risperidone, and sulpiride), fluphenazine and sulpiride had by far the smallest effect on mean nuclear lobularity, a measure of neutrophil immaturity. Total leukocyte and neutrophil counts in patients and controls were not significantly different (Delieu et al., 2001, 2006).

5.4.4   Blood Dyscrasia Other Than Neutropenia Associated With Antipsychotics

In addition to the transient leukocytosis that occurs commonly with clozapine (Fig. 5.1), neutrophilia, eosinophilia, thrombocytosis, anemia, lymphopenia, and thrombocytopenia have all been reported with this drug (Pirmohamed and Park, 1997; Box 5.9). Anemia has been identified in 25% of patients given clozapine over the first 2 years of treatment (Lee et al., 2015). The occurrence of a transient leukocytosis (Fig. 5.1) was reported in 41% of clozapine-treated patients (Hummer et al., 1994). Others have reported the incidence of transient leukocytosis to range from 0.6% to 7.7% (Lieberman et al., 1989; Lambertenghi Deliliers, 2000).

Variable rates of eosinophilia ranging from 2% to 62% (Banov et al., 1993; Chatterton, 1997; Lambertenghi Deliliers, 2000; Hummer et al., 1994) have been identified with clozapine treatment. There is an increased risk of eosinophilia (eosinophil count $> 0.7 \, nL^{-1}$), especially in women (23%, men 7%), associated with the use of clozapine (Banov et al., 1993). Typically this occurs after 3−5 weeks of treatment and resolves spontaneously (Hummer et al., 1994). There is concern that, on rare occasions, eosinophilia may be associated with myocarditis (Kortner et al., 2007). The recommendation is to consider stopping clozapine if the eosinophil count is >3 nL^{-1}, and not to restart clozapine until the eosinophil count is <1 nL^{-1} (Chatterton, 1997).

REFERENCES

Ahn, Y.M., Jeong, S.H., Jang, H.S., Koo, Y.J., Kang, U.G., Lee, K.Y., et al., 2004. Experience of maintaining clozapine medication in patients with 'red-alert zone' neutropenia: long-term follow-up results. Int. Clin. Psychopharmacol. 19, 97−101.

Ahokas, A., Elonen, E., 1999. Circadian rhythm of white blood cells during clozapine treatment. Psychopharmacology (Berl.) 144, 301−302.

Alvir, J.M., Lieberman, J.A., Safferman, A.Z., Schwimmer, J.L., Schaaf, J.A., 1993. Clozapine-induced agranulocytosis. Incidence and risk factors in the United States. N. Engl. J. Med. 329, 162−167.

Alvir, J.M., Lieberman, J.A., Safferman, A.Z., 1995. Do white-cell count spikes predict agranulocytosis in clozapine recipients? Psychopharmacol. Bull. 31, 311−314.

Andersohn, F., Konzen, C., Garbe, E., 2007. Systematic review: agranulocytosis induced by nonchemotherapy drugs. Ann. Intern. Med. 146, 657−665.

Anderson, R., Walters, L., Grabow, G., van der Merwe, M., van Rensburg, C.E., 1982. The effects of lithium on the functions of human neutrophils and lymphocytes in vitro and in vivo. S. Afr. Med. J. 62, 519−523.

Andrès, E., Noel, E., Kurtz, J.E., Henoun Loukili, N., Kaltenbach, G., Maloisel, F., 2004. Life-threatening idiosyncratic drug-induced agranulocytosis in elderly patients. Drugs Aging 21, 427−435.

Andrès, E., Federici, L., Weitten, T., Vogel, T., Alt, M., 2008. Recognition and management of drug-induced blood cytopenias: the example of drug-induced acute neutropenia and agranulocytosis. Expert Opin. Drug Saf. 7, 481−489.

Andrès, E., Zimmer, J., Mecili, M., Weitten, T., Alt, M., Maloisel, F., 2011. Clinical presentation and management of drug-induced agranulocytosis. Expert Rev. Hematol. 4, 143−151.

Athanasiou, M.C., Dettling, M., Cascorbi, I., Mosyagin, I., Salisbury, B.A., Pierz, K.A., et al., 2011. Candidate gene analysis identifies a polymorphism in HLA-DQB1 associated with clozapine-induced agranulocytosis. J. Clin. Psychiatry 72, 458−463.

Atkin, K., Kendall, F., Gould, D., Freeman, H., Lieberman, J., O'Sullivan, D., 1996. Neutropenia and agranulocytosis in patients receiving clozapine in the UK and Ireland. Br. J. Psychiatry 169, 483−488.

Balda, M.V., Garay, O.U., Papale, R.M., Bignone, I., Bologna, V.G., Brandolini, A., et al., 2015. Clozapine-associated neutropenia and agranulocytosis in Argentina (2007−2012). Int. Clin. Psychopharmacol. 30, 109−114.

Ballin, A., Lehman, D., Sirota, P., Litvinjuk, U., Meytes, D., 1998. Increased number of peripheral blood CD34 + cells in lithium-treated patients. Br. J. Haematol. 100, 219−221.

Banov, M.D., Tohen, M., Friedberg, J., 1993. High risk of eosinophilia in women treated with clozapine. J. Clin. Psychiatry 54, 466−469.

Barreto, J.N., Leung, J.G., Philbrick, K.L., Rasmussen, K.G., Thompson, C.A., 2015. Clozapine therapy throughout myelosuppressive chemotherapy: regulations without standardization. Psychooncology 24, 1581−1585.

Benedetti, F., Cavallaro, R., Smeraldi, E., 1999. Olanzapine-induced neutropenia after clozapine-induced neutropenia. Lancet 354, 567.

Berk, M., Fitzsimons, J., Lambert, T., Pantelis, C., Kulkarni, J., Castle, D., et al., 2007. Monitoring the safe use of clozapine: a consensus view from Victoria, Australia. CNS Drugs 21, 117–127.

Berliner, N., Horwitz, M., Loughran, T.P., 2004. Congenital and acquired neutropenia. Hematology Am. Soc. Hematol. Educ. Program 63–79.

Bhatt, V., Saleem, A., 2004. Review: drug-induced neutropenia—pathophysiology, clinical features, and management. Ann. Clin. Lab. Sci. 34, 131–137.

Blake, L.M., Marks, R.C., Luchins, D.J., 1992. Reversible neurologic symptoms with clozapine and lithium. J. Clin. Psychopharmacol. 12, 297–299.

Blier, P., Slater, S., Measham, T., Koch, M., Wiviott, G., 1998. Lithium and clozapine-induced neutropenia/agranulocytosis. Int. Clin. Psychopharmacol. 13, 137–140.

Bogers, J.P., 2007. Granulocytopenia while using clozapine: continuing or stopping treatment. Tijdschr. Psychiatr. 49, 575–579.

Bogers, J.P., Bui, H., Herruer, M., Cohen, D., 2015. Capillary compared to venous blood sampling in clozapine treatment: patients' and healthcare practitioners' experiences with a point-of-care device. Eur. Neuropsychopharmacol. 25, 319–324.

Boshes, R.A., Manschreck, T.C., Desrosiers, J., Candela, S., Hanrahan-Boshes, M., 2001. Initiation of clozapine therapy in a patient with preexisting leucopenia: a discussion of the rationale of current treatment options. Ann. Clin. Psychiatry 13, 233–237, Erratum 14: 141.

Bray, A., 2008. Ethnic neutropenia and clozapine. Aust. N. Z. J. Psychiatry 42, 342–345.

Brunoni, A.R., Kobuti Ferreira, L.R., Gallucci-Neto, J., Elkis, H., Velloso, E.D., Vinicius Zanetti, M., 2008. Lithium as a treatment of clozapine-induced neutropenia: a case report. Prog. Neuropsychopharmacol. Biol. Psychiatry 32, 2006–2007.

Buchanan, J.A., Oyer, R.J., Patel, N.R., Jacquet, G.A., Bornikova, L., Thienelt, C., et al., 2010. A confirmed case of agranulocytosis after use of cocaine contaminated with levamisole. J. Med. Toxicol. 6, 160–164.

Burckart, G.J., Snidow, J., Bruce, W., 1981. Neutropenia following acute chlorpromazine ingestion. Clin. Toxicol. 18, 797–801.

Cabral, C.G., de Castro, M., das Neves, L., Nicolato, R., Lauar, H., Salgado, J.V., 2007. Hematological alterations associated to olanzapine use after clozapine-induced neutropenia. Rev. Bras. Psiquiatr. 29, 93.

Capannolo, M., Fasciani, I., Romeo, S., Aloisi, G., Rossi, M., Bellio, P., et al., 2015. The atypical antipsychotic clozapine selectively inhibits interleukin 8 (IL-8)-induced neutrophil chemotaxis. Eur. Neuropsychopharmacol. 25, 413–424.

Centorrino, F., Baldessarini, R.J., Flood, J.G., Kando, J.C., Frankenburg, F.R., 1995. Relation of leukocyte counts during clozapine treatment to serum concentrations of clozapine and metabolites. Am. J. Psychiatry 152, 610–612.

Chatterton, R., 1997. Eosinophilia after commencement of clozapine treatment. Aust. N. Z. J. Psychiatry 31, 874–876.

Chaves, A.C., Yamauti, A.C., Timerman, N.J., 2008. Leucopenia and neutropenia secondary to a lymphoma in a patient exposed to several antipsychotics. Prog. Neuropsychopharmacol. Biol. Psychiatry 32, 901–902.

Chigaev, A., Winter, S.S., Sklar, L.A., 2011. Is prolonged stem cell mobilization detrimental for hematopoiesis? Med. Hypotheses 77, 1111–1113.

Chowdhury, N.I., Remington, G., Kennedy, J.L., 2011. Genetics of antipsychotic-induced side effects and agranulocytosis. Curr. Psychiatry Rep. 13, 156–165.

Cohen, D., Monden, M., 2013. White blood cell monitoring during long-term clozapine treatment. Am. J. Psychiatry 170, 366–369.

Cohen, D., Bogers, J.P., van Dijk, D., Bakker, B., Schulte, P.F., 2012. Beyond white blood cell monitoring: screening in the initial phase of clozapine therapy. J. Clin. Psychiatry 73, 1307–1312.

Conus, P., Nanzer, N., Baumann, P., 2001. An alternative to interruption of treatment in recurrent clozapine-induced severe neutropenia. Br. J. Psychiatry 179, 180.

Cordes, J., Streit, M., Loeffler, S., von Wilmsdorff, M., Agelink, M., Klimke, A., 2004. Reversible neutropenia during treatment with olanzapine: three case reports. World J. Biol. Psychiatry 5, 230–234.

Coşar, B., Taner, M.E., Eser, H.Y., Altınöz, A.E., Tarhan, R., 2011. Does switching to another antipsychotic in patients with clozapine-associated granulocytopenia solve the problem? Case series of 18 patients. J. Clin. Psychopharmacol. 31, 169–173.

Cowan, C., Oakley, C., 2007. Leucopenia and neutropenia induced by quetiapine. Prog. Neuropsychopharmacol. Biol. Psychiatry 31, 292–294.

Croarkin, P., Rayner, T., 2001. Acute neutropenia in a patient treated with quetiapine. Psychosomatics 42, 368.

Curtis, B.R., 2014. Drug-induced immune neutropenia/agranulocytosis. Immunohematology 30, 95–101.

Davis, M.C., Fuller, M.A., Strauss, M.E., Konicki, P.E., Jaskiw, G.E., 2014. Discontinuation of clozapine: a 15-year naturalistic retrospective study of 320 patients. Acta Psychiatr. Scand. 130, 30–39.

Deavall, D.G., Martin, E.A., Horner, J.M., Roberts, R., 2012. Drug-induced oxidative stress and toxicity. J. Toxicol. 2012, 645460.

Delieu, J.M., Badawoud, M., Williams, M.A., Horobin, R.W., Duguid, J.K., 2001. Antipsychotic drugs result in the formation of immature neutrophil leucocytes in schizophrenic patients. J. Psychopharmacol. 15, 191–194.

Delieu, J.M., Horobin, R.W., Duguid, J.K., 2006. Formation of immature neutrophil leucocytes in schizophrenic patients treated with various antipsychotic drugs: comparisons and predictions. J. Psychopharmacol. 20, 824–828.

Delieu, J.M., Horobin, R.W., Duguid, J.K., 2009. Exploring the relationship of drug-induced neutrophil immaturity & haematological toxicity to drug chemistry using quantitative structure-activity models. Med. Chem. 5, 7–14.

Demler, T.L., Trigoboff, E., 2011. Are clozapine blood dyscrasias associated with concomitant medications? Innov. Clin. Neurosci. 8, 35–41.

Demler, T.L., Morabito, N.E., Meyer, C.E., Opler, L., 2016. Maximizing clozapine utilization while minimizing blood dyscrasias: evaluation of patient demographics and severity of events. Int. Clin. Psychopharmacol. 31 (2), 76–83.

Dettling, M., Sachse, C., Muller-Oerlinghausen, B., Roots, I., Brockmoller, J., Rolfs, A., et al., 2000. Clozapine-induced agranulocytosis and hereditary polymorphisms of clozapine metabolizing enzymes: no association with myeloperoxidase and cytochrome $P_{450}2D6$. Pharmacopsychiatry 33, 218–220.

Dietrich-Muszalska, A., Olas, B., 2009. The changes of aggregability of blood platelets in schizophrenia. World J. Biol. Psychiatry 10, 171–176.

Duggal, H.S., Singh, I., 2005. Psychotropic drug-induced neutropenia. Drugs Today (Barc.) 41, 517–526.

Duggal, H.S., Gates, C., Pathak, P.C., 2004. Olanzapine-induced neutropenia: mechanism and treatment. J. Clin. Psychopharmacol. 24, 234–235.

Dunk, L.R., Annan, L.J., Andrews, C.D., 2006. Rechallenge with clozapine following leucopenia or neutropenia during previous therapy. Br. J. Psychiatry 188, 255–263.

Eseonu, C., Carlson, J., 2010. Clozapine rechallenge in refractory schizophrenia. Am. J. Psychiatry 167, 602–603.

Esposito, D., 2007. Comment on "lithium and clozapine rechallenge: a retrospective case analysis". J. Clin. Psychiatry 68, 635, author reply 635.

Esposito, D., Aouillé, J., Rouillon, F., Limosin, F., 2004. Two year follow-up of a patient with successful continuation of clozapine treatment despite morning pseudoneutropenia. J. Clin. Psychiatry 65, 1281.

Esposito, D., Corruble, E., Hardy, P., Chouinard, G., 2005a. Risperidone-induced morning pseudoneutropenia. Am. J. Psychiatry 162, 397.

Esposito, D., Rouillon, F., Limosin, F., 2005b. Continuing clozapine treatment despite neutropenia. Eur. J. Clin. Pharmacol. 60, 759–764.

Esposito, D., Chouinard, G., Hardy, P., Corruble, E., 2006. Successful initiation of clozapine treatment despite morning pseudoneutropenia. Int. J. Neuropsychopharmacol. 9, 489–491.

Fehsel, K., Loeffler, S., Krieger, K., Henning, U., Agelink, M., Kolb-Bachofen, V., et al., 2005. Clozapine induces oxidative stress and proapoptotic gene expression in neutrophils of schizophrenic patients. J. Clin. Psychopharmacol. 25, 419–426.

Fitzsimons, J., Berk, M., Lambert, T., Bourin, M., Dodd, S., 2005. A review of clozapine safety. Expert Opin. Drug Saf. 4, 731–744.

Focosi, D., Azzarà, A., Kast, R.E., Carulli, G., Petrini, M., 2009. Lithium and hematology: established and proposed uses. J. Leukocyte Biol. 85, 20–28.

Food and Drug Administration, 2015. Drug Safety Communication: FDA modifies monitoring for neutropenia associated with schizophrenia medicine clozapine; approves new shared REMS program for all clozapine medicines. <http://www.fda.gov/Drugs/DrugSafety/ucm461853.htm> (accessed 15.10.15.).

Gagliano, A., Masi, G., 2009. Clozapine-aripiprazole association in a 7-year-old girl with schizophrenia: clinical efficacy and successful management of neutropenia with lithium. J. Child Adolesc. Psychopharmacol. 19, 595–598.

Garbe, E., 2007. Non-chemotherapy drug-induced agranulocytosis. Expert Opin. Drug Saf. 6, 323–335.

Gardner, I., Popovic, M., Zahid, N., Uetrecht, J.P., 2005. A comparison of the covalent binding of clozapine, procainamide, and vesnarinone to human neutrophils in vitro and rat tissues in vitro and in vivo. Chem. Res. Toxicol. 18, 1384–1394.

Gerbino-Rosen, G., Roofeh, D., Tompkins, D.A., Feryo, D., Nusser, L., Kranzler, H., et al., 2005. Hematological adverse events in clozapine-treated children and adolescents. J. Am. Acad. Child Adolesc. Psychiatry 44, 1024–1031.

Gillman, K., 2000. Paradoxical pattern of haematological risk with clozapine. Br. J. Psychiatry 177, 88.

Gogtay, N., Rapoport, J., 2008. Clozapine use in children and adolescents. Expert Opin. Pharmacother. 9, 459–465.

Goldstein, J.I., Jarskog, L.F., Hilliard, C., Alfirevic, A., Duncan, L., Fourches, D., et al., 2014. Clozapine-induced agranulocytosis is associated with rare HLA-DQB1 and HLA-B alleles. Nat. Commun. 5, 4757.

Gomez-Estrada, H., Hernandez-Delgado, J., Diaz-Esquivel, P., 1984. Decreased myeloperoxidase activity of mice polymorphonuclear leukocytes by lithium carbonate treatment. Arch. Invest. Med. (Mex.) 15, 287–291.

Haddy, T.B., Rana, S.R., Castro, O., 1999. Benign ethnic neutropenia: what is a normal absolute neutrophil count? J. Lab. Clin. Med. 133, 15−22.

Hall, R.L., Smith, A.G., Edwards, J.G., 2003. Haematological safety of antipsychotic drugs. Expert Opin. Drug Saf. 2, 395−399.

Hasegawa, M., Cola, P.A., Meltzer, H.Y., 1994. Plasma clozapine and desmethylclozapine levels in clozapine-induced agranulocytosis. Neuropsychopharmacology 11, 45−47.

Hayes, R.D., Downs, J., Chang, C.K., Jackson, R.G., Shetty, H., Broadbent, M., et al., 2015. The effect of clozapine on premature mortality: an assessment of clinical monitoring and other potential confounders. Schizophr. Bull. 41, 644−655.

Herceg, M., Mužinić, L., Jukić, V., 2010. Can we prevent blood dyscrasia (leucopenia, thrombocytopenia) and epileptic seizures induced by clozapine. Psychiatr. Danub. 22, 85−89.

Hodgson, R.E., Mendis, S., 2010. Lithium enabling use of clozapine in a patient with pre-existing neutropenia. Br. J. Hosp. Med. (Lond.) 71, 535.

Hsuanyu, Y., Dunford, H.B., 1999. Oxidation of clozapine and ascorbate by myeloperoxidase. Arch. Biochem. Biophys. 368, 413−420.

Hughes, D., Morcos, M., 2008. Use of aripiprazole in treatment resistant schizophrenia. J. Psychopharmacol. 22, 927−928.

Hummer, M., Kurz, M., Barnas, C., Saria, A., Fleischhacker, W.W., 1994. Clozapine-induced transient white blood count disorders. J. Clin. Psychiatry 55, 429−432.

Husain, Z., Almeciga, I., Delgado, J.C., Clavijo, O.P., Castro, J.E., Belalcazar, V., et al., 2006. Increased FasL expression correlates with apoptotic changes in granulocytes cultured with oxidized clozapine. Toxicol. Appl. Pharmacol. 214, 326−334.

Igrutinović, Z., Obradović, S., Vuletić, B., Marković, S., 2008. Impact of valproates on haemostasis and blood cell count in children. Srp. Arh. Celok. Lek. 136, 267−273.

Imbarlina, M.J., Sarkar, S., Marwah, S., Parepally, H., Johnston, P.R., Brar, J.S., et al., 2004. Leucopenia in clozapine treated patients may be induced by other drugs: a case series. Eur. Psychiatry 19, 506−509.

Iverson, S., Kautiainen, A., Ip, J., Uetrecht, J.P., 2010. Effect of clozapine on neutrophil kinetics in rabbits. Chem. Res. Toxicol. 23, 1184−1191.

Jagadheesan, K., Mehrtens, J., 2007. Prolongation of clozapine-induced neutropenia with olanzapine. Aust. N. Z. J. Psychiatry 41, 192.

Jaquenoud Sirot, E., Knezevic, B., Morena, G.P., Harenberg, S., Oneda, B., Crettol, S., et al., 2009. ABCB1 and cytochrome P450 polymorphisms: clinical pharmacogenetics of clozapine. J. Clin. Psychopharmacol. 29, 319−326.

Jauss, M., Pantel, J., Werle, E., Schroder, J., 2000. G-CSF plasma levels in clozapine-induced neutropenia. Biol. Psychiatry 48, 1113−1115.

Joffe, G., Eskelinen, S., Sailas, E., 2009. Add-on filgrastim during clozapine rechallenge in patients with a history of clozapine-related granulocytopenia/agranulocytosis. Am. J. Psychiatry 166, 236.

Kanaan, R.A., Kerwin, R.W., 2006. Lithium and clozapine rechallenge: a retrospective case analysis. J. Clin. Psychiatry 67, 756−760.

Kelly, D.L., Kreyenbuhl, J., Dixon, L., Love, R.C., Medoff, D., Conley, R.R., 2007. Clozapine underutilization and discontinuation in African Americans due to leucopenia. Schizophr. Bull. 33, 1221−1224.

Kerwin, R.W., Osborne, S., Sainz-Fuertes, R., 2004. Heat stroke in schizophrenia during clozapine treatment: rapid recognition and management. J. Psychopharmacol. 18, 121−123.

Khan, A.A., Harvey, J., Sengupta, S., 2013. Continuing clozapine with granulocyte colony-stimulating factor in patients with neutropenia. Ther. Adv. Psychopharmacol. 3, 266−271.

Kim, Y., Kim, B.N., Cho, S.C., Kim, J.W., Shin, M.S., 2008. Long-term sustained benefits of clozapine treatment in refractory early onset schizophrenia: a retrospective study in Korean children and adolescents. Hum. Psychopharmacol. Clin. Exp. 23, 715−722.

King, D.J., Wager, E., 1998. Haematological safety of antipsychotic drugs. J. Psychopharmacol. 12, 283−288.

Kortner, K., Neuhaus, A.H., Schurer, F., Dettling, M., 2007. Eosinophilia indicating subclinical clozapine-induced pericarditis. J Clin Psychiatry 68, 1147−1148.

Lahdelma, L., Appelberg, B., 2012. Clozapine-induced agranulocytosis in Finland, 1982−2007: long-term monitoring of patients is still warranted. J. Clin. Psychiatry 73, 837−842.

Lahdelma, L., Oja, S., Korhonen, M., Andersson, L.C., 2010. Clozapine is cytotoxic to primary cultures of human bone marrow mesenchymal stromal cells. J. Clin. Psychopharmacol. 30, 461−463.

Lambertenghi Deliliers, G., 2000. Blood dyscrasias in clozapine-treated patients in Italy. Haematologica 85, 233−237.

Lander, M., Bastiamphillai, T., 2011. Neutropenia associated with quetiapine, olanzapine, and aripiprazole. Aust. N. Z. J. Psychiatry 45, 89.

Lee, J., Takeuchi, H., Fervaha, G., Powell, V., Bhaloo, A., Bies, R., et al., 2015. The effect of clozapine on hematological indices: a 1-year follow-up study. J. Clin. Psychopharmacol. 35, 510−516.

Levin, G.M., DeVane, C.L., 1992. A review of cyclic antidepressant-induced blood dyscrasias. Ann. Pharmacother. 26, 378−383.

Lieberman, J.A., Kane, J.M., Johns, C.A., 1989. Clozapine: guidelines for clinical management. J. Clin. Psychiatry 50, 329−338.

Lieberman, J.A., Yunis, J., Egea, E., Canoso, R.T., Kane, J.M., Yunis, E.J., 1990. HLA-B38, DR4, DQw3 and clozapine-induced agranulocytosis in Jewish patients with schizophrenia. Arch. Gen. Psychiatry 47, 945−948.

Lieschke, G.J., Burgess, A.W., 1992. Granulocyte colony-stimulating factor and granulocyte-macrophage colony-stimulating factor. N. Engl. J. Med. 327, 28−35.

Lim, M.H., Park, J.I., Park, T.W., 2013. A case report with neutropenia related with the use of various atypical antipsychotics. Psychiatr. Investig. 10, 428−431.

Majczenko, T.G., Stewart, J.T., 2008. Failure of filgrastim to prevent severe clozapine-induced agranulocytosis. South Med. J. 101, 639−640.

Manfredi, G., Solfanelli, A., Dimitri, G., Cuomo, I., Sani, G., Kotzalidis, G.D., et al., 2013. Risperidone-induced leukopenia: a case report and brief review of literature. Gen. Hosp. Psychiatry 35, 102. e3-6.

Manu, P., Sarpal, D., Muir, O., Kane, J.M., Correll, C.U., 2012. When can patients with potentially life-threatening adverse effects be rechallenged with clozapine? A systematic review of the published literature. Schizophr. Res. 134, 180−186.

Mathewson, K.A., Lindenmayer, J.P., 2007. Clozapine and granulocyte colony-stimulating factor: potential for long-term combination treatment for clozapine-induced neutropenia. J. Clin. Psychopharmacol. 27, 714−715.

Mattai, A., Fung, L., Bakalar, J., Overman, G., Tossell, J., Miller, R., et al., 2009. Adjunctive use of lithium carbonate for the management of neutropenia in clozapine-treated children. Hum. Psychopharmacol. 24, 584−589.

Meged, S., Stein, D., Sitrota, P., Melamed, Y., Elizur, A., Shmuelian, I., et al., 1999. Human leucocyte antigen typing, response to neuroleptics, and clozapine-induced agranulocytosis in Jewish Israeli schizophrenic patients. Int. Clin. Psychopharmacol. 14, 305−312.

Meyer, N., Gee, S., Whiskey, E., Taylor, D., Mijovic, A., Gaughran, F., et al., 2015. Optimizing outcomes in clozapine rechallenge following neutropenia: a cohort analysis. J. Clin. Psychiatry 76, 1410–1416.

Mintzer, D.M., Billet, S.N., Chmielewski, L., 2009. Drug-induced hematologic syndromes. Adv. Hematol. 2009, 495863.

Monga, V., Broucek, M., Amani, M., Ramaswamy, S., 2015. Clozapine and concomitant chemotherapy in a patient with schizophrenia and new onset esophageal cancer. Psychooncology 24, 971–972.

Montgomery, J., 2006. Ziprasidone-related agranulocytosis following olanzapine-induced neutropenia. Gen. Hosp. Psychiatry 28, 83–85.

Mosyagin, I., Dettling, M., Roots, I., Mueller-Oerlinghausen, B., Cascorbi, I., 2004. Impact of myeloperoxidase and NADPH-oxidase polymorphisms in drug-induced agranulocytosis. J. Clin. Psychopharmacol. 24, 613–617.

Müller-Oerlinghausen, B., Lewitzka, U., 2010. Lithium reduces pathological aggression and suicidality: a mini-review. Neuropsychobiology 62, 43–49.

Munro, J., O'Sullivan, D., Andrews, C., Arana, A., Mortimer, A., Kerwin, R., 1999. Active monitoring of 12,760 clozapine recipients in the UK and Ireland. Beyond pharmacovigilance. Br. J. Psychiatry 175, 576–580.

Murry, P., Laurent, A., 2001. Is it possible to distinguish between benign and malignant neutropenia in clozapine-treated patients by means of a hydrocortisone test? Psychopharmacology (Berl.) 158, 329–330.

Nielsen, J., Young, C., Ifteni, P., Kishimoto, T., Xiang, Y.T., Schulte, P.F., et al., 2016. Worldwide Differences in Regulations of Clozapine Use. CNS Drugs 30, 149–161.

Nykiel, S., Henderson, D., Bhide, G., Freudenreich, O., 2010. Lithium to allow clozapine prescribing in benign ethnic neutropenia. Clin. Schizophr. Relat. Psychoses 4, 138–140.

Opgen-Rhein, C., Dettling, M., 2008. Clozapine-induced agranulocytosis and its genetic determinants. Pharmacogenomics 9, 1101–1111.

Oyesanmi, O., Kunkel, E.J., Monti, D.A., Field, H.L., 1999. Hematologic side effects of psychotropics. Psychosomatics 40, 414–421.

Ozdemir, M.A., Sofuoglu, S., Tanrikulu, G., Aldanmaz, F., Esel, E., Dundar, S., 1994. Lithium-induced hematologic changes in patients with bipolar affective disorder. Biol. Psychiatry 35, 210–213.

Palominao, A., Kukoyi, O., Xiong, G.L., 2010. Leukocytosis after lithium and clozapine combination therapy. Ann. Clin. Psychiatry 22, 205–206.

Pantelis, C., Adesanya, A., 2001. Increased risk of neutropaenia and agranulocytosis with sodium valproate used adjunctively with clozapine. Aust. N. Z. J. Psychiatry 35, 544–545.

Papetti, F., Darcourt, G., Giordana, J.Y., Spreux, A., Thauby, S., Feral, F., et al., 2004. Treatment of clozapine-induced granulocytopenia with lithium (two observations). Encephale 30, 578–582.

Patel, N.C., Dorson, P.G., Bettinger, T.L., 2002. Sudden late onset of clozapine-induced agranulocytosis. Ann. Pharmacother. 36, 1012–1015.

Patel, N.C., Crismon, M.L., Miller, A.L., Johnsrud, M.T., 2005. Drug adherence: effects of decreased visit frequency on adherence to clozapine therapy. Pharmacotherapy 25, 1242–1247.

Pereira, A., Dean, B., 2006. Clozapine bioactivation induces dose-dependent, drug-specific toxicity of human bone marrow stromal cells: a potential in vitro system for the study of agranulocytosis. Biochem. Pharmacol. 72, 783–793.

Pessina, A., Turlizzi, E., Bonomi, A., Guizzardi, F., Cavicchini, L., Croera, C., et al., 2006. In vitro toxicity of clozapine, olanzapine, and quetiapine on granulocyte-macrophage progenitors (GM-CFU). Pharmacopsychiatry 39, 20–22, 39, 160.

Philipps, R.J., Lee Demler, T., Lee, C., 2012. Omeprazole-induced blood dyscrasia in a clozapine-treated patient. Innov. Clin. Neurosci. 9, 14–17.

Phillips, D., Rezvani, K., Bain, B.J., 2000. Exercise induced mobilisation of the marginated granulocyte pool in the investigation of ethnic neutropenia. J. Clin. Pathol. 53, 481–483.

Pinninti, N.R., Houdart, M.P., Strouse, E.M., 2010. Case report of long-term lithium for treatment and prevention of clozapine-induced neutropenia in an African American male. J. Clin. Psychopharmacol. 30, 219–221.

Pirmohamed, M., Park, K., 1997. Mechanism of clozapine-induced agranulocytosis. Current status of research and implications for drug development. CNS Drugs 7, 139–158.

Plesnicar, B.K., Plesnicar, A., 2008. Risperidone- and aripiprazole-induced leukopenia: a case report. J. Clin. Psychiatry 10, 482–483.

Pollmächer, T., Fenzel, T., Mullington, J., Hinze-Selch, D., 1997. The influence of clozapine treatment on plasma granulocyte colony-stimulating (G-CSF) levels. Pharmacopsychiatry 30, 118–121.

Pontikoglou, C., Papadaki, H.A., 2010. Idiosyncratic drug-induced agranulocytosis: the paradigm of deferiprone. Hemoglobin 34, 291–304.

Pope, H.G., Cole, J.O., Choras, P.T., Fulwiler, C.E., 1986. Apparent neuroleptic malignant syndrome with clozapine and lithium. J. Nerv. Ment. Dis. 174, 493–495.

Porter, R., Mohamed, A., 2006. Diurnal variation of neutropenia during clozapine treatment. Int. J. Neuropsychopharmacol. 9, 373–374.

Ragonnet, L., Abadie, P., Dollfus, S., 2010. Use of clozapine in an adolescent with refractory first-episode psychosis and neutropenia. J. Clin. Psychopharmacol. 30, 336–338.

Rahman, A., Mican, L.M., Fischer, C., Campbell, A.H., 2009. Evaluating the incidence of leukopenia and neutropenia with valproate, quetiapine, or the combination in children and adolescents. Ann. Pharmacother. 43, 822–830.

Rajagopal, S., 2005. Clozapine, agranulocytosis, and benign ethnic neutropenia. Postgrad. Med. J. 81, 545–546.

Rajagopal, G., Graham, J.G., Haut, F.F., 2007. Prevention of clozapine-induced granulocytopenia/agranulocytosis with granulocyte-colony stimulating factor (G-CSF) in an intellectually disabled patient with schizophrenia. J. Intellect. Disabil. Res. 51, 82–85.

Reich, D., Nalls, M.A., Kao, W.H., Akylbekova, E.L., Tandon, A., Patterson, N., et al., 2009. Reduced neutrophil count in people of African descent is due to a regulatory variant in the Duffy antigen receptor for chemokines gene. PLoS Genet. 5, e1000360.

Ronaldson, K.J., Taylor, A.J., Fitzgerald, P.B., Topliss, D.J., Elsik, M., McNeil, J.J., 2010. Diagnostic characteristics of clozapine-induced myocarditis identified by an analysis of 38 cases and 47 controls. J. Clin. Psychiatry 71, 976–981.

Rothstein, G., Clarkson, D.R., Larsen, W., Grosser, B.I., Athens, J.W., 1978. Effect of lithium on neutrophil mass and production. N. Engl. J. Med. 298, 178–180.

Sayin, A., Cosar, B., 2006. Prolongation of clozapine-induced leucopenia with olanzapine treatment. Prog. Neuropsychopharmacol. Biol. Psychiatry 30, 958–959.

Sedky, K., Lippmann, S., 2006. Psychotropic medications and leucopenia. Curr. Drug Targets 7, 1191–1194.

Sedky, K., Shaughnessy, R., Hughes, T., Lippmann, S., 2005. Clozapine-induced agranulocytosis after 11 years of treatment. Am. J. Psychiatry 162, 814.

Shander, A., Javidroozi, M., Ashton, M.E., 2011. Drug-induced anemia and other red cell disorders: a guide in the age of polypharmacy. Curr. Clin. Pharmacol. 6, 295−303.

Shankar, B.R., 2007. Quetiapine-induced leucopenia and thrombocytopenia. Psychosomatics 48, 530−531.

Sikora, A., Adamus, J., Marcinek, A., 2007. Disproportionation of clozapine radical: a link between one-electron oxidation of clozapine and formation of its nitrenium cation. Chem. Res. Toxicol. 20, 1093−1098.

Silvestrini, C., Arcangeli, T., Biondi, M., Pancheri, P., 2000. A second trial of clozapine in a case of granulocytopenia. Hum. Psychopharmacol. 15, 275−279.

Sissung, T.M., Mross, K., Steinberg, S.M., Behringer, D., Figg, W.D., Sparreboom, A., et al., 2006. Association of ABCB1 genotypes with paclitaxel-mediated peripheral neuropathy and neutropenia. Eur. J. Cancer 42, 2893−2896.

Sluys, M., Guzelcan, Y., Casteelen, G., de Haan, L., 2004. Risperidone-induced leucopenia and neutropenia: a case report. Eur. Psychiatry 19, 117.

Small, J.G., Klapper, M.H., Malloy, F.W., Steadman, T.M., 2003. Tolerability and efficacy of clozapine combined with lithium in schizophrenia and schizoaffective disorder. J. Clin. Psychopharmacol. 23, 223−228.

Sopko, M.A., Caley, C.F., 2010. Chronic leukocytosis associated with clozapine treatment. Clin. Schizophr. Relat. Psychoses 4, 141−144.

Spencer, B.W., Williams, H.R., Gee, S.H., Whiskey, E., Rodrigues, J.P., Mijovic, A., et al., 2012. Granulocyte colony stimulating factor (G-CSF) can allow treatment with clozapine in a patient with severe benign ethnic neutropaenia (BEN): a case report. J. Psychopharmacol. 26, 1280−1282.

Sporn, A., Gogtay, N., Ortiz-Aguayo, R., Alfaro, C., Tossell, J., Lenane, M., et al., 2003. Clozapine-induced neutropenia in children: management with lithium carbonate. J. Child Adolesc. Psychopharmacol. 13, 401−404.

Stephan, F., Podlipski, M.A., Kerleau, J.M., Petit, M., Guillin, O., 2009. Toxicité médullaire des phénothiazines: à propos d'un cas d'agranulocytose sous chlorpromazine. L'Encéphale 35, 173−175.

Stergiou, V., Bozikas, V.P., Garyfallos, G., Nikolaidis, N., Lavrentiadis, G., Fokas, K., 2005. Olanzapine-induced leucopenia and neutropenia. Prog. Neuropsychopharmacol. Biol. Psychiatry 29, 992−994.

Stip, E., Langlois, R., Thuot, C., Mancini-Marie, A., 2007. Fatal agranulocytosis: the use of olanzapine in a patient with schizophrenia and myelodysplasia. Prog. Neuropsychopharmacol. Biol. Psychiatry 31, 297−300.

Stoner, S.C., Deal, E., Lurk, J.T., 2008. Delayed-onset neutropenia with divalproex sodium. Ann. Pharmacother. 42, 1507−1510.

Stübner, S., Grohmann, R., Engel, R., Bandelow, B., Ludwig, W.D., Wagner, G., et al., 2004. Blood dyscrasias induced by psychotropic drugs. Pharmacopsychiatry 37 (Suppl. 1), S70−S78.

Suraweera, C., Hanwella, R., de Silva, V., 2014. Use of lithium in clozapine-induced neutropenia: a case report. BMC Res. Notes 7, 635.

Tang, H.C., Chung, K.H., 2014. Quetiapine-induced neutropenia in a bipolar patient with hepatocellular carcinoma. Int. J. Psychiatr. Med. 47, 255−261.

Taylor, D., Paton, C., Kapur, S., 2015. The Maudsley Prescribing Guidelines, 12th ed. Informa Healthcare, London.

Thangadurai, P., Jyothi, K.S., Gopalakrishnan, R., Kuruvilla, A., Jacob, K.S., 2006. Reversible neutropenia with olanzapine following clozapine-induced neutropenia. Am. J. Psychiatry 163, 1298.

Thinn, S.S., Liew, E., May, A.L., Chua, H.C., Sim, K., 2007. Reversible delayed onset olanzapine-associated leukopenia and neutropenia in a clozapine-naive patient on concomitant depot antipsychotic. J. Clin. Psychopharmacol. 27, 394−395.

Tiihonen, J., Lönnqvist, J., Wahlbeck, K., Klaukka, T., Niskanen, L., Tanskanen, A., et al., 2009. 11-year follow-up of mortality in patients with schizophrenia: a population-based cohort study (FIN11 study). Lancet 374, 620−627.

Tseng, K.C., Hwang, T.J., 2009. Rhabdomyolysis following dose increase of clozapine and combination therapy with lithium. J. Clin. Psychopharmacol. 29, 398−399.

Turkozkan, N., Durmus, O., Boran, N., 1993. Biochemical investigation of leukocyte functions during lithium therapy. Int. J. Biochem. 25, 1501−1504.

Urban, A.E., Wiglusz, M.S., Cubała, W.J., Landowski, J., Krysta, K., 2015. Rapid-onset agranulocytosis in a patient treated with clozapine and lamotrigine. Psychiatr. Danub. 27 (Suppl. 1), S459−S461.

Usta, N.G., Poyraz, C.A., Aktan, M., Duran, A., 2014. Clozapine treatment of refractory schizophrenia during essential chemotherapy: a case study and mini review of a clinical dilemma. Ther. Adv. Psychopharmacol. 4, 276−281.

Valevski, A., Klein, T., Gazit, E., Meged, S., Stein, D., Elizur, A., et al., 1998. HLA-B38 and clozapine-induced agranulocytosis in Israeli Jewish schizophrenic patients. Eur. J. Immunogenet. 25, 11−13.

Verbelen, M., Collier, D.A., Cohen, D., MacCabe, J.H., Lewis, C.M., 2015. Establishing the characteristics of an effective pharmacogenetic test for clozapine-induced agranulocytosis. Pharmacogenomics J. 15, 461−466.

Vila-Rodriguez, F., Tsang, P., Barr, A.M., 2013. Chronic benign neutropenia/agranulocytosis associated with non-clozapine antipsychotics. Am. J. Psychiatry 170, 1213−1214.

Wang, C., Li, L., 2012. Proper use of clozapine: experiences in China. Shanghai Arch. Psychiatry 24, 108−109.

Whiskey, E., Taylor, D., 2007. Restarting clozapine after neutropenia: evaluating the possibilities and practicalities. CNS Drugs 21, 25−35.

Whiskey, E., Olofinjana, O., Taylor, D., 2011. The importance of the recognition of benign ethnic neutropenia in black patients during treatment with clozapine: case reports and database study. J. Psychopharmacol. 25, 842−845.

Wu, S.Y., Liu, C.C., Hsieh, M.H., 2008. Successful re-exposure to clozapine following uneventful rechallenge with olanzapine in a patient with neutropenia related to both agents. Prog. Neuropsychopharmacol. Biol. Psychiatry 32, 1089−1090.

Yalcin, D.O., Goka, E., Aydemir, M.C., Kisa, C., 2008. Is aripiprazole the only choice of treatment of the patients who developed anti-psychotic agents-induced leucopenia and neutropenia? A case report. J. Psychopharmacol. 22, 333−335.

Yen, C.F., Chong, M.Y., Kuo, M.C., Chang, C.S., 1997. Severe granulocytopenia secondary to chlorpromazine despite concurrent lithium treatment: a case report. Kaohsiung J. Med. Sci. 13, 635−638.

Young, N.S., Scheinberg, P., Calado, R.T., 2008. Aplastic anemia. Curr. Opin. Hematol. 15, 162−168.

Zhou, S.F., Wang, B., Yang, L.P., Liu, J.P., 2010. Structure, function, regulation and polymorphism and the clinical significance of human cytochrome P450 1A2. Drug. Metab. Rev. 42, 268−354.

Part III

Antipsychotic-Related Pathology of the Digestive System

Chapter 6

Gastrointestinal Hypomotility and Dysphagia

Robert J. Flanagan[1] and Kathlyn J. Ronaldson[2]
[1]*King's College Hospital, London, United Kingdom,*
[2]*Monash University, Melbourne, VIC, Australia*

6.1 GASTROINTESTINAL HYPOMOTILITY

6.1.1 Introduction

Life-threatening adverse effects caused by impaired gastrointestinal motility, intestinal obstruction, fecal impaction, and paralytic ileus, have been associated with clozapine, and with other antipsychotics but much less so. Various forms of colitis in patients taking clozapine, apparently without constipation, have also been reported, albeit rarely. The case fatality for life-threatening cases of clozapine-induced gastrointestinal hypomotility may be as high as 28% (Palmer et al., 2008), but will depend on many factors, including the promptness and appropriateness of intervention. Gastrointestinal hypomotility with clozapine is a known adverse effect (Every-Palmer et al., 2016; see Table 6.1 for cases), but one that is not given sufficient proactive attention and one that may not be considered following a sudden death. It is also an effect exacerbated by the lifestyle of many patients with psychiatric disorders.

6.1.2 Epidemiology

In a multinational study recruiting 409 patients taking antipsychotic medication, 20% of men and 39% of women ($p < 0.001$) reported, at interview, constipation in varying degrees from very little to very much (Barbui et al., 2005). De Hert et al. (2011a) observed that, among 273 inpatients on antipsychotic treatment, 99 had at least one new pharmacological intervention for constipation, and by X-ray (data unclear, but assuming two

TABLE 6.1 Cases of Life-Threatening Gastrointestinal Hypomotility With Clozapine

Patient (Sex, Age)	Clozapine Dose (mg d⁻¹)	Clozapine Duration	Clinical Features	Investigations	Treatment	Outcome	References
M, 29	400	36 d	Aspirated vomit	Obstruction of the transverse colon		Died	Hayes and Gibler (1995)
F, 31	300–800	5 w		Large bowel obstruction with mucosal necrosis, pulmonary edema, shock		Died	Théret et al. (1995)
M, 49	500		Intermittent nausea, vomiting, indigestion, and chest pain for 3 w. Physical exam 13 d prior: Slight abdominal tenderness. Complaining of constipation for 11 d. Spurious diarrhea	Autopsy: Severe pulmonary edema from inhalation of feculent vomit. Extensive, severe fecal impaction of large bowel; feculent fluid extending to the stomach. Reflux esophagitis		Died unexpectedly	Drew and Herdson (1997)
M, 44	500			Pulmonary edema, visceral vascular congestion, esophagitis, paralytic ileus of the sigmoid colon, gastroenteritis, eosinophilia of ileocaecal valve region		Died (death wrongly attributed to fluoxetine inhibition of clozapine metabolism)	Ferslew et al. (1998)
M, 49	400	6 w	Prior to clozapine, untreated constipation	Colon perforation and feculent peritonitis	Emergency hemicolectomy	Survived, but perioperative dense cerebrovascular accident: dense hemiplegia	Freudenreich and Goff (2000)
M, 43	750	5.5 yr	History of ulcerative esophagitis. Vomiting, epigastric pain	Gastroscopy, abdominal CT: ulcerated esophagitis, constipation	Omeprazole 20 mg d⁻¹, psyllium		Levin et al. (2002)
			5 mo later: Vomiting, abdominal pain		Omeprazole 40 mg d⁻¹, psyllium		
			1 mo later: Unwell with abdominal pain, feculent vomiting. Cyanosis, tachycardia, confusion. Unrecordable BP	Laparotomy: Large bowel obstruction, secondary to fecal impaction of entire colon. Large intestine necrosis, dilation	Manual decompression, total colectomy and ileostomy	Died after 3 w from sepsis and multiple organ failure	

Patient	Dose	Duration	Clinical features	Diagnosis	Treatment	Outcome	Reference
F, 47	600			Large bowel infarct		Died	Flanagan et al. (2005)
M, 19	200 + morphine 65 mg d⁻¹	10 d	Abdominal pain, constipation, fever, shock (systolic BP 65 mm Hg)	Necrotizing enterocolitis	Right hemicolectomy and ilectomy	Recovery	Khaldi et al. (2005)
M, 20	900	1 yr	Constipation for 2 d, severe abdominal pain, collapse	Bowel infarction		Died	Townsend and Curtis (2006)
M, 34	300	4 mm	Constipation for 1 w, then acute abdominal pain/distension, fever, and nausea/vomiting. Raised creatinine and urea	X-ray: Massive fecal loading of large bowel (diameter of the colon >10 cm) with necrotizing colitis	Right hemicolectomy, IV crystalloids and antibiotics	Recovery; rechallenge, outcome not stated	Leong et al. (2007)
M, 45	400	5 mm	Constipation, abdominal distension, vomiting, fever, severe fecal impaction, megacolon for 3 w	Rectal exam: Fecaloma. Creatinine, urea, electrolytes normal. X-ray: Dilated loops of small, large bowel, megacolon with extensive fecal impaction	Clozapine dose reduced to 250 mg d⁻¹. Conservative treatment: IV fluids, Fleet enema, rectal washout	Regular bowel movements in 1 w with high fiber, adequate fluid, stool softeners, exercise	Pelizza et al. (2007)
M, 30	600		3 mo later: Gross abdominal distension, belching, flatus. No severe abdominal pain or vomiting	Obstruction: Meckel's diverticulum; Paralytic ileus	Small bowel resection; Clozapine dose reduced to 450 mg d⁻¹	Recovery; no recurrence at 3 mo	Rondla and Crane (2007)
F, 61	600	36 d	Constipation. Also prescribed bupropion, zuclopenthixol and methotrimeprazine	Colonic perforation, septic shock		Died	Rousseau and Charbonneau (2007)
M, 62	100 Olanzapine 30 mg d⁻¹, risperidone 8 mg d⁻¹ + 37.5 mg IM 4d prior		Vomiting, abdominal bloating. No prior complaints	Laparotomy: Marked distension of small bowel, filled with bowel and gastric juice. Large bowel not distended. No mechanical obstruction	Laparotomy: Small bowel decompression to stomach. Intubation, mechanical ventilation, parenteral nutrition, 4 d. Parenteral neostigmine 3 mg d⁻¹, metoclopramide 30 mg d⁻¹	Full recovery	Dome et al. (2007)

(Continued)

TABLE 6.1 (Continued)

Patient (Sex, Age)	Clozapine Dose (mg d⁻¹)	Clozapine Duration	Clinical Features	Investigations	Treatment	Outcome	References
M, 53	700 + olanzapine 20 mg d^{-1}	1 yr	Severe abdominal pain and bilious vomiting, tachycardia, hypotension. Raised WBC, normal urea, electrolytes, LFTs	X-ray: Severe fecal impaction in the large and small bowel. CT: Transverse, descending colon feces loaded. No mechanical obstruction. Sepsis from fecal impaction	Manual bowel disimpaction. Further episode of severe constipation with fecal impaction on olanzapine 20 mg d^{-1}, clozapine 350 mg d^{-1} despite laxatives. Resolved on clozapine withdrawal	Recovered, but requiring weekly enemas	Rege and Lafferty (2008)
M, 28	500		History of constipation and abdominal distension several w. Septic shock, multiorgan dysfunction	Colonoscopy: severe ischemic colitis without perforation or obstruction	Antibiotics. Enemas no effect, but responded to IV neostigmine; surgery not required	Full recovery	De Bruin et al. (2009)
M, 61	600	7 yr	History of constipation. No bowel sounds. Later distended abdomen, feculent vomiting	Abdominal CT: Severe fecal impaction, with edematous rectal mucosa and acute-on-chronic constipation		Died after developing pneumonia and sepsis	Hibbard et al. (2009)
M, 63	400	20 d	Constipation, collapse, severe fecal impaction with distention of the small and large bowel	CT: Near collapse of inferior vena cava from pressure in abdominal cavity, feces impaction in rectum and sigmoid	Decompression of large bowel obstruction	Died: Multiorgan failure	Hibbard et al. (2009)
F, 40	700		History of large bowel resections and colostomy due to clozapine treatment 8 and 7 yr before. Right-sided pain, nausea, vomiting bilious material, with aspiration. Septic shock		Surgery to remove long section of gangrenous bowel, ventilation for 2.5 w, dialysis for 6 w	Recovery. Clozapine reintroduced successfully at 75 mg d^{-1}	McKinnon et al. (2009)

M, 34	200	Episode of constipation for several d, acute abdominal pain, hypotension, and hematemesis	X-ray: Marked dilatation of intestinal loops. CT: Giant fecaloma, GI tract dilatation, intestinal wall pneumatosis, air in portal vein. Laparotomy: Bowel ischemia, inflammatory fluid in peritoneal cavity	Fecaloma extracted through the anus. Clozapine withdrawn	Full recovery 2 w later; no further surgery	Díaz-Caneja et al. (2010)
F, 53	70	Acute onset abdominal pain and nausea with constipation. Distended abdomen and tenderness. No abdominal masses were detected	Autopsy: Grossly distended intestine stomach to rectum. Feculent material throughout the GI tract. No mechanical obstruction	Stool softener and lactulose	Died 5 h post-admission	Abeyasinghe et al. (2010)
M, 41	750	Day before death reported feeling "bunged up." Neutrophilia, monocytosis, acidosis	Autopsy: Small bowel dilated, with blood-stained mucus, particularly in jejunum. Large bowel dilated with foul-smelling, blood stained fluid and a small amount of stool	4 × Movicol; failed to defecate. Next morning vomited copious quantities of tea-colored fluid. Given 2 × Movicol. Severe, uncontrollable diarrhea developed	Found collapsed and not breathing. Resuscitation attempt failed	Flanagan and Ball (2011)
M, 49	200 + quetiapine 500 mg d^{-1}	Emergency admission with discomfort, abdominal swelling, and vomiting that had been present and increasing for some 2 w	Autopsy: Dilatation of the small and large bowel with no obvious obstruction. Dilated, flabby heart (720 g) with left ventricular hypertrophy. Liver extensive centrilobular hepatic necrosis; 5.2 L of straw-colored ascitic fluid in abdomen		Died after 2 d	
M, 47	625	12 d history of constipation. Found collapsed; could not be resuscitated. 1 h before speech slurred	Autopsy: Massive gaseous distension of large bowel, fecal loading of the distal sigmoid and rectum. No stercoral ulceration, perforation, or toxic bowel changes		Died	

(Continued)

TABLE 6.1 (Continued)

Patient (Sex, Age)	Clozapine Dose (mg d^{-1})	Clinical Features	Investigations	Treatment	Outcome	References
M, 44	300	Dyspnea, cough, abdominal pain, nausea, vomiting, diarrhea, somnolence, abdominal distension, tenderness, and hypoactive intestinal sounds	X-ray: Dilated small bowel loops. CT scan: nonobstructive dilatation of small intestine and transverse colon. Chest X-ray: No pulmonary infiltrate	Clozapine withdrawn, IV nutrition, GI decompression. Normal GI function in 1 w. Clozapine 50 mg d^{-1} on day 9 post-admission; diarrhea, abdominal tenderness and pain	Made full recovery after clozapine discontinued	Abou Farha et al. (2012)
M, 65	100 Clozapine still being titrated; olanzapine 10 mg d^{-1}, docusate 200 mg d^{-1}	Malaise, anorexia, nausea, vomiting, and diarrhea, followed (at 9 d) by tachypnea and hypotension. History: Gastroesophageal reflux disease, small bowel obstruction on olanzapine	Abdominal CT: Adynamic ileus. Chest X-ray: Infiltrate suggestive of aspiration. Colonoscopy: Diverticulosis without malignancy	Stabilized after 3 w, but 10 d after restarting olanzapine developed diarrhea, tachypnea, and tachycardia requiring medical stabilization	Died 3 d later. No autopsy. Assumed cause complications of ileus	Fayad and Bruijnzeel (2012)
M, 56	500	Developed partial small bowel obstruction		Clozapine discontinued. Cautious reintroduction to 500 mg d^{-1} again led to partial small bowel obstruction after 5 w. Obstruction resolved; maintained on PEG, senna, and sorbitol, plus enemas; still constipated. Changed to bethanechol, PEG and senna	Survived. Continued successfully on clozapine 500 mg d^{-1} for 6 mo with 1–2 soft stools d^{-1}	Poetter and Stewart (2013)

M, 47	6 d	200	Poor appetite, vomiting, abdominal pain, generalized fatigue. Abdomen tympanic on percussion. Ileus, bacterial peritonitis	CT: Multiple dilated air/fluid loops in the small and large bowel and pneumointestine. No evidence of mechanical obstruction	Day 7 terminal ileum resection subtotal colectomy, Hartmann's procedure with ileostomy	Died day 8 after three attempts at resuscitation	Yu et al. (2013)
M, 46	14 mo	275	Constipation, mild abdominal discomfort. 3 d later: vomiting, persistent abdominal pain. Hard, distended abdomen	X-ray: Megacolon. CT: Colon distension, fecal compaction. Postoperative: pulmonary embolism	Clozapine stopped, enema, nil by mouth. 4 d later, colon perforation with free air and dilatation by CT. Emergency appendectomy, intraperitoneal drainage	Prolonged recovery. Rechallenge with clozapine 200 mg d^{-1} with laxatives, exercises, weekly abdominal exam, monthly X-ray for 5 mo	Ikai et al. (2013)
M, 28		200	Severe abdominal pain and distention, fever, raised leukocytes. Developed severe dyspnea, septic lung thromboembolism	At 12 h laparotomy: large bowel severely dilated, 4.5 kg compacted stools, areas of necrosis in transverse colon		Died 36 h post-admission	Baptista (2014)
M, 40		600	Mild abdominal ache and constipation	CT: Sigmoid inflammation with marked colonic dilation sigmoid to cecum. Flexible sigmoidoscopy: Severely impacted feces	Senna; within 12 h chest pain, respiratory distress. Intubated and ventilated after resuscitation from respiratory arrest. Chest CT confirmed pneumonia; IV antibiotics	Recovery over 11 d. Developed good bowel movements; inpatient for several w	Galappathie and Khan (2014)
M, 49	14 yr	500	History of constipation managed with laxatives; Sudden onset of severe abdominal pain, nausea, vomiting	CT: Small bowel obstruction from fecal impaction, ischemic small bowel	Surgery but no resection. Postoperative pneumonia and sepsis	9 mo later rechallenged clozapine 250 mg d^{-1} with lubiprostone, laxatives; no recurrence in 3 yr	Meyer and Cummings (2014)

(Continued)

TABLE 6.1 (Continued)

Patient (Sex, Age)	Clozapine Dose (mg d^{-1})	Clozapine Duration	Clinical Features	Investigations	Treatment	Outcome	References
M, 33	500 + Carbamazepine 800 mg d^{-1}			Colonic obstruction up to hepatic flexure	Nil by mouth, nasogastric decompression for days unsuccessful. Total colectomy, ileorectal anastomosis	On olanzapine 20 mg d^{-1} developed postoperative ileus. Recovered after switch to aripiprazole 15 mg d^{-1}	Lu and Shen (2014)
F, 25	225 Chlorpromazine 100 mg d^{-1}		Abdominal pain and constipation.	Autopsy: Deep vein and pulmonary emboli	Laxative and two glycerine suppositories	Collapsed and died on the toilet	Flanagan (unpublished)
M, 45	500		Breathlessness, distended abdomen. Recently stopped smoking. Constipation, vomiting. Hypertensive, ascites, mild hepatomegaly	Autopsy: Large bowel cecum to splenic flexure distended at maximum point. Hard feces throughout large bowel; no other cause for obstruction	Prescribed laxatives, clozapine stopped	Died day 5	
M, 44	450 chlorpromazine	10 yr	Hyperventilating, agitated and anxious. Repeated episodes of hypotension	Severe liver damage (INR 2.5); renal function deteriorating. Autopsy: Fecal loading in left colon		Collapsed and could not be resuscitated	
M, 47	600	>10 yr	Found lying on floor. Nausea, but not constipation. Examination: Soft abdomen, possibly slightly distended	Autopsy: Large intestines and sigmoid colon markedly dilated with firm feces. No other cause for obstruction		Found unconscious; could not be resuscitated	
M, 42	900	15 yr	History of constipation. Drowsy and agitated. Suddenly labored breathing, restless and unwell. BP 55/36 mm Hg	Autopsy: Marked fecal overloading of the colon with proximal bowel distension. No other cause for obstruction		Appeared to fit, then vomited blood, became unresponsive; could not be resuscitated	

BP, blood pressure; CT, computerized tomography; d, day(s); F, female; GI, gastrointestinal; h, hour(s); INR, international normalized ratio; IM, intramuscular; IV, intravenous; LFTs, liver function tests; mo, month(s); M, male; PEG, polyethyleneglycol; w, week(s); WBC, white blood cells; yr, year(s).

radiographs per patient) 13 had fecal accumulation and 34 fecal impaction. A study focusing on clozapine found a higher rate of constipation at 60%, and at least 12% required repeated enemas to obtain relief (Hayes and Gibler, 1995). In a nationwide study conducted in Denmark, the incidence of admission for ileus with clozapine was 0.8% (Nielsen and Meyer, 2012). From spontaneous reporting data in Australasia, for which the reporting will be incomplete, the calculated incidence of clozapine-related life-threatening hypomotility was 0.3% (Palmer et al., 2008).

Data suggest that life-threatening conditions associated with gastrointestinal hypomotility, fecal impaction, adynamic ileus, bowel obstruction and pseudoobstruction, are collectively more common with clozapine than other antipsychotic agents (De Hert et al., 2011b). In case-control analysis, the use of clozapine in schizophrenia was associated with a twofold increased risk of ileus (OR 1.99, 95% CI: 1.21−3.29), and a sevenfold increased risk of fatality from this cause (OR 6.73, 95% CI: 1.55−29.17) (Nielsen and Meyer, 2012). The risk of ileus was increased with first-generation antipsychotics of low ($p = 0.02$), medium ($p = 0.05$), and high (0.001) potency, but not with olanzapine, quetiapine, amisulpride, risperidone, or ziprasidone, and aripiprazole was found to be protective ($p = 0.001$) (Nielsen and Meyer, 2012). These authors explored risk factors for ileus and found the mean clozapine dose was higher among patients with ileus than among the control patients who were also receiving clozapine ($p = 0.008$). Palmer et al. (2008) also noted a dose effect (mean dose among cases 428 mg d^{-1}; mean dose among fatal cases 535 mg d^{-1}; mean dose among all New Zealand recipients of clozapine 369 mg d^{-1}; $p < 0.01$ and < 0.0001, respectively). In addition, Nielsen and Meyer (2012) found that among patients with schizophrenia, the risk of ileus increased with age (3% y^{-1}; 95% CI: 1−4%), with female sex (OR 1.60; 95% CI: 1.10−2.31), with concomitant use of other anticholinergics (1.48; 1.00−2.19), opioids (2.14; 1.36−3.36), and tricyclic antidepressants (2.29; 1.29−4.09). A study of gastrointestinal hypomotility with antipsychotics reported to the French pharmacovigilance program included 38 cases of ischemic colitis and gastrointestinal necrosis, both of which may occur as a consequence of severe constipation (Peyrière et al., 2009). In addition to clozapine, the first-generation antipsychotics, levomepromazine, cyamemazine, and haloperidol, were strongly represented. Fourteen patients died and 66% were taking other drugs with antimuscarinic or anticholinergic activity.

Constipation is a known adverse effect of some of the second-generation agents. For example, a Cochrane review observed that constipation occurred with aripiprazole monotherapy more frequently than with placebo: RR 1.75 (1.23−2.49) (Brown et al., 2013); a multicenter study of elderly nursing home residents found that 7% of those on olanzapine, but none of those taking risperidone, developed constipation (Frenchman, 2005); and 5 of 12 treatment-resistant patients given high dose quetiapine became constipated

(Boggs et al., 2008). If constipation occurs with these agents, serious consequences may ensue and some such cases are listed in Table 6.2.

Two reports involving clozapine, but also implicating other second-generation antipsychotics, have been published. In one case, fecal impaction developed after addition of aripiprazole to clozapine and resolved after withdrawal of aripiprazole (Table 6.2) (Legrand et al., 2013), in the other case, fatal bowel obstruction developed 10 days after initiation of olanzapine, following adynamic ileus during clozapine initiation (Table 6.1) (Fayad and Bruijnzeel, 2012).

Three cases of eosinophilic colitis with severe diarrhea occurring within 1 month of commencing clozapine, and thus within the typical timeframe for a hypersensitivity reaction (e.g., myocarditis which may occur with severe diarrhea; see Chapter 2, Myocarditis and Cardiomyopathy), have been described (Friedberg et al., 1995; Karmacharya et al., 2005). Further cases of colitis were of pseudomembranous colitis, without evidence of *Clostridium difficile*, but with necrosis requiring surgery (Sim et al., 2006); necrotizing colitis, which was fatal within hours of surgery (Shammi and Remington, 1997); and colitis with evidence of intraepithelial lymphocytosis on biopsy (Pelizza and Melegari, 2007). The last patient recovered, but had a recurrence of fever and diarrhea after two doses on rechallenge. The causal sequence for these cases is unknown, but they may have occurred as a consequence of constipation, although this was not described.

A review that included published cases and pharmacovigilance data from Australia and New Zealand noted a fatal outcome among 28% of 102 patients developing life-threatening conditions related to gastrointestinal hypomotility while taking clozapine (Palmer et al., 2008). On the one hand, this figure may be elevated due to reporting and publication bias, but on the other hand the apparently precipitate nature of cases among psychiatric patients may result in death without identified cause (Manu et al., 2011).

6.1.3 Pathobiology

All or most antipsychotics are associated with constipation, and Tan et al. (2013) have found changes in colonic architecture, specifically to be capacious, redundant, featureless, or megacolonic, to be associated with chronic use of these agents in an Asian population (adjusted odds ratio 5.5; 95% CI: $1.6-19$; $p = 0.007$).

Gastrointestinal motility is controlled by the parasympathetic, sympathetic and intrinsic nervous systems. In particular the parasympathetic system promotes intestinal motility. With this nervous system involvement, it is no surprise that drugs, such as antipsychotics, which inhibit neurotransmitters, decrease motility (Hiranyakas et al., 2011). Thus all drugs with anticholinergic activity will impair gastrointestinal motility. However, clozapine has more severe effects on gastrointestinal motility than other antipsychotics,

TABLE 6.2 Reports of Gastrointestinal Hypomotility During Treatment With Antipsychotics Other Than Clozapine

Patient (Sex, Age)	Drugs (mg d⁻¹)	Clinical Presentation	Investigations	Treatment	Outcome	References
F, 46	Chlorpromazine, loxapine, trihexyphenidyl, tropatepine	Abdominal pain, vomiting 4 d. No electrolyte imbalance	Chest X-ray, abdominal CT: Gaseous distension of stomach and whole intestinal tract, with hepatodiaphragmatic interposition of the large bowel	Surgical decompression and segmental colonic resection of infarcted intestinal loops. No evidence of mechanical bowel obstruction	Not stated	Lemyze et al. (2009)
F, 42	Chlorpromazine 300	Generalized abdominal pain for 2 d, then collapse	Examination: Advanced peritonitis, peripheral circulatory failure. X-ray: Gross colonic dilatation with gas-fluid. Laparotomy: turbid, foul-smelling fluid in peritoneal cavity; necrotizing colitis	Resuscitative procedures. Hemicolectomy	Recovered	Hay (1978)
M, 27	Cyamemazine (cyamepromazine)	Found unresponsive. Abdomen distended, extremely hard, no bowel sounds. BP 80/60 mm Hg, HR 110 min⁻¹, hypothermia. Electrolyte imbalance, creatinine 280 μmol/L.	Abdominal CT: Small bowel, colonic dilatation with aortic compression; ischemia of the abdominal viscera under origin of renal arteries	Emergency laparotomy confirmed severe distension of the bowel	Fatal cardiac arrest after surgery. Multiple organ failure	Jambet et al. (2012)

(Continued)

TABLE 6.2 (Continued)

Patient (Sex, Age)	Drugs (mg d^{-1})	Clinical Presentation	Investigations	Treatment	Outcome	References
M, 65	Bromperidol 24 Chlorpromazine 75 Trihexyphenidyl 12	History of dilated intestine with stool impaction treated with laxatives	Paralytic ileus. Dilation of colon, but no obstruction	Hyperbaric oxygen	Recovered with bromperidol 4 mg d^{-1}, lower doses of chlorpromazine and trihexyphenidyl	Suzuki et al. (2007)
F, 35	Haloperidol prn, olanzapine 40, perphenazine 48, risperidone 12, benzatropine 3	Abdominal pain, distension. Long history of constipation; lacked a bowel regimen	X-ray: Paralytic ileus	Nil by mouth; Golytely by nasogastric tube; reduced benzatropine to 1 mg d^{-1}, risperidone to 8 mg d^{-1}	Discharged on polyethylene glycol	Kwiatkowski et al. (2011)
M, 27	Benzatropine, bupropion, olanzapine	Constipation, abdominal pain, nausea, vomiting for 6 d. HR >100 min^{-1}, BP 151/88 mm Hg. Developed fever	CT: Colitis from the splenic flexure to the sigmoid colon, without perforation. Diagnosis: Ischemic colitis	Treated with antibiotics and managed supportively; antipsychotics withdrawn	Discharged on docusate and PEG and new antipsychotic regimen prescribed	Park et al. (2012)
M, 59	Olanzapine, lorazepam, biperidene chlorohydrate	Stupor, abdominal distension; no bowel sounds	Abdominal CT: Enlarged sigmoid colon, fecal impaction, intraperitoneal free air. Laparotomy: 2 mm perforation; feces in the peritoneal cavity	Left hemicolectomy and colostomy	Recovered from surgery, but died 16 d later of unrelated cause	Toro et al. (2014)

M, 39	Quetiapine 300, tropatepine 20, lactulose	Abdominal pain and constipation	CT: Distension of the colon including the cecum	Subtotal colectomy. Histology: Necrotizing ischemic colitis	Survived	De Beaurepaire et al. (2015)
M, 44	Risperidone 3.5	Abdominal distension, overflow diarrhea; Usual bowel habit once in 3–5 d	X-ray: Fecal shadowing of entire large intestines, gross proximal dilatation	No response to Fleet enema, risperidone dose reduction (2 mg d^{-1}). Surgical decompression plus lactulose	Recovered; maintained on risperidone 1 mg d^{-1} without recurrence	Lim and Mahendran (2002)
M, 32	Risperidone 4, lorazepam, nasogastric nutrition	Bloated abdomen, vomiting	Paralytic ileus diagnosed	Conservative management, risperidone withdrawn	Recovered	Ramamourthy et al. (2013)
M, 25	Clozapine 500, aripiprazole 5. Problem occurred 1 w after addition of aripiprazole	Constipation with fecal vomiting and abdominal distension	X-ray: Widespread fecal impaction with partial bowel obstruction	Intensive treatment with purgatives for 2 w: obstruction severity increased	Recovery followed 2 w after aripiprazole withdrawal	Legrand et al. (2013)

BP, blood pressure; *CT*, computerized tomography; *d*, day(s); *F*, female; *h*, hour(s); *HR*, heart rate; *mo*, month(s); *M*, male; *PEG*, polyethyleneglycol; *w*, week(s).

and these effects extend the length of the gastrointestinal tract (Van Veggel et al., 2013), although they are more frequently observed in the lower area. Clozapine does not act on dopamine D_2 receptors, as do the first-generation antipsychotics, and has potent antiserotonergic and anticholinergic effects, the latter mediated by antimuscarinic activity (Bullock et al., 2007). Specifically, the effect of clozapine on gastrointestinal motility has been attributed to its peripheral anticholinergic effects, to delay colonic transit and relax intestinal smooth muscle, and to its antiserotonergic properties, to compound the inhibiting effects on smooth muscle contraction (Palmer et al., 2008; Hibbard et al., 2009; Dome et al., 2007). In addition, clozapine impairs blood glucose control, and the development of diabetes itself can impair gut motility as a result of diabetic neuropathy (Bishara and Taylor, 2014).

Intestinal obstruction or hypomotility affects the systemic fluid and electrolyte balance, first by interfering with fluid absorption, and second by fluid loss from vomiting and diarrhea (Jackson and Raiji, 2011). Gastrointestinal stasis encourages overgrowth of intestinal flora with two serious outcomes: feculent vomiting and bacterial migration across the bowel wall causing sepsis. Proximal obstruction is another cause of emesis (Jackson and Raiji, 2011). Intestinal dilation and fecal impaction may eventually result in reduced local arterial circulation, causing ischemia, necrosis, and perforation of the intestinal walls (Jackson and Raiji, 2011). Patients with a reduced level of consciousness, agitation or restlessness are at risk of aspiration of vomit, feculent or otherwise, which may cause pneumonia (Table 6.1) (Hayes and Gibler, 1995; Drew and Herdson, 1997; McKinnon et al., 2009).

The direct effects of clozapine and other agents impairing gastrointestinal motility are exacerbated by the lifestyle of patients with mental illness, which typically involves poor diet, limited fluid intake, and little exercise, all of which contribute to the risk of constipation (Lambert et al., 2003). In addition, those with mental illness usually have poor self-care and poor self-monitoring of bodily functions. In the presence of pain from any source, they may have a higher pain threshold and difficulty expressing that they have a problem (Lambert et al., 2003). The epidemiological data point to dose-, sex-, and age-related effects on risk. Motility of the entire gastrointestinal tract slows with age, resulting in increased absorption of medication through longer contact with gastric mucosa and also to exacerbation of medication-related impairment of motility (Newton, 2005; Bowskill et al., 2012; Bishara and Taylor, 2014). Further, the rate of drug metabolism may be reduced. On the other hand fecal impaction and intestinal obstruction may impair absorption of medication, resulting in reduced efficacy, and use of laxatives may also affect drug absorption (Altree and Galletly, 2013; Bregman et al., 2014). Rostami-Hodjegan et al. (2004) have documented the increase in clozapine plasma concentration with female gender and with increasing age.

Greater dose will, in general, result in greater pharmacodynamic effect, including increased inhibition of cholinergic and serotonergic receptors.

However, there are several factors influencing bioavailability besides dose. Smoking substantially increases the rate of metabolism of clozapine (Rostami-Hodjegan et al., 2004), and patients ceasing smoking should have their dose down titrated, to avoid direct toxicity, as well as an increased risk of constipation and other anticholinergic effects. Smoking cessation of itself may be associated with constipation (Hajek et al., 2003). In one case, the trigger for fatal fecal impaction in a patient on long-term clozapine appears to have been smoking cessation (Flanagan, unpublished data; see Table 6.1, 45-year-old man). Inflammation and infection may impair clozapine metabolism and result in increased clozapine and norclozapine (N-desmethylclozapine) plasma concentrations (de Leon, 2004; Pfuhlmann et al., 2009). Clozapine is primarily metabolized by CYP1A2, but also by CYP3A4 and CYP2D6, and drugs inhibiting these enzymes may increase the clozapine concentration in plasma. Norclozapine also has anticholinergic and antiserotonergic activity (Lameh et al., 2007). Hence, plasma clozapine and norclozapine are better measures of systemic clozapine activity, including anticholinergic activity, than is dose.

Other medication causing constipation, such as opiates, and other anticholinergic medication, other antipsychotics, benzatropine (benztropine), tricyclic antidepressants, anticonvulsants, antispasmodics, calcium channel blockers, antihistamines, and antiemetics, have an additive effect on gastrointestinal hypomotility, and should be avoided if possible (Wald, 2016).

In addition, patients taking antipsychotics may have prolongation of postoperative ileus. In one case the ileus resolved on postoperative day 13 (Erickson et al., 1995). Once the ileus had resolved the patient was able to continue clozapine without recurrence or extraordinary preventive measures. The additive effects of opiates and antipsychotics administered for pain and psychotic symptoms, respectively, postsurgery may also precipitate ileus (Sirois, 2005).

6.1.4   Clinical and Laboratory Features

Among 102 cases, Palmer et al. (2008) noted a time to onset of life-threatening hypomotility with clozapine of 3 days to 15 years, with 36% occurring in the first 4 months of treatment, but with almost 50% of cases occurring more than 1 year after commencing clozapine. Frequently cases occur suddenly without apparent warning of a developing life-threatening situation (Table 6.1) (Dome et al., 2007; Rege and Lafferty, 2008; Abeyasinghe et al., 2010; Flanagan and Ball, 2011) but, for several days or weeks, some have had symptoms, including nausea, vomiting, indigestion, chest pain, constipation, abdominal pain, and swelling, which have not been addressed or only inadequately so (Drew and Herdson, 1997; Freudenreich and Goff, 2000; Leong et al., 2007; Díaz-Caneja et al., 2010; Flanagan and Ball, 2011). Episodes of diarrhea may confound the diagnosis (Drew and Herdson, 1997; Abou Farha et al., 2012; Fayad and Bruijnzeel, 2012).

The presentation of cases involving fecal impaction may include feculent vomiting, fever, tachycardia, hypotension, abdominal distension, and pain. Inhalation of feculent vomit causes intractable pneumonia from the physical and infectious assault on the lungs. For any case of severe gastrointestinal hypomotility, tachycardia and hypotension may be the consequence of dehydration and fever of sepsis (Jackson and Raiji, 2011). In the more serious cases the patient may collapse and require resuscitation (Dome et al., 2007).

Laboratory investigation should include a complete blood screen, electrolytes, and liver and kidney function tests. An elevated white blood cell count may indicate sepsis, and hypokalemia, hypochloremia, and metabolic acidosis are likely to accompany severe emesis and prolonged chronic constipation. Severe dehydration may be indicated by increased hematocrit, urea, and creatinine (Hucl, 2013; Jackson and Raiji, 2011). Elevated liver function parameters may indicate an alternative cause or the progression of the illness to multiorgan compromise (Box 6.1).

6.1.5 Imaging Studies

Hucl (2013) recommends conducting a plain upright abdominal X-ray as part of the initial evaluation of patients with symptoms of intestinal obstruction. This has high sensitivity for high grade obstruction, but is less effective for a more minor condition. Dilation of many bowel loops will indicate small bowel obstruction and distal obstruction will be revealed by dilation of the colon and a decompressed small bowel. If the X-ray is negative and clinical suspicion remains, computerized tomography (CT) should be conducted. A CT scan may suggest ischemia (thickened intestinal wall), or necrosis and perforation (hemorrhagic mesenteric changes, pneumatosis, and free intraperitoneal air), or colitis (with inflammatory indicators) (Jackson and Raiji, 2011). X-ray or CT may reveal fecal impaction, though neither is 100% sensitive. Magnetic resonance imaging (MRI) may be more sensitive than CT, but it is not usually recommended because of the ease and cost-effectiveness of CT (Jackson and Raiji, 2011). In addition, in the published case reports, laparotomy has been employed to complete the diagnosis and collect biopsy samples, and has confirmed the presence of fecal impaction (Levin et al., 2002; Baptista, 2014).

BOX 6.1 Consequences of Gastrointestinal Hypomotility

- Fecal impaction, paralytic ileus
- Acute colonic obstruction or pseudo-obstruction and colonic dilation
- Ischemia, necrosis, colitis, and perforation
- Bacterial overgrowth resulting in sepsis and feculent vomit
- Dehydration, electrolyte imbalance, and acidosis

6.1.6   Differential Diagnosis

Alternative diagnoses to antipsychotic-induced gastrointestinal hypomotility include ascites from liver disease. In the absence of evidence of intestinal abnormalities from X-ray, CT, or laparotomy, liver function testing will indicate the presence of primary hepatic dysfunction (Jackson and Raiji, 2011). Malignancy is another cause of intestinal obstruction and the development of an intestinal tumor may be associated with bleeding and loss of weight. The routine visualizing techniques will reveal the presence of a tumor.

If a motility disorder is confirmed, it is worth considering alternative causes, besides clozapine or other antipsychotics, including other medication, neurological diseases, and metabolic disturbances (Wald, 2016). Defecation disorders, caused by an anatomical abnormality, dyssynergic defecation, or inadequate propulsive forces, are also possible and diagnosis would involve a colon transit study using a radio-opaque marker or a wireless capsule (Wald, 2016).

6.1.7   Complications and Significant Sequelae

In addition to the complications mentioned above, ischemia, necrosis, perforation, colitis, sepsis, dehydration, acidosis, aspiration pneumonia, and severe gastrointestinal hypomotility can result in a range of other complications. Three of the cases listed in Table 6.1 also had pulmonary embolism (Ikai et al., 2013; Baptista, 2014; Flanagan, unpublished, 25-year-old woman). It is unclear whether the pulmonary embolism was coincidental or causally related to the syndrome precipitated by severe constipation. Hagg et al. (2009) cite a case of venous thromboembolism with first-generation antipsychotics in the context of fecal impaction and dehydration. The addition of dehydration to other risk factors for venous thromboembolism may have precipitated these cases.

Fecal impaction can exert physical pressure on essential organs. In one case near complete collapse of the vena cava occurred and in another aortic compression developed (Hibbard et al., 2009; Jambet et al., 2012). In a further case, such pressure was exerted on the diaphragm that pneumonia developed due to compromised respiratory function (Galappathie and Khan, 2014).

In addition, one patient, following removal of a long section of gangrenous bowel, required ventilation for 2.5 weeks and dialysis for kidney failure for 6 weeks (McKinnon et al., 2009). A further patient (a 49-year-old man), survived, but suffered the long-term consequences of a cerebrovascular accident during emergency surgery for hemicolectomy (Freudenreich and Goff, 2000). Another case with paralytic ileus experienced acute cardiac decompensation and respiratory failure (Dome et al, 2007). These last three cases illustrate how severely ill patients may become with the acute effects of constipation.

6.1.8 Management

The first objectives of treatment of life-threatening constipation are to remove the obstruction or impacted feces and correct physiological derangement. The initial measure is to cease, or at least reduce the dose of, any potentially causative medication. In two cases reducing the clozapine dose was efficacious (Pelizza et al., 2007; Rondla and Crane, 2007), and in another the patient responded to purgative treatment only after aripiprazole was withdrawn (Legrand et al., 2013).

Conservative management, involving bowel rest (nil by mouth) together with intravenous fluid, correction of any electrolyte imbalance and mechanical ventilation, if required, may be sufficient for full recovery if the patient is clinically stable (Pelizza et al., 2007; Jackson and Raiji, 2011; Galappathie and Khan, 2014; Kwiatkowski et al., 2011).

Administration of enemas may assist resolution of fecal impaction (Pelizza et al., 2007), but frequently mechanical intervention is required. Provided obstruction is incomplete, decompression of the small intestines is conducted by nasogastric tube and colonic decompression by colonoscopy (Silen, 2012). Adynamic ileus is usually responsive to decompression without surgery and in one such case the intestinal contents were cleared by laparotomy (Silen, 2012; Dome et al., 2007). If there is evidence of complete obstruction, intestinal stimulation or decompression may exacerbate the condition, leading to ischemia (Jackson and Raiji, 2011). In these cases immediate surgery is indicated (Box 6.2).

The importance of reversing dehydration with intravenous isotonic fluid cannot be over-emphasized. There may be a tendency to evaluate the likelihood of dehydration on the basis of severity of symptoms, specifically diarrhea and vomiting, but dehydration occurs as a consequence of intestinal

---

BOX 6.2 Management of Life-Threatening Constipation

- Withdraw potentially causative medication, or at least reduce dose
- Institute nil by mouth regime, with administration of IV isotonic fluid
- Correct any electrolyte imbalance and provide support for vital organs as required
- Conduct decompression by nasogastric tube for small intestines or colonoscopy for colon, provided obstruction is incomplete
- Administer antibiotics, if evidence or immediate risk of infection
- In the presence of clinical instability, abdominal sepsis or complete obstruction conduct urgent surgery
- If no adequate response to conservative measures in 48 h, schedule emergency surgery

obstruction and fecal impaction, as well as being a contributing cause. Few case reports describe administration of fluids (Pelizza et al., 2007; Leong et al., 2007; Abou Farha et al., 2012). Two cases treated apparently only with laxatives resulted in death within hours of admission (Abeyasinghe et al., 2010; Flanagan and Ball, 2011).

In the presence of renal impairment or severe dehydration putting renal function at risk, a bladder catheter will aid monitoring of urine output. Respiratory support and support of other organs should be given as required.

Fever and leukocytosis are indicators of infection, and fecal impaction is a risk factor. In the presence of these features, treatment with IV antibiotics with coverage against gram-negative and anaerobic bacteria should be initiated (Jackson and Raiji, 2011). Peritonitis, clinical instability, or unexplained leuko-cytosis or acidosis may indicate the presence of abdominal sepsis, intestinal ischemia, or perforation, and should prompt immediate surgery. If conservative management is opted for, but the abdominal obstruction does not resolve within 48 hours, urgent surgery is warranted (Jackson and Raiji, 2011).

Administration of systemic prokinetic agents may be beneficial, but data in support are limited for any clinical context involving the acute conse-quences of gastrointestinal hypomotility. A Cochrane review of trials of patients with postoperative ileus concluded that lidocaine and neostigmine might be beneficial, but more study is needed (Traut et al., 2008). Neostigmine is a cholinergic agent (cholinesterase inhibitor) that increases intestinal tone, and it has been used successfully in cases of severe hypomo-tility caused by clozapine (Dome et al., 2007; de Bruin et al., 2009; Galappathie and Khan, 2014). Bethanechol, used for maintenance prokinesis in one case (Poetter and Stewart, 2013), has muscarinic agonism and a selec-tive stimulant effect on smooth muscle. Alvimopan and methylnaltrexone antagonize μ-opioid receptors without crossing the blood-barrier and thus are used for opioid-induced constipation, but they have been found to stimu-late intestinal transit in general and may have efficacy in gastrointestinal motility disorders from other causes (Holzer, 2007; Thompson and Magnuson, 2012; Nelson and Camilleri, 2015).

Despite the catastrophic consequences and the potential for a fatal out-come of severe constipation with clozapine, there have been instances of rechallenge, including some which were apparently successful in the long term. Rechallenge was implemented because of the substantial mental health advantage of clozapine over other alternatives. In one case, diarrhéa with abdominal tenderness developed within hours of rechallenge (Abou Farha et al., 2012). Two other cases experienced a further episode of fecal impac-tion or bowel obstruction after clozapine re-initiation (Rege and Lafferty, 2008; Poetter and Stewart, 2013), but in one of these cases treatment with clozapine at the same dose as previously (500 mg d^{-1}) was successfully con-tinued for more than six months with aggressive gastrointestinal motility assistance (bethanechol, polyethylene glycol, and senna) (Poetter and Stewart, 2013). Two others were rechallenged with substantially lower doses of clozapine and one report states that exercise, as well as laxatives, was part of the management strategy (McKinnon et al., 2009; Ikai et al., 2013). In addition, weekly physical abdominal examinations and monthly or bimonthly abdominal X-rays were conducted (Ikai et al., 2013).

6.1.9 Prevention

Before prescription of clozapine, a thorough medical history should be taken and abdominal examination conducted. Any patients found to have constipation should receive treatment and resolution of the problem should be confirmed before clozapine is initiated. Patients commencing clozapine, and their family members and/or carers should be advised of the risk of life-threatening constipation. Steps should be taken to ensure clozapine recipients have adequate fluid intake, dietary fruit and vegetables, as well as sufficient exercise. The ideal amount of fiber in this context has not been determined and Palmer et al. (2008) have warned that high fiber without adequate fluid may increase the risk of intestinal obstruction (Box 6.3).

Clozapine should be titrated to the minimum effective dose, bearing in mind that response improves with time (Xiang et al., 2006). Clozapine and

---

BOX 6.3 Prevention or Management of Constipation in Patients Taking Antipsychotic Medication

- Take a thorough medical history and treat any preexisting constipation before prescribing
- Advise patient, family members, and carers of the need to prevent constipation
- Advise of the importance of:
  - Fruit and vegetable intake
  - Fluid intake
  - Exercise
- Titrate to the lowest effective dose and minimize use of other constipating medication
- Be aware of factors changing bioavailability of the antipsychotic and check plasma concentrations to avoid excessive exposure
- Consider use of a stool softener and a stimulant for prevention
- Conduct weekly bowel performance review in first 4 weeks of therapy and monthly thereafter
- In those at high risk of constipation conduct colon transit time studies to determine adequacy of intervention

norclozapine plasma concentrations should be monitored at frequent regular intervals and checked following smoking cessation, addition of medication interfering with clozapine metabolism, use of laxatives, and in the presence of inflammatory illness (de Leon, 2004; Pfuhlmann et al., 2009). Dose should be adjusted if plasma concentrations are too high or too low, based on knowledge of appropriate concentrations for the patient.

Since almost 40% of cases of life-threatening hypomotility develop within the first 4 months of clozapine therapy (Palmer et al., 2008), reviewing patients weekly for bowel function for the first 4 months may serve to reduce case severity. Ongoing monitoring, including a regular physical examination, should be conducted, and changes which may increase the risk of constipation should prompt increased vigilance. Patients with difficulties could be referred to practitioners with expertise in the management of constipation, such as pain specialists managing opiate-induced constipation. Such monitoring may reduce the risk of severe constipation later in therapy, as patients with problems would receive suitable early interventions.

Any patients with confirmed constipation should be referred to a gastroenterologist before symptoms develop. The presence of symptoms, abdominal pain and distension, diarrhea, and vomiting, means the hypomotility has reached a critical stage.

Bulking agents are not recommended as laxatives in this setting, but a combination of a stool softener and a stimulant, for example, docusate or polyethylene glycol and senna, is thought to be suitable (Palmer et al., 2008). In a review article, Wald (2016) has advised that stimulant laxatives are underused, and when used appropriately, they are both safe and effective in the long-term prevention of constipation, and carry no risk of harm.

Other preventive strategies require further investigation. Gum chewing elicits release of gastrin, pancreatic polypeptide, and neurotensin all of which promote gastrointestinal motility (Hiranyakas et al., 2011), and results of a preliminary study suggested that orlistat may reduce constipation in clozapine recipients, but whether it significantly blunts the risk of severe constipation in either the short, or long term is unknown (Chukhin et al., 2013). Recently, lubiprostone and linaclotide, which are secretory drugs, have become available (Wald, 2016). Lubiprostone 48 μg d^{-1}, with lactulose and docusate, permitted a patient with previous bowel obstruction with clozapine to have a successful clozapine rechallenge (Table 6.1) (Meyer and Cummings, 2014). Where there is a high risk of constipation, constipation proving difficult to treat adequately, or the intention to rechallenge with clozapine after severe hypomotility, colon transit-time studies using a radio-opaque marker, radionuclide scintigraphy or a wireless motility capsule will assist in the assessment of the efficacy of treatment and help to shape an efficacious management regimen (Kim and Rhee, 2012).

6.1.10 Conclusion

Although life-threatening hypomotility with antipsychotic drugs, particularly clozapine, has been a recognized adverse reaction for two decades (Hayes and Gibler, 1995), there is only a flimsy evidence base for pharmacological strategies (both topical and systemic) to prevent or treat this problem. Clinicians are left with treating empirically using their knowledge of the mechanism of action of the various options and the history of interventions given to the individual patient.

6.2 DYSPHAGIA AND SIALORRHEA

6.2.1 General Considerations

Antipsychotic-induced dysphagia and sialorrhea are gastrointestinal system adverse effects with potentially life-threatening consequences, namely, aspiration pneumonia, asphyxia, and choking (Aldridge and Taylor, 2012; Visser et al., 2014; Trigoboff et al., 2013). There is some overlap in possible mechanism, complications and treatment, between sialorrhea and dysphagia. Clozapine, in particular, is associated with hypersalivation (Praharaj et al., 2006), but it has also been described with olanzapine and risperidone (Boyce and Bakheet, 2005; Freudenreich, 2005). Having an excess of saliva is vexing to the patient, causing drooling, and at night, a choking sensation and a wet pillow.

In three published reports, a patient developed life-threatening pneumonia in the context of sialorrhea associated with clozapine and the cause was thought to be aspiration of saliva (Hinkes et al., 1996; Saenger et al., 2013; Trigoboff et al., 2013). Although in these cases there was no firm evidence that aspiration had occurred, this remains a clinical risk in patients with sialorrhea, particularly if they become severely sedated or consciousness is impaired or in the presence of dysphagia. Aspiration pneumonia is a known adverse effect in schizophrenia and antipsychotic drug use (Hatta et al., 2014).

6.2.2 Pathobiology

Dysphagia may have a neuropsychiatric cause (i.e., be disease-related), but the swallowing mechanism involves smooth coordination of muscular activity and could be impaired by anticholinergic medication (Visser et al. 2014). Alternatively, dysphagia could be a manifestation of extrapyramidal effects or tardive dyskinesia, or a consequence of eating too quickly (Bazemore et al., 1991). After four patients died of asphyxia in a 400-bed psychiatric hospital in 1 year, Bazemore et al. (1991) documented 32 instances of choking the following year and identified five causes of dysphagia: bradykinetic, dyskinetic, paralytic, fast eating, and medical, with the first three potentially related to antipsychotic medication. Dysphagia has been associated with first- and second-generation antipsychotics (haloperidol, loxapine, trifluperazine, aripiprazole, clozapine, olanzapine, quetiapine, and risperidone) (Sokoloff and Pavlakovic, 1997; Dziewas et al., 2007; Rudolph et al., 2008; Lin et al., 2012).

Salivary flow is known to be mediated by cholinergic activity, particularly the M3 muscarinic receptors. Thus sialorrhea with clozapine appears paradoxical; clozapine would be expected to reduce saliva generation. However, the cause of excessive saliva may be disruption of the swallowing reflex, rather than overproduction, or the cause may lie in the anticholinergeric effect of clozapine on esophageal motility (Fitzsimons et al., 2005; Kruger, 2014). In addition, an inability to seal the lips will contribute to the overflow effect (Silvestre-Donat and Silvestre-Rangil, 2014).

6.2.3 Prevention and Management

Sialorrhea frequently develops during clozapine titration and, as some degree of tolerance may occur, a slower titration scheme may reduce severity. Similarly, for a patient stabilized on clozapine reducing the dose may help, provided it does not lead to worsening psychiatric symptoms. Alternatively, augmenting clozapine with an antipsychotic not associated with sialorrhea, such as amisulpride or sulpiride, may allow the dose of clozapine to be reduced without risking a deterioration in mental health (Cook and Hoogenboom, 2004; Kreinin et al., 2006; Kreinin et al., 2005; Croissant et al., 2005). Administration of anticholinergics (e.g., atropine spray, benzatropine tablets) has been used to minimize the distress caused by excessive saliva (Camp-Bruno et al., 1989), but systemic anticholinergics will increase the risk and severity of constipation, and will not be beneficial if esophageal hypomotility is involved in the etiology of the condition. Cautious use of amitriptyline ($75-100$ mg d^{-1}) has been suggested to treat not only hypersalivation, but also clozapine-induced nocturnal enuresis (Praharaj and Arora, 2007). Alternatively, α2-adrenergic agonists such as clonidine and lofexidine have also been tried to minimize clozapine-induced hypersalivation (Sockalingam et al., 2007). Patients being treated with clonidine should have their blood pressure checked, due to the antihypertensive properties of this drug (Fitzsimons et al., 2005).

The use of chewing gum may help minimize the saliva problem during the day. At night, raising the height of pillows and covering them with a towel may make the problem more tolerable. At the same time it is important to maintain hydration.

For dysphagia, the obvious options are to reduce the dose or switch to another antipsychotic. Alternatively, for both sialorrhea and dysphagia, instruction in swallowing without inhaling, and repeated swallowing exercises may be beneficial (Silvestre-Donat and Silvestre-Rangil, 2014). Further, in the presence of either dysphagia or hypersalivation, it may be

---

BOX 6.4 Sialorrhea and Dysphagia

- Sialorrhea and dysphagia may be associated with aspiration pneumonia, asphyxia, and choking
- Sialorrhea may be caused by excessive saliva production, impaired swallowing reflex, or esophageal hypomotility
- Dysphagia could be related to anticholinergic, extrapyramidal, or tardive dyskinesic effects
- Treatment options for sialorrhea include anticholinergics, α2-adrenergic agonists, and antipsychotic dose reduction with or without augmentation with an alternative antipsychotic
- Patients with sialorrhea or dysphagia may benefit from referral to a speech therapist

---

worth investigating the swallowing mechanism using barium esophagram, manometry or videofluoroscopy and referring the patient to a speech therapist with expertise in stroke or Parkinson's disease (Kruger, 2014; Aldridge and Taylor, 2012) (Box 6.4).

ACKNOWLEDGMENT

The authors wish to thank Professor Dan Dumitrascu, Professor of Medicine (Gastroenterology), University of Medicine and Pharmacy, Cluj, Romania, for checking the manuscript.

REFERENCES

Gastrointestinal Hypomotility

Abeyasinghe, N., Gunathilake, T.B., Gambheera, H., 2010. Death due to intestinal obstruction in a patient treated with clozapine. Sri Lankan J. Psychiatr. 1, 64–66.

Abou Farha, K., van Vliet, A., Knegtering, H., Bruggeman, R., 2012. The value of desmethylclozapine and serum CRP in clozapine toxicity: a case report. Case Rep. Psychiatr. 2012, 592784.

Altree, T.J., Galletly, C., 2013. Laxative use and altered drug absorption. Aust. N. Z. J. Psychiatr. 47, 686.

Baptista, T., 2014. A fatal case of ischemic colitis during clozapine administration. Rev. Bras. Psiquiatr. 36, 358.

Barbui, C., Nose, M., Bindman, J., Schene, A., Becker, T., Mazzi, M.A., et al., 2005. Sex differences in the subjective tolerability of antipsychotic drugs. J. Clin. Psychopharmacol. 25, 521–526.

Bishara, D., Taylor, D., 2014. Adverse effects of clozapine in older patients: epidemiology, prevention and management. Drugs Aging 31, 11–20.

Boggs, D., Kelly, D.L., Feldman, S., McMahon, R.P., 2008. Quetiapine at high doses for the treatment of refractory schizophrenia. Schizophr. Res. 101, 347–348.

Bowskill, S., Couchman, L., MacCabe, J.H., Flanagan, R.J., 2012. Plasma clozapine and norclozapine in relation to prescribed dose and other factors in patients aged 65 years and over: data from a therapeutic drug monitoring service, 1996–2010. Hum. Psychopharmacol. 27, 277–283.

Bregman, A., Fritz, K., Xiong, G.L., 2014. Lactulose-associated lithium toxicity: a case series. J. Clin. Psychopharmacol. 34, 742–743.

Brown, R., Taylor, M.J., Geddes, J., 2013. Aripiprazole alone or in combination for acute mania. Cochrane Database Syst. Rev. 12, CD005000.

Bullock, S., Manias, E., Galbraith, A., 2007. Antipsychotic drugs. In: Fundamentals of Pharmacology, fifth ed. Pearson Education Australia, Frenchs Forest, NSW, pp. 355–368. (Chapter 34).

Chukhin, E., Takala, P., Hakko, H., Raidma, M., Putkonen, H., Räsänen, P., et al., 2013. In a randomized placebo-controlled add-on study orlistat significantly reduced clozapine-induced constipation. Int. Clin. Psychopharmacol. 28, 67–70.

de Beaurepaire, R., Trinh, I., Guirao, S., Taieb, M., 2015. Colitis possibly induced by quetiapine. BMJ Case Rep. Feb 26, Available from: http://dx.doi.org/10.1136/bcr-2014-207912.

de Bruin, G.J., Bac, D.J., van Puijenbroek, E.P., van der Klooster, J.M., 2009. Ogilvie Syndrome induced by clozapine. Ned. Tijdschr. Geneeskd. 153, B437.

De Hert, M., Dockx, L., Bernagie, C., Peuskens, B., Sweers, K., Leucht, S., et al., 2011a. Prevalence and severity of antipsychotic related constipation in patients with schizophrenia: a retrospective descriptive study. BMC. Gastroenterol. 11, 17.

De Hert, M., Hudyana, H., Dockx, L., Bernagie, C., Sweers, K., Tack, J., et al., 2011b. Second-generation antipsychotics and constipation: a review of the literature. Eur. Psychiat. 26, 34–44.

de Leon, J., 2004. Respiratory infections rather than antibiotics may increase clozapine levels: a critical review of the literature. J. Clin. Psychiatry 65, 1144–1145.

Díaz-Caneja, C.M., González-Molinier, M., Conejo Galindo, J., Moreno Iñiguez, M., 2010. Severe bowel ischemia due to clozapine with complete remission after withdrawal. J. Clin. Psychopharmacol. 30, 463–465.

Dome, P., Teleki, Z., Kotanyi, R., 2007. Paralytic ileus associated with combined atypical antipsychotic therapy. Prog. Neuropsychopharmacol. Biol. Psychiatr. 31, 557–560.

Drew, L., Herdson, P., 1997. Clozapine and constipation: a serious issue. Aust. N. Z. J. Psychiatr. 31, 149–150.

Erickson, B., Morris, D.M., Reeve, A., 1995. Clozapine-associated postoperative ileus: case report and review of the literature. Arch. Gen. Psychiatry. 52, 508–509.

Every-Palmer, S., Nowitz, M., Stanley, J., Grant, E., Huthwaite, M., Dunn, H., et al., 2016. Clozapine-treated patients have marked gastrointestinal hypomotility, the probable basis of life-threatening gastrointestinal complications: a cross sectional study. EBioMedicine 5, 25–34.

Fayad, S.M., Bruijnzeel, D.M., 2012. A fatal case of adynamic ileus following initiation of clozapine. Am J Psychiatr 169, 538–539.

Ferslew, K.E., Hagardorn, A.N., Harlan, G.C., McCormick, W.F., 1998. A fatal drug interaction between clozapine and fluoxetine. J. Forensic. Sci. 43, 1082–1085.

Flanagan, R.J., Ball, R.Y., 2011. Gastrointestinal hypomotility: an under-recognised life-threatening adverse effect of clozapine. Forensic. Sci. Int. 206, e31–e36.

Flanagan, R.J., Spencer, E.P., Morgan, P.E., Barnes, T.R., Dunk, L., 2005. Suspected clozapine poisoning in the UK/Eire, 1992-2003. Forensic. Sci. Int. 155, 91–99.

Frenchman, I.B., 2005. Atypical antipsychotics for nursing home patients: a retrospective chart review. Drugs Aging 22, 257–264.

Freudenreich, O., Goff, D.C., 2000. Colon perforation and peritonitis associated with clozapine. J. Clin. Psychiatr. 61, 950−951.

Friedberg, J.W., Frankenburg, F.R., Burk, J., Johnson, W., 1995. Clozapine-caused eosinophilic colitis. Ann. Clin. Psychiatr. 7, 97−98.

Galappathie, N., Khan, S., 2014. Clozapine-associated pneumonia and respiratory arrest secondary to severe constipation. Med. Sci. Law. 54, 105−109.

Hagg, S., Jonsson, A.K., Spigset, O., 2009. Risk of venous thromboembolism due to antipsychotic drug therapy. Expert. Opin. Drug. Saf. 8, 537−547.

Hajek, P., Gillison, F., McRobbie, H., 2003. Stopping smoking can cause constipation. Addiction 98, 1563−1567.

Hay, A.M., 1978. Association between chlorpromazine therapy and necrotizing colitis: report of a case. Dis. Colon. Rectum. 21, 380−382.

Hayes, G., Gibler, B., 1995. Clozapine-induced constipation. Am J Psychiatr 152, 298.

Hibbard, K.R., Propst, A., Frank, D.E., Wyse, J., 2009. Fatalities associated with clozapine-related constipation and bowel obstruction: a literature review and two case reports. Psychosomatics 50, 416−419.

Hiranyakas, A., Bashankaev, B., Seo, C.J., Khaikin, M., Wexner, S.D., 2011. Epidemiology, pathophysiology and medical management of postoperative ileus in the elderly. Drugs Aging 28, 107−118.

Holzer, P., 2007. Treatment of opioid-induced gut dysfunction. Expert. Opin. Investig. Drugs. 16, 181−194.

Hucl, T., 2013. Acute GI obstruction. Best. Pract. Res. Clin. Gastroenterol. 27, 691−707.

Ikai, S., Suzuki, T., Uchida, H., Mimura, M., Fujii, Y., 2013. Reintroduction of clozapine after perforation of the large intestine—a case report and review of the literature. Ann Pharmacother 47, e31.

Jackson, P.G., Raiji, M., 2011. Evaluation and management of intestinal obstruction. Am. Fam. Physician. 83, 159−165.

Jambet, S., Guiu, B., Olive-Abergel, P., Grandvuillemin, A., Yeguiayan, J.M., Ortega-Deballon, P., 2012. Psychiatric drug-induced fatal abdominal compartment syndrome. Am. J. Emerg. Med. 30, 513.e5-7.

Karmacharya, R., Mino, M., Pirl, W.F., 2005. Clozapine-induced eosinophilic colitis. Am. J. Psychiatr. 162, 1386−1387.

Khaldi, S., Gourevitch, R., Matmar, M., Llory, A., Olié, J.P., Chauvelot-Moachon, L., 2005. Necrotizing enterocolitis after antipsychotic treatment involving clozapine and review of severe digestive complications—a case report. Pharmacopsychiatry 38, 220−221.

Kim, E.R., Rhee, P.L., 2012. How to interpret a functional or motility test—colon transit study. J Neurogastroenterol Motil 18, 94−99.

Kwiatkowski, M., Denka, Z.D., White, C.C., 2011. Paralytic ileus requiring hospitalization secondary to high-dose antipsychotic polypharmacy and benztropine. Gen. Hosp. Psychiatr. 33, 200.e5-7.

Lambert, T.J.R., Velakoulis, D., Pantellis, C., 2003. Medical comorbidity in schizophrenia. Med J Aust 178, S67−S70.

Lameh, J., Burstein, E.S., Taylor, E., Weiner, D.M., Vanover, K.E., Bonhaus, D.W., 2007. Pharmacology of N-desmethylclozapine. Pharmacol. Ther. 115, 223−231.

Legrand, G., May, R., Richard, B., Kernisant, M., Jalenques, I., 2013. A case report of partial bowel obstruction after aripiprazole addition to clozapine in a young male with schizophrenia. J. Clin. Psychopharmacol. 33, 571−572.

Lemyze, M., Chaaban, R., Collet, F., 2009. Psychotic woman with painful abdominal distension. Life-threatening psychotropic drug-induced gastrointestinal hypomotility. Ann. Emerg. Med. 54, 756–759.

Leong, Q.M., Wong, K.S., Koh, D.C., 2007. Necrotising colitis related to clozapine? A rare but life threatening side effect. World. J. Emerg. Surg. 2, 21.

Levin, T.T., Barrett, J., Mendelowitz, A., 2002. Death from clozapine-induced constipation: case report and literature review. Psychosomatics 43, 71–73.

Lim, D.K., Mahendran, R., 2002. Risperidone and megacolon. Singapore. Med. J. 43, 530–532.

Lu, C.L., Shen, Y.C., 2014. Aripiprazole for the treatment of a manic patient with clozapine-related colonic obstruction receiving total colectomy. J. Neuropsychiatry. Clin. Neurosci. 26, E58–E59.

Manu, P., Kane, J.M., Correll, C.U., 2011. Sudden deaths in psychiatric patients. J. Clin. Psychiatry 72, 936–941.

McKinnon, N.D., Azad, A., Waters, B.M., Joshi, K.G., 2009. Clozapine-induced bowel infarction: a case report. Psychiatry (Edgmont) 6, 30–35.

Meyer, J.M., Cummings, M.A., 2014. Lubiprostone for treatment-resistant constipation associated with clozapine use. Acta Psychiatr. Scand. 130, 71–72.

Nelson, A.D., Camilleri, M., 2015. Chronic opioid induced constipation in patients with nonmalignant pain: challenges and opportunities. Therap. Adv. Gastroenterol. 8 (4), 206–220. Available from: http://dx.doi.org/10.1177/1756283X15578608.

Newton, J.L., 2005. Effect of age-related changes in gastric physiology on tolerability of medications for older people. Drugs Aging 22, 655–661.

Nielsen, J., Meyer, J.M., 2012. Risk factors for ileus in patients with schizophrenia. Schizophr. Bull. 38, 592–598.

Palmer, S.E., McLean, R.M., Ellis, P.M., Harrison-Woolrych, M., 2008. Life-threatening clozapine-induced gastrointestinal hypomotility: an analysis of 102 cases. J. Clin. Psychiatr. 69, 759–768.

Park, S.J., Gunn, N., Harrison, S.A., 2012. Olanzapine and benztropine as a cause of ischemic colitis in a 27-year-old man. J. Clin. Gastroenterol. 46, 515–517.

Pelizza, L., De Luca, P., La Pesa, M., Borella, D., 2007. Clozapine-induced intestinal occlusion: a serious side effect. Acta Biomed. 78, 144–148.

Pelizza, L., Melegari, M., 2007. Clozapine-induced microscopic colitis: a case report and review of the literature. J. Clin. Psychopharmacol. 27, 571–574.

Peyrière, H., Roux, C., Ferard, C., Deleau, N., Kreft-Jais, C., Hillaire-Buys, D., et al., 2009. French Network of the Pharmacovigilance Centers. Antipsychotics-induced ischaemic colitis and gastrointestinal necrosis: a review of the French pharmacovigilance database. Pharmacoepidemiol. Drug. Saf. 18, 948–955.

Pfuhlmann, B., Hiemke, C., Unterecker, S., Burger, R., Schmidtke, A., Riederer, P., et al., 2009. Toxic clozapine serum levels during inflammatory reactions. J. Clin. Psychopharmacol. 29, 392–394.

Poetter, C.E., Stewart, J.T., 2013. Treatment of clozapine-induced constipation with bethanechol. J. Clin. Psychopharmacol. 33, 713–714.

Ramamourthy, P., Kumaran, A., Kattimani, S., 2013. Risperidone associated paralytic ileus in schizophrenia. Indian J. Psychol. Med. 35, 87–88.

Rege, S., Lafferty, T., 2008. Life-threatening constipation associated with clozapine. Australas. Psychiatry 16, 216–219.

Rondla, S., Crane, S., 2007. A case of clozapine-induced paralytic ileus. Emerg. Med. J. 24, e12.

Rostami-Hodjegan, A., Amin, A.M., Spencer, E.P., Lennard, M.S., Tucker, G.T., Flanagan, R.J., 2004. Influence of dose, cigarette smoking, age, sex and metabolic activity on plasma clozapine concentrations: a predictive model and nomograms to aid clozapine dose adjustment and to assess compliance in individual patients. J. Clin. Psychopharmacol. 24, 70–78.

Rousseau, A., Charbonneau, M., 2007. Severe fecal impaction under clozapine, resulting in death. J. Assn. Med. Psychiatr. Quebec 11, 16–18.

Shammi, C.M., Remington, G., 1997. Clozapine-induced necrotizing colitis. J. Clin. Psychopharmacol. 17, 230–232.

Silen W (2012) Acute intestinal obstruction. In: Longo D.L., Fauci A.S., Kasper D.L., Hauser S. L., Jameson J., Loscalzo J. (Eds.), Harrison's Principles of Internal Medicine, eighteenth ed. New York, NY: McGraw-Hill. <http://accessmedicine.mhmedical.com.ezproxy.lib.monash. edu.au/content.aspx?bookid=331&Sectionid=40727093> (accessed 19.01.2016) (Chapter 299).

Sim, K., Yong, T.W., Liew, E., Choon, C.H., 2006. Clozapine-associated pseudomembranous colitis: a case report and review of the literature. J. Clin. Psychopharmacol. 26, 89.

Sirois, F.J., 2005. Haloperidol-induced ileus. Psychosomatics 46, 275–276.

Suzuki, T., Uchida, H., Watanabe, K., Kashima, H., 2007. Minimizing antipsychotic medication obviated the need for enema against severe constipation leading to paralytic ileus: a case report. J. Clin. Pharm. Ther. 32, 525–527.

Tan, E.J., Soh, K.C., Ngiam, K.Y., 2013. Colonic architectural change on colonoscopy in patients taking psychotropic medications. Surg. Endosc. 27, 1601–1606.

Théret, L., Germain, M.L., Burde, A., 1995. Current aspects of the use of clozapine in the Châlons-sur-Marne Psychiatric Hospital: intestinal occlusion with clozapine. Ann. Med. Psychol (Paris) 153, 474–477.

Thompson, M., Magnuson, B., 2012. Management of postoperative ileus. Orthopedics 35, 213–217.

Toro, A., Cappello, G., Mannino, M., Di Carlo, I., 2014. Could the complications of megacolon be avoided by monitoring the risk patients? Cases report. Chirurgia (Bucur) 109, 550–554.

Townsend, G., Curtis, D., 2006. Case report: rapidly fatal bowel ischaemia on clozapine treatment. BMC Psychiatry 6, 43.

Traut, U., Brugger, L., Kunz, R., Pauli-Magnus, C., Haug, K., Bucher, H.C., et al., 2008. Systemic prokinetic pharmacologic treatment for postoperative adynamic ileus following abdominal surgery in adults. Cochrane Database Syst Rev. 1, CD004930.

Van Veggel, M., Olofinjana, O., Davies, G., Taylor, D., 2013. Clozapine and gastro-oesophageal reflux disease (GORD)—an investigation of temporal association. Acta Psychiatr. Scand. 127, 69–77.

Wald, A., 2016. Constipation. Advances in diagnosis and treatment. J. Am. Med. Assoc. 315, 185–191.

Xiang, Y.Q., Zhang, Z.J., Weng, Y.Z., et al., 2006. Serum concentrations of clozapine and norclozapine in the prediction of relapse of patients with schizophrenia. Schizophr. Res. 83, 201–210.

Yu, S.C., Chen, H.K., Lee, S.M., 2013. Rapid development of fatal bowel infarction within 1 week after clozapine treatment: a case report. Gen. Hosp. Psychiatr. 35, 679. e5–6.

Dysphagia and Sialorrhea

Aldridge, K.J., Taylor, N.F., 2012. Dysphagia is a common and serious problem for adults with mental illness: a systematic review. Dysphagia 27, 124–137.

Bazemore, P.H., Tonkonogy, J., Ananth, R., 1991. Dysphagia in psychiatric patients: clinical and videofluoroscopic study. Dysphagia 6, 2–5.

Boyce, H.W., Bakheet, M.R., 2005. Sialorrhea: a review of a vexing, often unrecognized sign of oropharyngeal and esophageal disease. J. Clin. Gastroenterol. 39, 89−97.

Camp-Bruno, J.A., Winsberg, B.G., Green-Parsons, A.R., Abrams, J.P., 1989. Efficacy of benztropine therapy to drooling. Dev. Med. Child Neurol. 31, 309−319.

Cook, B., Hoogenboom, G., 2004. Combined use of amisulpride and clozapine for patients with treatment-resistant schizophrenia. Australas. Psychiatry 12, 74−76.

Croissant, B., Hermann, D., Olbrich, R., 2005. Reduction of side effects by combining clozapine with amisulpride: case report and short review of clozapine-induced hypersalivation—a case report. Pharmacopsychiatry 38, 38−39.

Dziewas, R., Warnecke, T., Schnabel, M., Ritter, M., Nabavi, D.G., Schilling, M., et al., 2007. Neuroleptic-induced dysphagia: case report and literature review. Dysphagia 22, 63−67.

Fitzsimons, J., Berk, M., Lambert, T., Bourin, M., Dodd, S., 2005. A review of clozapine safety. Expert. Opin. Drug. Saf. 4, 731−744.

Freudenreich, O., 2005. Drug-induced sialorrhea. Drugs Today (Barc) 41, 411−418.

Hatta, K., Kishi, Y., Wada, K., Odawara, T., Takeuchi, T., Shiganami, T., et al., 2014. Antipsychotics for delirium in the general hospital setting in consecutive 2453 inpatients: a prospective observational study. Int. J. Geriatr. Psychiatry. 29, 253−262.

Hinkes, R., Quesada, T.V., Currier, M.B., Gonzalez-Blanco, M., 1996. Aspiration pneumonia possibly secondary to clozapine-induced sialorrhea. J. Clin. Psychopharmacol. 16, 462−463.

Kreinin, A., Epshtein, S., Sheinkman, A., Tell, E., 2005. Sulpiride addition for the treatment of clozapine-induced hypersalivation: preliminary study. Isr J Psychiatr Relat Sci 42, 61−63.

Kreinin, A., Novitski, D., Weizman, A., 2006. Amisulpride treatment of clozapine-induced hypersalivation in schizophrenia patients: a randomized, double-blind, placebo-controlled cross-over study. Int. Clin. Psychopharmacol. 21, 99−103.

Kruger, D., 2014. Assessing esophageal dysphagia. J. Am. Acad. Physician. Assist. 27, 23−30.

Lin, T.W., Lee, B.S., Liao, Y.C., Chiu, N.Y., Hsu, W.Y., 2012. High dosage of aripiprazole-induced dysphagia. Int. J. Eat. Disord. 45, 305−306.

Praharaj, S.K., Arora, M., Gandotra, S., 2006. Clozapine-induced sialorrhea: pathophysiology and management strategies. Psychopharmacology (Berl) 185, 265−273.

Praharaj, S.K., Arora, M., 2007. Amitriptyline for clozapine-induced nocturnal enuresis and sialorrhoea. Br. J. Clin. Pharmacol. 63, 128−129.

Rudolph, J.L., Gardner, K.F., Gramigna, G.D., McGlinchey, R.E., 2008. Antipsychotics and oropharyngeal dysphagia in hospitalized older patients. J. Clin. Psychopharmacol. 28, 532−535.

Saenger, R.C., Finch, T.H., Francois, D., 2013. Aspiration pneumonia due to clozapine-induced sialorrhea. Clin. Schizophr. Relat. Psychoses 1−7, Jun 17.

Silvestre-Donat, F.J., Silvestre-Rangil, J., 2014. Drooling. Monogr. Oral. Sci. 24, 126−134.

Sockalingam, S., Shammi, C., Remington, G., 2007. Clozapine-induced hypersalivation: a review of treatment strategies. Can. J. Psychiatr. 52, 377−384.

Sokoloff, L.G., Pavlakovic, R., 1997. Neuroleptic-induced dysphagia. Dysphagia 12, 177−179.

Trigoboff, E., Grace, J., Szymanski, H., Bhullar, J., Lee, C., Watson, T., 2013. Sialorrhea and aspiration pneumonia: a case study. Innov. Clin. Neurosci. 10, 20−27.

Visser, H.K., Wigington, J.L., Keltner, N.L., Kowalski, P.C., 2014. Biological perspectives: Choking and antipsychotics: is this a significant concern? Perspect. Psychiatr. Care 50, 79−82.

Chapter 7

Liver Failure

Katie F.M. Marwick
University of Edinburgh, Edinburgh, United Kingdom

7.1 DEFINITION

Acute liver failure is rapid onset hepatic necrosis leading to a severe impairment of liver function associated with multiorgan failure (Bernal et al., 2010). It is generally understood as arising in the absence of preexisting liver disease, although some authors suggest preexisting autoimmune hepatitis, Wilson's disease, or hepatitis B infection would not exclude the diagnosis (Punzalan and Barry, 2015). It is a rare syndrome caused predominantly by drugs in high income countries and by viral infection in lower income countries (Bernal et al., 2010). Very rarely, antipsychotics can cause acute liver failure, but are not a drug class commonly associated with severe drug-induced liver injury (antimicrobials are the commonest) (Andrade et al., 2005). Far more often, antipsychotics are associated with asymptomatic elevations in liver function tests (LFT). Above certain thresholds these altered laboratory parameters are termed drug-induced liver injury, whether or not they are associated with symptoms of liver dysfunction (Navarro and Senior, 2006). Rarely, drug-induced liver injury can progress to liver failure, and for this reason LFT elevations are now the leading cause of drug withdrawal due to safety concerns (Bakke et al., 1995). This chapter will focus on the rare but life-threatening antipsychotic side effect of acute liver failure, but will also review the literature on what is much more likely to be encountered in clinical practice, that is, asymptomatically elevated LFT in adults taking regular antipsychotics.

7.2 SEARCH STRATEGY

The contents of this chapter are based largely on data extracted in a recent systematic review (Marwick et al., 2012), with the search updated to include subsequently published studies (to week 15, 2015). The original review screened 878 articles and found 10 group studies and 91 case reports/series to be eligible. The updated search screened 430 subsequently published articles, of which 16 case reports were eligible. This chapter is therefore based on data

Life-Threatening Effects of Antipsychotic Drugs. DOI: http://dx.doi.org/10.1016/B978-0-12-803376-0.00007-1
© 2016 Elsevier Inc. All rights reserved.

synthesized from 10 group studies and 107 case reports/series. LFTs were considered to include those in current widespread use: serum glutamic pyruvic transaminase (SGPT)/alanine transaminase/alanine aminotransferase (ALT); serum glutamic oxaloacetic transaminase (SGOT)/aspartate transaminase/aspartate aminotransferase (AST); gamma-glutamyltransferase/gamma-glutamyl transpeptidase (GGT); alkaline phosphatase (ALP); and total bilirubin (Bil).

7.3 EPIDEMIOLOGY

7.3.1 Acute Liver Failure

Acute liver failure occurs rarely, with an annual incidence of around six cases per million people in high income countries where paracetamol (acetaminophen) overdose is common (Bretherick et al., 2011; Bower et al., 2007) and around one case per million people per year in countries where it is not (Brandsœter et al., 2002; Escorsell et al., 2007). Excluding paracetamol (acetaminophen) overdose, drug-induced liver failure accounts for around 0.1—0.3 cases per million people per year (Escorsell et al., 2007; Brandsœter et al., 2002; Bretherick et al., 2011). Drug-induced liver failure is more common in older adults, in contrast to other etiologies (Bower et al., 2007; Andrade et al., 2005), and more common in women (Reuben et al., 2010). Severe drug-induced liver injury (defined as liver injury sufficient to require referral to hospital—in most cases not acute liver failure) is more common, at around 17 cases per million people per year (Andrade et al., 2005). Symptomatic drug-induced liver injury (generally not requiring referral to hospital) is commoner still, at around 140 cases per million people per year (Sgro et al., 2002). Females with drug-induced liver injury have been found to be more likely to progress to liver failure than men (Andrade et al., 2005). In general, drug-induced liver injury is more common in those taking more than one potentially hepatotoxic medication (de Abajo et al., 2004).

Acute liver failure associated with antipsychotics is rare and it is not possible to draw out epidemiological risk factors specific to it. However, some work has been done on the epidemiology of antipsychotic-induced severe liver injury. The antipsychotic about which most is known is chlorpromazine, in part because it has a long history of common use. Analyses of UK primary care databases in the 1980s and 1990s found that risk of chlorpromazine-induced severe liver injury was around 1 in 1000 users (de Abajo et al., 2004; Derby et al., 1993). Risk was greatest in older adults (aged >70 years), symptoms were most likely to arise within 30 days of commencing the drug, risk was not influenced by dose or by sex, and all cases initially presented with jaundice (de Abajo et al., 2004; Derby et al., 1993).

The systematic search identified 107 case reports/series reporting an association between antipsychotic use and symptomatic liver injury, of which a minority progressed to acute liver failure (Table 7.1). The information from

TABLE 7.1 Case Reports Linking Antipsychotics to Symptomatic Liver Injury

Drug	Severe Injury/ Outcome Not Reported (n)	Fatal Injury (n)
Phenothiazines		
Chlorpromazine	>350 (reviewed in[1] also[2-13])	8[14-21]
Prochlorperazine	12[1,22-30]	1[31]
Thioridazine	7[32-38]	-
Promazine	2[39,40]	-
Trifluoperazine	2[41,42]	-
Trifluoperazine then Thioridazone	-	1[43]
Fluphenazine	3[44-46]	-
Perazine	1[47]	-
Other Antipsychotic Classes		
Clozapine	23[48-67]	3[68-70]
Quetiapine	4[71-74]	2[75,76]
Risperidone	14[72,77-87]	-
Olanzapine	9[88-96]	-
Sulpiride	4[97-100]	-
Bromperidol	1[101]	-
Chlorprothixene	1[102]	-
Haloperidol	1[103]	-
Molindone	1[104]	-
Ziprasidone	1[105]	-

1. Ishak, K.G. Irey, N.S., 1972. Hepatic injury associated with the phenothiazines. Clinicopathologic and follow-up study of 36 patients. Arch. Pathol. Lab. Med. 93, 283–304.
2. Ahmed, A., 1972. Hepatitis and phenothiazines. J. Indian Med. Assoc. 58, 300.
3. Bach, N., Thung, S.N., Schaffner, F., Tobias, H., 1989. Exaggerated cholestasis and hepatic fibrosis following simultaneous administration of chlorpromazine and sodium valproate. Dig. Dis. Sci. 34, 1303–1307.
4. Ben-Yehuda, A., Bloom, A., Lijovetzky, G., Flusser, D., Tur-Kaspa, R., 1990. Chlorpromazine-induced liver and bone marrow granulomas associated with agranulocytosis. Isr. J. Med. Sci. 26, 449–451.
5. Bolton, B., 1967. Prolonged chlorpromazine jaundice. Am. J. Gastroenterol. 48, 497–503.
6. Cheongvee, E.M., Hurst, L., Smith, R.H., 1967. Agranulocytosis and jaundice associated with chlorpromazine. Br. J. Clin. Pract. 21, 95–96.
7. Chlumska, A., Curik, R., Boudova, L., Mukensnabl, P. Klvana, P., 2001. Chlorpromazine-induced cholestatic liver disease with ductopenia. Cesk. Patol. 37, 118–122.
8. Johnson, E., Lanford, R., Solomon, K., 1979. Chlorpromazine, eosinophilia and hepatotoxicity. Va. Med. 106, 683–684.

(Continued)

TABLE 7.1 (Continued)

9. Levine, R.A., Briggs, G.W., Lowell, D.M., 1966. Chronic chlorpromazine cholangiolitic hepatitis. Report of a case with immunofluorescent studies. Gastroenterology 50, 665–670.
10. Moradpour, D., et al., 1994. Chlorpromazine-induced vanishing bile duct syndrome leading to biliary cirrhosis. Hepatology 20, 1437–1441.
11. Russell, R.I., Allan, J.G., Patrick, R., 1973. Active chronic hepatitis after chlorpromazine ingestion. Br. Med. J. 1, 655–656.
12. Sidi, Y., Douer, D., Pinkhas, J., 1989. Simultaneous appearance of agranulocytosis and cholestatic jaundice following chlorpromazine treatment. Med. Interne. 27, 69–71.
13. Swett, C.J., 1975. Adverse reactions to chlorpromazine in medical patients: a report from the Boston Collaborative Drug Surveillance Program, Boston University Medical Center. Curr. Ther. Res. Clin. Exp. 18, 199–206.
14. Isaacs, B., MacArthur, J.G., Taylor, R.M., 1955. Jaundice in relation to chlorpromazine therapy. Br. Med. J. 2, 1122–1124.
15. Cammack, K.V, Hoffman, J.W., Dodds, M., 1958. Thorazine jaundice. J. Mich. State Med. Soc. 57, 582–586.
16. Boardman, R.H., 1954. Fatal case of toxic hepatitis implicating chlorpromazine. Br. Med. J. 2, 579.
17. Murphy, J.D., Ofner, F., 1956. A case of chlorpromazine jaundice. Med. J. Aust. 43, 504–505.
18. Elliott, R.N., Schrut, A.H., Marra, J.J., 1956. Fatal acute aseptic necrosis of the liver associated with chlorpromazine. Am. J. Psychiatry 112, 940.
19. Rodin, A.E., Robertson, D.M., 1958. Fatal toxic hepatitis following chlorpromazine therapy; report of a case with autopsy findings. A.M.A. Arch. Pathol. 66, 170–175.
20. Gruber, L.N., Chapman, W.W., Pratt-Thomas, H.R., 1963. Fatal toxic reaction to chlorpromazine (Thorazine). Case report and brief review of literature. J. S. C. Med. Assoc. 59, 203–204.
21. Walker, C.O., Combes, B., 1966. Biliary cirrhosis induced by chlorpromazine. Gastroenterology 51, 631–640.
22. Weinstein, A., Alper, B.J., Dade, J.R., 1959. Cholestasis due to prochlorperazine. J. Am. Med. Assoc. 170, 1663–1664.
23. Deller, D.J., Brodziak, I.A., Phillips, A.D., 1959. Jaundice during Prochlorperazine Therapy. Br. Med. J. 2, 93.
24. Crandell, A., Ma, J.Y., 1959. Jaundice precipitated by prochlorperazine (compazine) in the treatment of alcoholic psychiatric disturbance. J. Med. Soc. N. J. 56, 553–554.
25. Levine, B., Bergman, B.B., 1960. Prochlorperazine cholestatic hepatitis: report of a case. J. Newark Beth Isr. Hosp. 11, 85.
26. Solomon Jr., F.A., Campagna, F.A., 1959. Jaundice due to prochlorperazine (compazine). Am. J. Med. 27, 840–843.
27. Chatterji, N.N., 1962. Treatment of chronic schizophrenia with prochlorperazine. J. Indian Med. Assoc. 38, 225–226.
28. Lok, A.S., Ng, I.O., 1988. Prochlorperazine-induced chronic cholestasis. J. Hepatol. 6, 369–373.
29. Mechanic, R.C., Meyers, L., 1958 Chlorpromazine-type cholangitis; report of a case occurring after the administration of prochlorperazine. N. Engl. J. Med. 259, 778–780.
30. Mindikoglu, A.L., et al., 2003. Prochlorperazine-induced cholestasis in a patient with alpha-1 antitrypsin deficiency. Hepatogastroenterology 50, 1338–1340.
31. Mcfarland, R.B., 1963. Fatal drug reaction associated with prochlorperazine (Compazine). Report of a case characterized by Jaundice, Thrombocytopenia, and Agranulocytosis. Am. J. Clin. Pathol. 40, 284–290.
32. Barancik, M., Brandborg, L.L., Albion, M.J., 1967. Thioridazine-induced cholestasis. JAMA 200, 69–70.
33. Reinhart, M.J., Benson, R.M., Kwass, S.K., Storey, W.F., 1966. Suggestive evidence of hepatotoxicity concomitant with thioridazine hydrochloride use. JAMA 197, 767–769.
34. Urberg, M., 1990. Thioridazine-induced non-icteric hepatotoxicity. Report of a case. J. Fam. Pract. 30, 342–343.
35. Weiden, P.L., Buckner, C.D., 1973. Thioridazine toxicity. Agranulocytosis and hepatitis with encephalopathy. JAMA 224, 518–520.
36. Winkelmayer, R., 1966. Subicterus following the administration of thioridazine and chlordiazepoxide. Del. Med. J. 38, 334–336.
37. Block, S.L., 1962. Jaundice following thioridazine administration. Am. J. Psychiatry 119, 77.

(*Continued*)

TABLE 7.1 (Continued)

38. Tanikawa, K., Tanaka, M., 1966. Electron microscopic observation of thioridazine-induced hepatitis. Kurume Med. J. 13, 15−21.
39. Kemp, J.A., 1957. Jaundice occurring during administration of promazine. Gastroenterology 32, 937−938.
40. Waitzkin, L., 1957. Hepatic dysfunction during promazine therapy. N. Engl. J. Med. 257, 276−277.
41. Kohn, N., Myerson, R.M., 1961. Cholestatic hepatitis associated with trifluoperazine. N. Engl. J. Med. 264, 549−550.
42. Margulies, A.I., Berris, B., 1968. Jaundice associated with the administration of trifluoperazine. Can. Med. Assoc. J. 98, 1063−1064.
43. Hull, M., Jones, R., Bendall, M., 1994. Fatal hepatic necrosis associated with trazodone and neuroleptic drugs. Br. Med. J. 309, 378.
44. Holt, R., 1984. Fluphenazine decanoate-induced cholestatic jaundice and thrombocytopenia. Pharmacotherapy 4, 227−229.
45. Snyder, S., 1980. Fluphenazine jaundice. Report of a case. Am. J. Gastroenterol. 73, 336−340.
46. Kennedy, P., 1983. Liver cross-sensitivity to antipsychotic drugs. Br. J. Psychiatry 143, 312.
47. Pantel, J., Schroder, J., 1996. Acute hepatitis, rhabdomyolisis and pancytopenia associated with perazine therapy. Pharmacopsychiatry 29, 43.
48. Barrons, E., Johnson, E., Nynkowski, P., 1996. Restarting clozapine: a case report. Psychiatr. Serv. 47, 92.
49. Bauer, M., 1995. Concurrent agranulocytosis and acute hepatitis resulting from combination of classic neuroleptics and subsequent successful clozapine treatment. Pharmacopsychiatry 28, 29−31.
50. Contoreggi, C., Cheskin, L.J., Lange, W.R., 1996. Acute hepatitis after clozapine administration: a case report and review. Am. J. Addict. 5, 5−11.
51. Eggert, A.E., Crismon, M.L., Dorson, P.G., Taylor, R.L., 1994. Clozapine rechallenge after marked liver enzyme elevation. J. Clin. Psychopharmacol. 14, 425−426.
52. Erdogan, A., Kocabasoglu, N., Yalug, I., Ozbay, G., Senturk, H., 2004. Management of marked liver enzyme increase during clozapine treatment: a case report and review of the literature. Int. J. Psychiatry Med. 34, 83−89.
53. Fong, S.Y.Y., Yeung, K.L.A., Tosh, J.M.Y., Wing, Y.K., 2005. Clozapine-induced toxic hepatitis with skin rash. J. Psychopharmacol. 19, 107.
54. Keane, S., Lane, A., Larkin, T., Clarke, M., 2009. Management of clozapine-related hepatotoxicity. J. Clin. Psychopharmacol. 29, 606−607.
55. Kellner, M., Wiedemann, K., Krieg, J.C., Berg, P.A., 1993. Toxic hepatitis by clozapine treatment. Am. J. Psychiatry 150, 985−986.
56. Markowitz, J.S., Grinberg, R., Jackson, C., 1997. Marked liver enzyme elevations with clozapine. J. Clin. Psychopharmacol. 17, 70−71.
57. Thatcher, G.W., Cates, M., Bair, B., 1995. Clozapine-induced toxic hepatitis. Am. J. Psychiatry 152, 296−297.
58. Wirshing, W.C., Ames, D., Bisheff, S., Pierre, J.M., 1997. Hepatic encephalopathy associated with combined clozapine and divalproex sodium treatment. J. Clin. Psychopharmacol. 17, 120−121.
59. Worrall, R., Wilson, A., Cullen, M., 1995. Dystonia and drug-induced hepatitis in a patient treated with clozapine. Am. J. Psychiatry 152, 647−648.
60. Panagiotis, B., 1999. Grand mal seizures with liver toxicity in a case of clozapine treatment. J. Neuropsychiatry Clin. Neurosci. 11, 117−118.
61. Chou, A.I.W., Lu, M., Shen, W.W., 2014. Hepatotoxicity induced by clozapine: a case report and review of literature. Neuropsychiatr. Dis. Treat. 1585−1587.
62. Kang, S.H., Lee, J.I.L., 2013. Eosinophilia, pleural effusion, hepatitis, and jaundice occurring early in clozapine treatment. Clin. Psychopharmacol. Neurosci. 11, 103−105.
63. Jang, S., Yi, H., Paek, J., Lee, S., 1999. Clozapine-induced acute hepatitis. J. Korean Neuropsychiatr. Assoc. 38, 227−233.
64. Hong, H., Kim, C., Song, D., Lee, S., Lee, H., 1999. A case of clozapine-induced eosinophilia combined with bilateral pleural effusion, ascites, cholecysctitis, and hepatitis. Korean J. Psychopharmacol. 10, 191−195.
65. Quevedo, B.C., Salgado, M.M., 2010. Neuroleptic-induced toxic hepatitis. Actas Esp. Psiquiatr. 39, 79−80.
66. Tucker, P., 2013. Liver toxicity with clozapine. Aust. N. Z. J. Psychiatry 47, 975−976.

(Continued)

TABLE 7.1 (Continued)

67. Brown, C., Telio, S., Warnock, C., Wong, A., 2013. Clozapine toxicity and hepatitis. J. Clin. Psychopharmacol. 33, 2013.
68. Chang, A., Krygier, D.S., Chatur, N., Yoshida, E.M., 2009. Clozapine-induced fatal fulminant hepatic failure: a case report. Can. J. Gastroenterol. 23, 376–378.
69. Macfarlane, B., et al., 1997. Fatal acute fulminant liver failure due to clozapine: a case report and review of clozapine-induced hepatotoxicity. Gastroenterology 112, 1707–1709.
70. Chaplin, A., Curley, M., Wanless, I. Re: Chang, A., Krygier. D., Chatur, N., Yoshida, E.M., 2010. Clozapine induced fatal fulminant hepatic failure. Can. J. Gastroenterol. 24, 739–740.
71. Shpaner, A., Li, W., Ankoma-Sey, V., Botero, R.C., 2008. Drug-induced liver injury: hepatotoxicity of quetiapine revisited. Eur. J. Gastroenterol. Hepatol. 20, 1106–1109.
72. Wright, T.M., Vandenberg, A.M., 2007. Risperidone- and quetiapine-induced cholestasis. Ann. Pharmacother. 41, 1518–1523.
73. Al Mutairi, F., Dwivedi, G., Al Ameel, T., 2012. Fulminant hepatic failure in association with quetiapine: a case report. J. Med. Case Reports 6, 418.
74. Naharci, M., et al., 2011. Fatal hepatotoxicity in an elderly patient receiving low-dose quetiapine. Am. J. Psychiatry 168, 212–213.
75. El Hajj, I., Sharara, A.I., Rockey, D.C., 2004. Subfulminant liver failure associated with quetiapine. Eur. J. Gastroenterol. Hepatol. 16, 1415–1418.
76. Lin, C.H., Liu, C.M., Huang, W.L., 2012. Quetiapine-induced hepatocellular damage. Psychosomatics 53, 601–602.
77. Benazzi, F., 1998. Risperidone-induced hepatotoxicity. Pharmacopsychiatry 31, 241.
78. Cordeiro, Q.J., Elkis, H., 2001. Pancreatitis and cholestatic hepatitis induced by risperidone. J. Clin. Psychopharmacol. 21, 529–530.
79. Esposito, D., et al., 2005. Risperidone-induced immunoallergic hepatitis. Am. J. Psychiatry 162, 1984.
80. Fuller, M.A., Simon, M.R., Freedman, L., 1996. Risperidone-associated hepatotoxicity. J. Clin. Psychopharmacol. 16, 84–85.
81. Krebs, S., et al., 2001. Risperidone-induced cholestatic hepatitis. Eur. J. Gastroenterol. Hepatol. 13, 67–69.
82. Oyewole, D., Skerritt, U., Montgomery, S., 1996. Jaundice associated with the use of risperidone in a case of presenile dementia. Int. J. Geriatr. Psychiatry 11, 177.
83. Paulzen, M., Orfanos, S., Grunder, G., 2010. Remission of drug-induced hepatitis after switching from risperidone to paliperidone. Am. J. Psychiatry 167, 351–352.
84. Llinares Tello, F., et al., 2005. Acute cholestatic hepatitis probably associated with risperidone. Int. J. Psychiatry Med. 35, 189–205.
85. Whitworth, A.B., Liensberger, D., Fleischhacker, W.W., 1999. Transient increase of liver enzymes induced by risperidone: two case reports. J. Clin. Psychopharmacol. 19, 475–476.
86. Phillips, E.J., Liu, B.A., Knowles, S.R., 1998. Rapid onset of risperidone-induced hepatotoxicity. Ann. Pharmacother. 32, 843.
87. Lopez-Torresa, E., et al., 2014. Liver enzyme abnormalities during antipsychotic treatment: a case report of risperidone-associated hepatotoxicity. Drug Metabol. Drug Interact. 29, 123–126.
88. Hung, C., Wei, I.H., Huang, C., 2009. Late-onset cholestatic hepatitis induced by olanzapine in a patient with schizophrenia. Prog. Neuropsychopharmacol. Biol. Psychiatry 33, 1574–1575.
89. Jadallah, K.A., Limauro, D.L., Colatrella, A.M., 2003. Acute hepatocellular-cholestatic liver injury after olanzapine therapy. Ann. Intern. Med. 138, 357–358.
90. Lui, S.Y., Tso, S., Lam, M., Cheung, E.F., 2009. Possible olanzapine-induced hepatotoxicity in a young Chinese patient. Hong Kong Med. J. 15, 394–396.
91. Ozcanli, T., et al., 2006. Severe liver enzyme elevations after three years of olanzapine treatment: a case report and review of olanzapine associated hepatotoxicity. Prog. Neuropsychopharmacol. Biol. Psychiatry 30, 1163–1166
92. Raz, A., Bergman, R., Eilam, O., Yungerman, T., Hayek, T., 2001. A case report of olanzapine-induced hypersensitivity syndrome. Am. J. Med. Sci. 321, 156–158.
93. Tchernichovsky, E., Sirota, P., 2004. Hepatotoxicity, leucopenia and neutropenia associated with olanzapine therapy. Int. J. Psychiatry Clin. Pract. 8, 173–177.
94. Waage, C., Carlsson, H., Nielsen, E.W., 2004. Olanzapine-induced pancreatitis: a case report. J. Pancreas 5, 388–391.

(Continued)

TABLE 7.1 (Continued)

95. Malli, A., Trikudanathan, G., 2013. Acute liver failure following olanzapine use in anorexia nervosa: a case report. Am. J. Gastroenterol. 108, S106–S161.
96. Dominguez-Jimenez, J., Puente-Gutierrez, J., Pelado-Garcia, E., Cuesta-Cubillas, D., Garcia-Moreno, A., 2012. Liver toxicity due to olanzapine. Rev. Esp. Enferm. Dig. 104, 617–618.
97. Melzer, E., Knobel, B., 1987. Severe cholestatic jaundice due to sulpiride. Isr. J. Med. Sci. 23, 1259–1260.
98. Ohmoto, K., Yamamoto, S., Hirokawa, M., 1999. Symptomatic primary biliary cirrhosis triggered by administration of sulpiride. Am. J. Gastroenterol. 94, 3660–3661.
99. Sarfraz, A., Cook, M., 1996. Sulpiride-induced cholestalic jaundice. Aust. N. Z. J. Psychiatry 30, 701–702.
100. Villari, D., et al., 1995. Bile ductopenia following therapy with sulpiride. Virchows Arch. 427, 223–226.
101. Van Bellinghen, M., Peuskens, J., Appelmans, A., 1989. Hepatotoxicity following treatment with bromperidol. J. Clin. Psychopharmacol. 9, 389–390.
102. Ruddock, D.G., Hoenig, J., 1973. Chlorprothixene and obstructive jaundice. Br. Med. J. 1, 231.
103. Fuller, C.M., Yassinger, S., Donlon, P., Imperato, T.J., Ruebner, B., 1977. Haloperidol-induced liver disease. West. J. Med. 127, 515–518.
104. Bhatia, S.C., Banta, L.E., Ehrlich, D.W., 1985. Molindone and hepatotoxicity. Drug Intell. Clin. Pharm. 19, 744–746.
105. Tsai, C.-F., Tsai, S.-J., Hwang, J.-P., 2005. Ziprasidone-induced hypersensitivity syndrome in an aged schizophrenia patient. Int. J. Geriatr. Psychiatry 20, 797–799.

case reports needs to be treated with caution as not all provided strong causal evidence implicating the antipsychotic prescribed in the hepatic injury suffered—it is possible that some are spurious associations. Further, case reports cannot be used reliably to compare the safety of different antipsychotics as the frequency of prescription varies widely between drugs, and older medications have had more time to give rise to case reports than newer drugs. With these caveats in mind, it can be seen that chlorpromazine is associated with by far the largest number of published cases of drug-induced liver injury. Beyond this, no other one antipsychotic or class stands out as being particularly safe or particularly associated with drug-induced liver injury.

7.3.2 Asymptomatic Antipsychotic-Induced Liver Injury and Lesser Elevations in LFT

Ten group studies evaluated the prevalence of abnormal LFT in adults receiving regular antipsychotics. These studies comprised four chart reviews (Pae et al., 2005; Atasoy et al., 2007; Gaertner et al., 2001; Gaertner et al., 1989), four prospective naturalistic studies (Marinkovic et al., 1994; Hummer et al., 1997; Kirkegaard et al., 1982; Kirkegaard and Jensen, 1979), and two prospective safety and efficacy studies (Kim et al., 2010; Mesotten et al., 1989). Results from these studies need to be interpreted with care as only one study included a control group, and most studies did not give details of concurrent medication or have a washout period for previous antipsychotic medication.

The studies show that abnormal LFT in adults receiving a range of antipsychotics are very common (median percentage on any antipsychotic 32%, with a range of 5–78%; Table 7.2). The majority of these elevations did not meet criteria for drug-induced liver injury, but clinically significant elevations were still common (median 4%, range 0–15%) (clinically significant defined as an increase greater than twofold above the upper limit of normal for ALP or greater than threefold above the upper limit of normal for ALT or AST; Verma and Kaplowitz, 2009). The prevalence of LFT abnormalities is higher than that generally found in asymptomatic populations—ranging from 0.5% in US Air Force recruits (Kundrotas and Clement, 1993), 15% in US employees with executive health insurance (Patt et al., 2003) to 22% in German construction workers (Arndt et al., 1998).

TABLE 7.2 Prevalence of LFT Abnormalities Associated with Antipsychotics

Study	Sample Size	Treatment Duration when LFT Tested	Any LFT Abnormality	Clinically Significant Abnormality
Second-Generation Antipsychotics				
Clozapine				
Kirkegaard et al. (1982)	17	3 years	24%	6% (1 patient)
Kirkegaard and Jensen (1979)	24	17 weeks	33%	8%
Marinkovic et al. (1994)	100	>1 week	36%	Nil
Gaertner et al. (1989)	290 (330 treatments)	8 weeks	49%	Not reported (20% > twofold elevation)
Hummer et al. (1997)	167	1–18 weeks	67%	Not reported (37% > twofold elevation)
Gaertner et al. (2001)	1280 treatments	Not reported	78%	15%
Olanzapine				
Pae et al. (2005)	145	1–9 weeks	27%	8%
Atasoy et al. (2007)	33	2–4 weeks	30%	6%

(Continued)

TABLE 7.2 (Continued)

Study	Sample Size	Treatment Duration when LFT Tested	Any LFT Abnormality	Clinically Significant Abnormality
Risperidone				
Mesotten et al. (1989)	15	4 weeks	7% (1 patient)	Nil
Pae et al. (2005)	289	7 weeks	14%	3%
Atasoy et al. (2007)	29	2—4 weeks	28%	Nil
Quetiapine				
Atasoy et al. (2007)	48	2—4 weeks	27%	Nil
Aripiprazole				
Kim et al. (2010)	19[a]	35 weeks	16%	Not reported
Ziprasidone				
Kim et al. (2010)	19[a]	12 weeks	5% (1 patient)	Not reported
First-Generation Antipsychotics				
Haloperidol				
Hummer et al. (1997)	71	1—18 weeks	46%	Not reported (17% >twofold elevation)
Gaertner et al. (2001)	2661 Treatments	Not reported	50%	2%
Perphenazine				
Gaertner et al. (2001)	917 Treatments	Not reported	62%	4%
Perazine				
Gaertner et al. (2001)	2398 Treatments	Not reported	59%	8%

Clinically significant defined as an increase greater than twofold above the upper limit of normal for ALP or greater than threefold above the upper limit of normal for ALT or AST.
Where overlap of abnormalities not reported, LFT with highest percentage abnormality reported.
[a]*Same patients, Kim et al. (2010) was a crossover trial. For further details of studies please see Marwick et al. (2012).*

Comparison between most of the antipsychotics is difficult because of differences in study design. However, two studies reporting on clozapine alongside other antipsychotics found that clozapine was the antipsychotic most commonly associated with abnormal LFT (Gaertner et al., 2001; Hummer et al., 1997). There was no clear difference between first- and second-generation antipsychotics.

7.3.3   Genetic Vulnerability

Polymorphisms or deletions of drug metabolizing enzymes have been found to influence the risk of experiencing a drug-induced liver injury in general (Huang et al., 2007; Lucena et al., 2008) and of experiencing liver injury due to specific drugs: antituberculosis agents (Huang et al., 2007) or sodium valproate (Stewart et al., 2010). Interestingly, a particular HLA haplotype has been found to greatly increase the risk of liver injury due to a range of medications (Kim and Naisbitt, 2016), implicating the host immune response in the pathophysiology of drug-induced liver injury. No studies have addressed the pharmacogenomics of drug-induced acute liver failure, due to the scarcity of the event, although it is plausible that genetic variations influence the risk of progression from liver injury to liver failure. It is also plausible that as yet unidentified genetic variations in drug metabolic pathways or immune response pathways influence the risk of antipsychotic-induced liver injury and failure.

7.4   PATHOBIOLOGY

Drug-induced liver injury is split into that which is "intrinsic" or predictable (the tiny minority) and that which is idiosyncratic, or unpredictable (Kim and Naisbitt, 2016). An example of predictable injury is that induced by paracetamol (acetaminophen), which is predictably metabolized into a hepatotoxic metabolite in a dose-dependent fashion. In contrast, idiosyncratric drug-induced liver injury is not thought to be due to direct toxicity of the drug or its metabolites, but due to an abnormal host immune response (Dara et al., 2015).

The liver is normally highly tolerant of foreign antigens, commensurate with its exposure to a diverse range of ingested antigens and those originating in the gut microbiome (Dara et al., 2015). Even when an immune response is stimulated, this is generally not amplified over time but rather reduced (clinical adaptation) (Dara et al., 2015), as is seen in practice when minor LFT abnormalities resolve despite continuing treatment. However, T cells can become maladaptively and excessively activated by a drug, its metabolite, or a drug covalently bound to a protein (a hapten) (Kim and Naisbitt, 2016), and a damaging hypersensitivity reaction result. The risk factors for this include genetic factors such as a person's HLA haplotype (which determines antigenic recognition by immune cells) (Kim and Naisbitt, 2016), but also more modifiable factors such as the extent of existing inflammation in the liver (e.g., viral infection), the liver's capacity for regeneration (e.g., damage from alcohol), diet, and the gut microbiome (Dara et al., 2015).

It is also possible that some of the LFT abnormalities seen in those taking regular antipsychotics are not true drug-induced liver injuries but rather reflect the consequence of some other side effect of antipsychotic medication, for example an increased risk of metabolic syndrome (De Hert et al., 2009) associated with an increased risk of nonalcoholic fatty liver disease (Vanni et al., 2010). In support of this possibility, elevated transaminases have been found to predict metabolic syndrome in those with schizophrenia (Kim et al., 2014). Further, a computer record study in Taiwan which identified a slight increased prevalence of chronic liver disease in those with schizophrenia compared to the general population found that chronic liver disease diagnosis was associated with treatment for diabetes, but not with antipsychotic treatment alone (Hsu et al., 2014).

7.5 CLINICAL AND LABORATORY FEATURES

Symptoms of liver dysfunction range from the nonspecific (malaise, fatigue, nausea, anorexia, right upper quadrant discomfort) to the more overtly concerning (jaundice—potentially with dark urine, pale stool and pruritus—ascites, abnormal bleeding, and altered mental state). The key clinical features marking the transition from dysfunction to failure are encephalopathy (any alteration in mental state) and coagulopathy (international normalized ratio >1.5) (Lee, 2012). Signs of multiorgan failure will soon follow: altered consciousness level, hypoxia, hypotension, tachycardia, and oliguria (Bernal et al., 2010). Laboratory tests in acute liver failure are likely to show dramatically elevated transaminases and bilirubin (although in drug-induced liver failure transaminases are less markedly elevated than in other etiologies at around $500-600$ IU L^{-1}; Reuben et al., 2010), coagulopathy, hypoglycemia, elevated lactate, elevated ammonia, and elevated urea and creatinine (Bernal et al., 2010).

Drug-induced liver injury may be associated with some or none of the symptoms of liver dysfunction. By definition, drug-induced liver injury requires the presence of transaminases elevated to above three times the upper limit of normal, and bilirubin raised above twice the upper limit of normal (Navarro and Senior, 2006). Milder, asymptomatic elevations in LFT associated with antipsychotics most commonly show a hepatocellular pattern of injury, with transaminases found to be elevated by all the group studies identified in the systematic review (Table 7.3). In contrast to other antipsychotics, chlorpromazine-induced liver injury is generally cholestatic, with predominant elevations in bilirubin and ALP (Navarro and Senior, 2006).

TABLE 7.3 Maximum Severity of LFT Abnormalities Associated with Different Antipsychotics

Antipsychotic	Maximum Factor of Increase Above Upper Limit Normal (One- (x), Two- (xx) or ≥ Three (xxx) fold Increase)			
	Transaminases	ALP	GGT	Bilirubin
Haloperidol	xxx	xxx	xx	xx
Olanzapine	xxx	xx	x	x
Risperidone	xxx	x	x	x
Quetiapine	x	x	x	x
Clozapine	xxx	xx	xxx	-
Perphenazine	xxx	xx	-	-
Perazine	xxx	xx	-	-
Aripiprazole	x	-	-	-
Ziprasidone	x	-	-	-

The group studies which reported on latency of LFT abnormality following commencement of antipsychotics found that the shortest time until onset of abnormality was 1 week, and most arose within 6 weeks (see Table 7.4).

7.5.1 Differential Diagnosis

Acute liver failure is hard to distinguish from other causes of multiorgan failure, such as sepsis. Once liver failure is confirmed, the main etiological differentials are drug-induced, viral hepatitis, autoimmune hepatitis, metabolic disorders (e.g., Wilson's disease), ischemia (due to systemic hypotension or occlusion of hepatic venous outflow—Budd–Chiari syndrome), poisoning by other toxins (e.g., fungal toxins), hyperthermic injury, neoplasia, and pregnancy-related (Bernal et al., 2010).

When considering a differential diagnosis for drug-induced liver injury it is important to exclude the causes above, and in addition to consider alcohol use and metabolic disorders such as hemochromatosis. For minor elevations in LFTs, there is an even wider differential for their etiology. In addition to all the potential causes of acute liver failure and drug-induced liver injury, consider fatty liver disease, gallstones, celiac disease, hypothyroidism, Addison's, and, in the case of an isolated hyperbilirubinemia, Gilbert's disease (Limdi and Hyde, 2003).

TABLE 7.4 Latency of LFT Abnormalities Associated with Different Antipsychotics

Study	Antipsychotic(s)	Abnormal LFT (*n*)	Monitoring Frequency	Time From Starting Treatment Until LFT Abnormality
Pae et al. (2005)	Olanzapine	39	Fortnightly (weekly if abnormal)	23 days (mean)
	Risperidone	41		19 days (mean)
Gaertner et al. (2001)	Haloperidol	35	Fortnightly (majority)	12 days (mean)
	Clozapine, Perphenazine, Perazine	188		32–37 days (mean)
Hummer et al. (1997)	Clozapine, Haloperidol	145	Weekly	Majority within 1–6 weeks
Atasoy et al. (2007)	Olanzapine, Quetiapine, Risperidone	30	Not reported	Majority within 4 weeks
Marinkovic et al. (1994)	Clozapine	36	Weekly	Majority within 4–6 weeks

7.5.2 Complications and Significant Sequelae

The mortality for acute liver failure is high, particularly when drug-induced: a recent series in the USA reported 27% spontaneous survival and 66% post transplantation survival at 3 weeks after study entry (Reuben et al., 2010). Many patients with acute liver failure do not receive a transplant: around 70% meet criteria for transplantation, but at most half are transplanted (Punzalan and Barry, 2015). Drug-induced liver injury has a better prognosis, with 2% requiring transplantation and an overall 6 months mortality of 8%, of which half the deaths were deemed due to nonhepatic causes (Chalasani et al., 2008). Asymptomatic LFT elevations in those taking regular antipsychotics were not associated with death or significant sequelae in any of the studies reporting them.

7.5.3 Risk Stratification for Death or Permanent Disability

Established poor prognostic factors in drug-induced acute liver failure include high bilirubin levels, prolonged prothrombin times, and severe encephalopathy (Reuben et al., 2010; Punzalan and Barry, 2015). In the future it is possible that serum markers more closely linked to the pathogenesis of the injury may be useful for risk stratification. For example, a recent study of drug-induced liver failure found that the level on admission of an inflammatory mediator released by liver macrophages was able to predict later systemic inflammatory response syndrome and mortality, adding predictive value beyond the risk scales in current everyday use (Rosen et al., 2015). Poor prognostic factors in drug-induced liver injury are raised transaminases and bilirubin, which have been found to be independent predictors of progression to liver failure (Andrade et al., 2005; Bjornsson and Olsson, 2005).

7.6 MANAGEMENT

If a patient is suspected to be in acute liver failure, antipsychotics should be stopped whether or not they are thought to have caused the condition in order to minimize sedation and allow better monitoring of the mental state. A prompt referral to a specialist hepatology team will be needed and if the diagnosis is confirmed the patient will require admission to an intensive care setting for organ support, specific treatment if available (e.g., *N*-acetyl cysteine for paracetamol (acetaminophen) overdose) and consideration of transplantation (Lee, 2012).

When a drug-induced liver injury is suspected based on markedly elevated LFT, first check for symptoms or signs of liver dysfunction. If these are present, stop the drug and promptly refer to a hepatologist. If the patient is asymptomatic it is important to screen for other differentials before finalizing the diagnosis and probably safe to continue the drug meanwhile. Take a history to include alcohol consumption, any suggestion of hemodynamic compromise (e.g., syncope, chest pain), and a thorough drug history including over the counter and herbal remedies. Performing a "liver screen" is recommended, including checking viral serology (surface antibody for hepatitis A, B, C, E, possibly HIV—which can worsen the consequences of viral hepatitis), checking autoantibodies (antinuclear antibody, smooth muscle antibody, and gamma globulins), and checking for metabolic disorders (ferritin, iron, total iron binding capacity, ceruloplasmin, α-1 antitrypsin level). Image the biliary tree to exclude biliary obstruction, by ultrasound and/or computerized tomography or magnetic resonance imaging (Navarro and Senior, 2006).

Minor asymptomatic abnormalities below the thresholds for potential drug-induced liver injury do not require discontinuation of medication, although in borderline cases account should be taken of other risk factors for liver disease such as alcohol and substance use. Given the association between transaminase elevations and metabolic syndrome (Kim et al., 2014) it may also be worth screening the patient for other evidence of metabolic syndrome (obesity, hypertension, dyslipidemia, hyperglycemia) and managing appropriately.

If an antipsychotic has been discontinued because of a suspected liver injury, it is not generally recommended to try a rechallenge because the reactions can increase in severity, particularly if there are features of immune involvement (rash, fever, eosinophilia) (Navarro and Senior, 2006). In the case of treatment-resistant schizophrenia, however, there may be strong clinical grounds to retry clozapine. Clozapine has been successfully rechallenged following asymptomatic liver injury (Erdogan et al., 2004; Eggert et al., 1994) but has also led to a return of liver injury (Markowitz et al., 1997). Before initiating a rechallenge it is important to consider the severity of the initial reaction, the likelihood of the antipsychotic being the causative agent, and the severity of psychotic illness. The idiosyncratic nature of the reactions mean it is not necessary to avoid all antipsychotics after a probable antipsychotic-induced liver injury.

7.7   PREVENTION

The rarity and idiosyncrasy of drug-induced liver injury and failure make these disorders hard to predict and prevent. Consortia are currently seeking new, more selective markers of liver injury to allow early detection of those developing a severe reaction, with candidates such as mitochondrial enzymes and micro RNAs under investigation (Kim and Naisbitt, 2016). What follows are good practice recommendations, based mainly on a respected UK prescribing handbook (Taylor et al., 2009).

Before starting an antipsychotic it is recommended to perform a baseline set of LFTs (Golebiewski 2006). If this demonstrates hepatic impairment, use of lower doses or antipsychotics with minimal hepatic metabolism may be advisable (e.g., sulpiride and amisulpride). Phenothiazines are not advised where there is preexisting liver disease. Caution is also advised for drugs with common side effects which may worsen symptoms of hepatic impairment (i.e., those that are particularly sedating or constipating). After commencing a patient with hepatic impairment on an antipsychotic, frequent monitoring is advised with weekly LFTs initially.

If a patient has normal hepatic function prior to commencing an antipsychotic, there is no clear consensus on how frequently LFTs should be checked thereafter. Checking annually (and also after 6 months for clozapine) (Taylor et al., 2009) has been recommended, but other centers suggest more frequent evaluation in the first year. More frequent monitoring and a lower threshold for concern is likely to be advisable in those who are heavy users of alcohol or illicit substances. Signs of hepatic impairment should prompt LFTs at any time.

7.8   CONCLUSION

LFT elevations in adults receiving regular antipsychotics are common, mild, and often transient, arise early in treatment, and are generally hepatocellular in pattern. The adverse effect may rarely progress to symptomatic liver injury and extremely rarely to acute liver failure.

REFERENCES

Andrade, R.J., et al., 2005. Drug-induced liver injury: an analysis of 461 incidences submitted to the Spanish registry over a 10-year period. Gastroenterology 129 (2), 512–521.

Arndt, V., et al., 1998. Elevated liver enzyme activity in construction workers: prevalence and impact on early retirement and all-cause mortality. Int. Arch. Occup. Environ. Health. 71 (6), 405–412.

Atasoy, N., et al., 2007. A review of liver function tests during treatment with atypical antipsychotic drugs: a chart review study. Prog. Neuropsychopharmacol. Biol. Psychiatry. 31 (6), 1255–1260.

Bakke, O.M., et al., 1995. Drug safety discontinuations in the United Kingdom, the United States, and Spain from 1974 through 1993: a regulatory perspective. Clin. Pharmacol. Ther. 58 (1), 108–117.

Bernal, W., et al., 2010. Acute liver failure. Lancet 376 (9736), 190–201.

Bjornsson, E., Olsson, R., 2005. Outcome and prognostic markers in severe drug-induced liver disease. Hepatology 42 (2), 481–489.

Bower, W.A., et al., 2007. Population-based surveillance for acute liver failure. Am. J. Gastroenterol. 102 (11), 2459–2463.

Brandsœter, B., et al., 2002. Fulminant hepatic failure: outcome after listing for highly urgent liver transplantation—12 Years experience in the Nordic countries. Liver Transpl 8 (11), 1055–1062.

Bretherick, A.D., et al., 2011. Acute liver failure in Scotland between 1992 and 2009; incidence, aetiology and outcome. Qjm 104 (11), 945–956.

Chalasani, N., et al., 2008. Causes, clinical features, and outcomes from a prospective study of drug-induced liver injury in the United States. Gastroenterology 135 (6), 1924–1934.

Dara, L., Liu, Z.-X., Kaplowitz, N., 2015. Mechanisms of adaptation and progression in idiosyncratic drug induced liver injury, clinical implications. Liver Int 36 (2), 158–165, p.n/a–n/a.

de Abajo, F.J., et al., 2004. Acute and clinically relevant drug-induced liver injury: a population based case-control study. Br. J. Clin. Pharmacol. 58 (1), 71–80.

De Hert, M., et al., 2009. Metabolic syndrome in people with schizophrenia: a review. World Psychiatry 8 (1), 15–22.

Derby, L.E., et al., 1993. Liver disorders in patients receiving chlorpromazine or isoniazid. Pharmacotherapy 13 (4), 353–358.

Eggert, A.E., et al., 1994. Clozapine rechallenge after marked liver enzyme elevation. J. Clin. Psychopharmacol. 14 (6), 425–426.

Erdogan, A., et al., 2004. Management of marked liver enzyme increase during clozapine treatment: a case report and review of the literature. Int. J. Psychiatry. Med. 34 (1), 83–89.

Escorsell, A., Mas, A., de la Mata, M., 2007. Acute liver failure in Spain: analysis of 267 cases. Liver Transpl 13, 1389–1395.

Gaertner, H.J., Fischer, E., Hoss, J., 1989. Side effects of clozapine. Psychopharmacology (Berl) 99 (Supl), S97–100.

Gaertner, I., et al., 2001. Relevance of liver enzyme elevations with four different neuroleptics: a retrospective review of 7,263 treatment courses. J. Clin. Psychopharmacol. 21 (2), 215–222.

Golebiewski, K., 2006. Antipsychotic Monitoring. Graylands Hosp Drug Bull 14 (3), 4.

Hsu, J.-H., et al., 2014. Increased risk of chronic liver disease in patients with schizophrenia: a population-based cohort study. Psychosomatics 55 (2), 163−171.

Huang, Y.-S., et al., 2007. Genetic polymorphisms of manganese superoxide dismutase, NAD(P) H:quinone oxidoreductase, glutathione S-transferase M1 and T1, and the susceptibility to drug-induced liver injury. J. Hepatol. 47 (1), 128−134.

Hummer, M., et al., 1997. Hepatotoxicity of clozapine. J. Clin. Psychopharmacol. 17 (4), 314−317.

Kim, E.Y., et al., 2014. Aminotransferase levels as a prospective predictor for the development of metabolic syndrome in patients with schizophrenia. Psychopharmacology 231 (23), 4479−4487.

Kim, S., Naisbitt, D.J., 2016. Update on advances in research on idiosyncratic drug-induced liver injury. Allergy Asthma Immunol Res 8 (1), 3−11.

Kim, S.-W., et al., 2010. Effectiveness of switching from aripiprazole to ziprasidone in patients with schizophrenia. Clin. Neuropharmacol. 33 (3), 121−125.

Kirkegaard, A., Jensen, A., 1979. An investigation of some side effects in 47 psychotic patients during treatment with clozapine and discontinuing of the treatment. Arzneimittel-forschung 29 (5), 851−858.

Kirkegaard, A., Hammershoj, E., Ostergard, P., 1982. Evaluation of side effects due to clozapine in long-term treatment of psychosis. Arzneimittelforschung 32 (4), 465−468.

Kundrotas, L.W., Clement, D.J., 1993. Serum alanine aminotransferase (ALT) elevation in asymptomatic US Air Force basic trainee blood donors. Dig. Dis. Sci. 38 (12), 2145−2150.

Lee, W., 2012. Acute Liver Failure. Semin. Respir. Crit. Care. Med. 33, 36−45.

Limdi, J., Hyde, G., 2003. Evaluation of abnormal liver function tests. Postgrad. Med. J. 79, 307−312.

Lucena, M.I., et al., 2008. Glutathione S-transferase m1 and t1 null genotypes increase susceptibility to idiosyncratic drug-induced liver injury. Hepatology 48 (2), 588−596.

Marinkovic, D., et al., 1994. The side-effects of clozapine: a four year follow-up study. Prog. Neuropsychopharmacol. Biol. Psychiatry. 18 (3), 537−544.

Markowitz, J.S., Grinberg, R., Jackson, C., 1997. Marked liver enzyme elevations with clozapine. J. Clin. Psychopharmacol. 17 (1), 70−71.

Marwick, K.F.M., Taylor, M., Walker, S.W., 2012. Antipsychotics and abnormal liver function tests: systematic review. Clin. Neuropharmacol. 35 (5), 244−253.

Mesotten, F., et al., 1989. Therapeutic effect and safety of increasing doses of risperidone (R 64766) in psychotic patients. Psychopharmacology 99 (4), 445−449.

Navarro, V.J., Senior, J.R., 2006. Drug-related hepatotoxicity. N Engl J Med 354 (7), 731−739.

Pae, C.U., et al., 2005. Naturalistic observation on the hepatic enzyme changes in patients treated with either risperidone or olanzapine alone. Int. Clin. Psychopharmacol. 20 (3), 173−176.

Patt, C.H., et al., 2003. Prevalence of transaminase abnormalities in asymptomatic, healthy subjects participating in an executive health-screening program. Dig. Dis. Sci. 48 (4), 797−801.

Punzalan, C.S., Barry, C.T., 2015. Acute liver failure: diagnosis and management. J Intensive Care Med. 1−12 [Epub ahead of print].

Reuben, A., et al., 2010. Drug-induced acute liver failure: results of a US multicenter, prospective study. Hepatology 52 (6), 2065−2076.

Rosen, H.R., et al., 2015. Association between plasma level of Galectin-9 and survival of patients with drug-induced acute liver failure. Clin Gastroenterol Hepatol 14 (4), 606−612.

Sgro, C., et al., 2002. Incidence of drug-induced hepatic injuries: a French population-based study. Hepatology 36 (2), 451−455.

Stewart, J.D., Horvath, R., Baruffini, E., Ferrero, I., Bulst, S., Watkins, P.B., Fontana, R.J., Day, C.P., Chinnery, P.F., 2010. Polymerase γ gene POLG determines the risk of sodium valproate-induced liver toxicity. Hepatology 52 (5), 1791−1796.

Taylor, D., Paton, C., Kapur, S., 2009. Maudsley Prescribing Guidelines 10th Edition. Informa Healthcare, London.

Vanni, E., et al., 2010. From the metabolic syndrome to NAFLD or vice versa? Dig Liver Dis 42 (5), 320−330.

Verma, S., Kaplowitz, N., 2009. Diagnosis, management and prevention of drug-induced liver injury. Gut 58 (11), 1555−1564.

Chapter 8

Pancreatitis

Peter Manu[1,2], Matisyahu Shulman[3] and Kathlyn J. Ronaldson[4]

[1]*Hofstra Northwell School of Medicine, Hempstead, NY, United States,* [2]*South Oaks Hospital, Amityville, NY, United States,* [3]*Zucker Hillside Hospital, Glen Oaks, NY, United States,* [4]*Monash University, Melbourne, VIC, Australia*

8.1 EPIDEMIOLOGY

A recent Swedish study of nationwide diagnoses of pancreatitis with current use of antipsychotics found a crude odds ratio (OR) of 1.4 (95% CI 1.1−1.6) compared with no antipsychotic use (Bodén et al., 2012). When the analysis was adjusted for factors associated with pancreatitis, including alcohol-related diagnoses, obesity, diabetes, and gall stone disease, the OR was 0.8 (0.6−0.9), indicating a protective effect from antipsychotic use. The antipsychotic medications act by differing mechanisms and an overall OR does not indicate the risk with individual classes of agent or individual drugs. Bodén et al. (2012) also found that olanzapine or clozapine did not change the risk of pancreatitis in the adjusted analysis: OR 0.9 (0.6−1.4). The null result does not exclude rare idiosyncratic events. An earlier analysis suggested that the risk of pancreatitis is elevated with first-generation antipsychotics and is higher with low potency (e.g., chlorpromazine) than with high potency agents (e.g., flupenthixol, haloperidol) (adjusted rate ratio 2.8; 2.0−3.8 vs 1.2; 0.7−2.0) (Gasse et al., 2008).

A survey of 192 cases of pancreatitis associated with clozapine, olanzapine, risperidone, and haloperidol in the literature and in the Medwatch database of the Food and Drug Administration, found that 39 cases occurred without any history of alcohol abuse, but 16 clozapine-related cases had newly diagnosed hyperglycemia (Koller et al., 2003). Valproate, a known cause, had been taken concurrently by 23% of cases. Twenty-two (11.5%) of the cases were fatal, and in four of these the time to onset was within 8 days (Box 8.1).

Life-Threatening Effects of Antipsychotic Drugs. DOI: http://dx.doi.org/10.1016/B978-0-12-803376-0.00008-3
© 2016 Elsevier Inc. All rights reserved.

BOX 8.1 Pancreatitis

- Only 2% of cases of acute pancreatitis are drug-related and antipsychotic-related cases may be idiosyncratic.
- Cases presenting in patients taking antipsychotics should be assessed for risk factors including alcohol abuse, gall stones, hypertriglyceridemia, and auto-immune disease.
- Pancreatitis may follow as a result of metabolic disease with the second-generation antipsychotics.
- Cases with hemoconcentration or local or systemic complications should receive aggressive fluid resuscitation and supportive treatment.

Overall, prescribed drugs taken in recommended dosages explain, at most, 2% of all cases of acute pancreatitis (Jones et al., 2015). In addition, there may be a causal relationship with any concomitant medication, particularly sodium valproate, and selective serotonin reuptake inhibitors (SSRI) antidepressants, as well as nonsteroidal anti-inflammatory drugs (NSAIDs), metformin, statins, angiotensin-converting enzyme (ACE) inhibitors, and thiazide diuretics, to name a few with recognized association with pancreatitis (Jones et al., 2015). Additive effects of more than one factor are possible.

8.2 PATHOBIOLOGY

Acute pancreatitis should be attributed to the use of an antipsychotic only after consideration of other causes and risk factors, primarily gall stones, alcohol abuse, smoking, hypertriglyceridemia, and autoimmune disease (Yadav and Lowenfels, 2013). The mechanisms by which antipsychotic medication leads to acute pancreatitis have not been elucidated, but in relation to clozapine an inflammatory response involving the immune system has been suggested based on the presence of eosinophilia in several case reports (Frankenburg and Kando, 1992; Garlipp et al., 2002; Bayard et al., 2005). A direct toxic effect on the pancreas, by the unaltered drug molecule or one of its metabolites, as has been proposed for sodium valproate, diuretics, and statins (Jones et al., 2015), is also possible.

Acute pancreatitis represents the pathologic outcome of premature activation of zymogens and the failure of pancreatic enzymatic defense mechanisms. These enzymatic precursors, of which trypsinogen is the best known, are normally activated when they bind with the duodenal enterokinase, a process that releases trypsin and initiates a complex proteolytic process (Jones et al., 2015). If the activation occurs before the zymogens are secreted in the duodenum, the resulting enzymes lead to pancreatic autodigestion. Intrapancreatic activation of zymogens has been proposed in biliary stasis and ethanol abuse (Jones et al., 2015). The presence of 759 C/T poly-morphism of the HTR2C gene, known to be associated with increased risk for metabolic syndrome, was observed in a case of olanzapine-related pancreatitis and suggests that abnormalities in triglyceride production may initiate the adverse drug effect (Rizos et al., 2015).

One case which developed following three years of clozapine was associated with very high triglycerides (5740 mg dL^{-1}) (Cerulli, 1999). Rising triglycerides and body mass index were noted during clozapine treatment and pancreatitis may have developed through this sequence of events, rather than as a direct effect of clozapine. In another case initially attributed to clozapine, the patient was found to have gallstones and clozapine was successfully recommenced with favorable psychiatric response (Schmitz-Hubsch et al., 2009).

8.3 CLINICAL AND LABORATORY FEATURES

Abdominal pain, increased blood levels of lipase and/or amylase, and abnormal findings on contrast-enhanced computed tomographic examination of the abdomen are the main diagnostic features of acute pancreatitis. The pain is located in the periumbilical area or in the epigastrium, is persistent, and may radiate to the back. Nausea, vomiting, and mild-to-moderate abdominal distention are not uncommon. In uncomplicated cases, the abdomen is soft, there is no rebound tenderness and bowel sounds are present. Increased lipase levels to three times greater than the upper limit of the normal range support the diagnosis. A patchy appearance indicative of necrotizing process, peripancreatic fat stranding, or changes indicating acute interstitial pancreatic edema on computed tomography are strongly suggestive of acute pancreatitis even if enzyme levels do not reach the diagnostic cut-off (Banks et al., 2013). Acute pancreatitis may be associated with new onset or worsening of preexistent respiratory, cardiovascular, and renal failure and the prognosis is worse if these abnormalities persist after the first week of illness (Banks et al., 2013). The risk of complications is greater in obese individuals (Frossard et al., 2009).

Pancreatitis may also occur together with other life-threatening adverse effects of antipsychotic treatment. In a recent report, acute pancreatitis developed in a 53-year-old male patient treated with clozapine (150 mg twice daily) and amisulpride (400 mg twice daily) for three years (Bonnet et al., 2015). The great severity of the condition was indicated by the presence of ketoacidosis, pleural effusion, and systemic inflammatory response syndrome. Admitted for intensive care, the patient developed generalized seizures, rhabdomyolysis, fever, and muscular rigidity consistent with neuroleptic malignant syndrome (NMS). The antipsychotics were discontinued and the patient recovered after treatment with dantrolene, diazepam, intravenous fluid hydration, and broad-spectrum antibiotics. He was rechallenged with clozapine (200 mg twice daily) without recurrence of pancreatitis, NMS, or seizure activity.

8.4 MANAGEMENT

The discontinuation of the potentially offending drug(s) is a cornerstone of the management of drug-induced pancreatitis (Jones et al., 2015). Patients who have systolic blood pressure greater than 100 mm Hg, respiratory rate less than 20 min^{-1}, heart rate less than 100 min^{-1}, normal oxygen saturation, and a serum creatinine level of less than 1.4 mg dL^{-1} may be treated in the psychiatric setting with analgesics for pain and fluid maintenance. The patient should be transferred to a medical ward for aggressive fluid resuscitation in the presence of markers of severity, such as obesity or hemoconcentration, clinical findings suggestive of local or systemic complications (e.g., fever, hypotension, leukocytosis, unremitting, or worsening abdominal pain), or persistent organ failure (Banks et al., 2013; Andersson et al., 2009; Muddana et al., 2009). In these severe cases additional supportive care should be given as required.

REFERENCES

Andersson, R., Sward, A., Tingstedt, B., Akerberg, O., 2009. Treatment of acute pancreatitis: focus on medical care. Drugs 69, 505−514.

Banks, P.A., Bollen, T.L., Dervenis, C., Gooszen, H.G., Johnson, C.D., Sarr, M.G., et al., 2013. Classification of acute pancreatitis − 2012: revision of the Atlanta classifications and definitions by international consensus. Gut 62, 102−111.

Bayard, J.M., Descamps, O.S., Evrard, S., et al., 2005. Case report: acute pancreatitis induced by clozapine. Acta Gastroenterol. Belg. 68, 92−94.

Bodén, R., Bexelius, T.S., Mattsson, F., et al., 2012. Antidopaminergic drugs and acute pancreatitis: a population-based study. BMJ Open 2, e000914.

Bonnet, U., Taazimi, B., Montag, M., Ronge, R., Gespers, H., Kuhlmann, R., et al., 2015. Severe acute pancreatitis, neuroleptic malignant syndrome and grand mal seizures associated with elevated amisulpride and low clozapine serum levels. Psychiatr. Danub. 27 (4), 424−425.

Cerulli, T.R., 1999. Clozapine-associated pancreatitis. Harv. Rev. Psychiatry 7, 61−63.

Frankenburg, F.R., Kando, J., 1992. Eosinophilia, clozapine, and pancreatitis. Lancet 340, 251.

Frossard, J.L., Lescuyer, P., Pastor, C.M., 2009. Experimental evidence of obesity as a risk factor for severe acute pancreatitis. World J. Gastroenterol. 15, 5260−5265.

Garlipp, P., Rosenthal, O., Haltenhof, H., et al., 2002. The development of a clinical syndrome of asymptomatic pancreatitis and eosinophilia after treatment with clozapine in schizophrenia: implications for clinical care, recognition and management. J. Psychopharmacol. 16, 399−400.

Gasse, C., Jacobsen, J., Pedersen, L., Mortensen, P.B., Norgaard, M., Sorensen, H.T., et al., 2008. Risk of hospitalization for acute pancreatitis associated with conventional and atypical antipsychotics: a population-based case-control study. Pharmacotherapy 28, 27−34.

Jones, M.A., Hall, O.M., Kaye, A.M., Kaye, A.D., 2015. Drug-induced pancreatitis: a review. Ochsner. J. 15, 45−51.

Koller, E.A., Cross, J.T., Doraiswamy, P.M., Malozowski, S.N., 2003. Pancreatitis associated with atypical antipsychotics: from the Food and Drug Administration's MedWatch surveillance system and published reports. Pharmacotherapy 23, 1123−1130.

Muddana, V., Whitcomb, D.C., Papachristou, G.I., 2009. Current management and novel insights in acute pancreatitis. Expert Rev. Gastroenterol. Hepatol. 3, 435–444.

Rizos, E., Tournikioti, K., Alevyzakis, E., Peppa, M., Papazaxos, K., Zorbas, G., et al., 2015. Acute necrotizing pancreatitis following olanzapine treatment and 759C/T polymorphism of HTR2C gene: a case report. In Vivo 29 (5), 529–531.

Schmitz-Hubsch, T., Schlaepfer, T.E., Westheide, J., et al., 2009. Clozapine: acquittal of the usual suspect. World J. Biol. Psychiatr. 10, 981–984.

Yadav, D., Lowenfels, A.B., 2013. The epidemiology of pancreatitis and pancreatic cancer. Gastroenterology 144, 1252–1261.

Part IV

Major Neurological and Neuromuscular Adverse Effects of Antipsychotic Drugs

Chapter 9

Seizures

Tilman Steinert and Walter Fröscher
Ulm University, Ulm, Germany

9.1 EPIDEMIOLOGY

An epileptic seizure is a transient occurrence of signs and/or symptoms due to abnormal excessive or synchronous neuronal activity in the brain (Fisher et al., 2005). Epilepsy is a disease of the brain defined by at least two unprovoked seizures occurring >24 hours apart; or one unprovoked seizure and a high probability of further seizures; or diagnosis of an epilepsy syndrome (Fisher et al., 2014).

In the general population, the frequency of unprovoked seizures is about 50 per 100,000 person-years according to a recent systematic review (Ngugi et al., 2011). However, in licensing studies for psychotropic agents, the incidence of seizures was over 1000 per 100,000 person-years in patients with depressive disorders, 784 in patients with psychotic disorders, and 433 in patients with obsessive-compulsive disorder (Alper et al., 2007). According to these data, the incidence of seizures is increased in comparison to the general population more than 10-fold in drug-naïve patients with schizophrenia. Even if the exact figures would require confirmation from more and broader samples, an increased incidence of seizures in patients with mental disorders has been confirmed repeatedly (Hyde and Weinberger, 1997; Swinkels et al., 2005), but not in all studies (Gelisse et al., 1999). The origin could be a common neurobiological substance responsible for the susceptibility to both types of disorders.

9.1.1 Seizures Occurring in Patients Receiving Therapeutic Dosages of Antipsychotic Drugs

For nearly all antipsychotics, case reports on the occurrence of seizures under therapeutic dosages can be found, the first being reported by Anton-Stephens

Life-Threatening Effects of Antipsychotic Drugs. DOI: http://dx.doi.org/10.1016/B978-0-12-803376-0.00009-5
© 2016 Elsevier Inc. All rights reserved.

(1954) after treatment with chlorpromazine. This fact is well-known and the respective case reports are not referenced here. In such cases, it is often difficult to determine in which proportion individual susceptibility, the prescribed drug, and occasional circumstances account for the occurrence of a seizure. In a review of observational studies, the highest incidence of seizures under antipsychotics was found for clozapine (1–4.4%) and chlorpromazine (0.5–9%); for the other substances, the incidence was considerably lower (Pisani et al., 2002). Some studies reported significantly higher percentages of patients with seizures. In a study of 129 patients under zotepine, seizures occurred in 22 (17.1%) after a duration of treatment of 48 days on average (Hori et al., 1992). Predictors were higher dosages, combinations with phenothiazines, and history of head trauma. However, an analysis of the findings of such observational studies shows that the incidence of seizures seems to be always higher in smaller samples. The reasons are unclear. Possibly the explanation is a publication bias with increased probability of noteworthy results being published. Yet it is also conceivable that in studies with higher numbers a lower level of scrutiny was applied to exploring the patients' histories.

In an evaluation of the WHO data base on medication side effects between 1968 and 2006 over 7 million reports were found for CNS-active agents, about 1% of them referring to seizures (Kumlien and Lundberg, 2009). The proportion of reports describing seizures was highest with maprotiline (14%), followed by escitalopram (10%), bupropion (9.5%), clozapine (9%), chlorprothixene (8.5%), amoxapine (8.5%), donepezil (8.4%), rivastigmine (6.4%), quetiapine (5.9%), and trimipramine (5.7%). However, it has to be taken into account that these figures do not necessarily reflect the absolute incidence of seizures with these substances and are subject to the biases inherent in spontaneous adverse reaction reporting. A systematic review and meta-analysis of the off-label use of atypical antipsychotics in elderly patients with dementia demonstrated that patients taking olanzapine had greater odds of having a neurological feature, such as confusion, dizziness, headaches, light-headedness, orthostatic dizziness, seizure, or tinnitus, than those taking risperidone (Maher et al., 2011). There is evidence that risperidone is safe and does not worsen the frequency of seizures in adolescents with epilepsy (Gonzalez-Heydrich et al., 2004). An analysis of data from the Spanish Pharmacovigilance System from 1984 to 2011 revealed that the reporting rate of seizures under second-generation antipsychotics (SGAs) was significantly higher than under first-generation antipsychotics (FGAs). If clozapine was excluded, the reporting odds ratio for seizures under SGAs compared to FGAs was 2.1 (confidence interval (CI) 1.4–3.1) (Lertxundi et al., 2013). However, reporting of seizures is unlikely to be uniform over time and may have been biased toward greater reporting with more recently introduced agents.

In an attempt to establish a ranking of the ictogenic potential of drugs based on published observational studies, Lee et al. (2003) identified a higher risk to the antipsychotics clozapine, olanzapine, and phenothiazines, and a lower risk to the others. Pisani et al. (2002) similarly ascribed a higher risk to the antipsychotics clozapine and chlorpromazine, and a lower risk to the others. They concluded that strong sedating effects are associated with an increased risk for seizures while strong extrapyramidal side effects are associated with a lower risk. Similar conclusions were drawn in the 1980s based on clinical experiences with high potency and low potency antipsychotics frequently used at that time (Itil and Soldatos, 1980). A question that would be of high practical relevance is the incidence of seizures under combinations of psychotropic agents as often happens in practice. However, to our knowledge no meaningful epidemiological data have been published in this respect. Based on a case report, Lee et al. (2003) discussed an increased risk of inducing seizures when combining antipsychotic agents.

A meta-analysis of data generated in clinical trials (phase II and III) has been presented in the Summary Basis of Approval Reports and are accessible to the public through the US Freedom of Information Act of 1996. Alper et al. (2007) analyzed data on over 20,000 patients in the licensing studies of all antipsychotics licensed between 1985 and 2004 in the United States, specifically clozapine, olanzapine, quetiapine, ziprasidone, aripiprazole, ziprasidone, and risperidone. Before 1985, the occurrence of seizures was not reported systematically, meaning no data are available on FGAs. After correcting for duration of observation, standardized incidence rates compared to placebo were calculated. These standardized incidence rates were 9.5 (95% CI 7.3−12.2) for clozapine, 2.5 (1.6−3.7) for olanzapine, 2.1 (1.2−3.2) for quetiapine, and 1.0 (0.77−1.35) for all other antipsychotics. This ranking of the ictogenic potency is well in line with the findings of the observational studies mentioned above. Generally, the incidence of seizures was higher in shorter than in longer observation periods, suggesting that seizures occur predominantly at the beginning of treatment and after increase of dosage.

Clozapine-associated seizures have been particularly vexing, as the drug has superior therapeutic efficacy and produces few, if any, extrapyramidal motor side effects. The incidence of seizures is dose-dependent and is reported as 1.0% at dosages under 300 mg, 2.5% at 300−600 mg, and about 4.4% at dosages above 600 mg, and there may be an increased risk with rapid dose titration (Devinsky et al., 1991). Serum concentrations can considerably increase, in some cases over $1000 \, \mu g \, L^{-1}$, after smoking cessation, and within a period of several months (Cormac et al., 2010). In a recent study on 222 patients who initiated treatment with clozapine, 6% developed seizures, but it was 38% in those receiving >500 mg per day (Grover et al., 2015). Clozapine is the only psychotropic agent which received a "black box" warning by the American Food and Drug Administration (FDA) referring to epileptic seizures (Alper et al., 2007). At least a quarter of observed seizures are myoclonic or astatic seizures. Myocloni can be associated with subsequent tonic−clonic seizures. Also stuttering can be induced by clozapine and in such cases seems to be of myoclonic origin (Wong and Delva, 2007).

9.1.2 Seizures After Intoxications With Antipsychotic Drugs

Many case studies report the prolonged occurrence of seizures, mostly generalized tonic−clonic seizures, up to 24 hours after accidental or intentional overdose of antipsychotics. In a case series of 31 intoxications with risperidone, partly in combination with other substances, a seizure was observed in only one patient (Acri and Henretig, 1998). In a series of 83 cases of an overdose (>1 g) of amisulpride, seizures occurred in only 2 cases (Isbister et al., 2010). In a retrospective cohort study of 20 acute quetiapine overdoses, 4 (20%) developed seizures, suggesting a higher risk for seizures compared to the two aforementioned substances, although only 6 of the 20 ingested only quetiapine (Eyer et al., 2011). Taken together, seizures play only a minor role among clinical complications of overdoses with antipsychotics, while coma, pulmonary depression, and cardiac arrhythmias are the most challenging clinical features.

9.1.3 Genetic Vulnerability

Among new cases of epilepsy, only around 1% have a clear family history and simple inheritance (Ottman, 1997). The first report describing a mutation causing epilepsy was published in 1995 (Steinlein et al., 1995). Since then, many hundreds of genes have been suggested to be associated with epilepsy. However, most cases of epilepsy are sporadic and at least partly caused by environmental factors. Family studies have yielded evidence that these sporadic cases also have a genetic component (Bianchi et al., 2003). Consequently, individual propensity to develop seizures during treatment with antipsychotic medication (or other drugs) depends among other factors on the individually inherited seizure threshold (Landowski and Cubala, 2007; Pisani et al., 2002). The presence of a previous history of epilepsy in the patient and/or the patient's family is the most frequently reported predisposing factor toward drug-induced seizures (Pisani et al., 1999).

The architecture of the genetic elements in common forms of epilepsy is not yet thoroughly understood. Definitely, the genetic components of sporadic epilepsy are complex. It is probable that multiple variants of weak effects combine to predispose individuals to epilepsy as well as there being a smaller number of variants with relatively strong effects. Cross-national case control studies could identify a set of single nucleotide polymorphisms which considerably contribute to disease predisposition, however in an apparently population-specific manner (Cavalleri et al., 2007). Thus, from the current research perspective, the genetic vulnerability for epilepsy is rather similar to that of other complex CNS disorders such as schizophrenia and autism, with a small percentage of disease cases being accountable to definitely identifiable single genetic factors, but the much bigger remainder to the contribution of multiple genetic variants that seem to differ between populations. These genetic determinants do not keep to the borders of the categories as defined by the current classification systems such as DSM-5 and ICD-10, but seem to be rather similar for major CNS disorders with different clinical features. At present, the set of genes of interest in this respect is becoming increasingly clearer. However, it is still unclear how they interact and which environmental factors contribute in which way to the manifestation of a specific disorder and why many individuals with a considerable number of these risk genes stay mentally healthy for their life time.

9.2 PATHOBIOLOGY

A seizure results when a sudden imbalance occurs between the excitatory and inhibitory forces within the network of cortical neurons in favor of a sudden-onset net excitation (Ko and Benbadis, 2014). Seizures can start with a focal onset or with a generalized onset. Focal epileptic seizures are conceptualized as originating within networks limited to one hemisphere. They may be discretely localized or more widespread. Generalized epileptic seizures are conceptualized as originating at some point within, and rapidly engaging, bilaterally distributed networks (Berg et al., 2010). Many studies have also reported so-called focal features among patients with idiopathic generalized epilepsy (Seneviratne et al., 2014). The pathophysiology of focal-onset seizures differs from the mechanisms underlying generalized-onset seizures. Overall, cellular excitability is increased, but the mechanisms of synchronization appear to substantially differ between these two types. The following mechanisms may coexist in different combinations to cause focal-onset seizures: decreased inhibition, defective activation of gamma-aminobutyric acid (GABA) neurons, and increased activation (Ko and Benbadis, 2014).

Antipsychotics are capable of increasing the incidence of seizures in persons with chronic epilepsy or of evoking seizures in susceptible individuals without epilepsy. Provoked or acute symptomatic seizures occur within close temporal proximity of a triggering event (drug intake in this case) and are considered distinct from epilepsy because they tend to recur only with a recurrence of the precipitant (Neligan et al., 2012). The presence of predisposing factors, such as history of epilepsy, brain damage, being elderly, reduced drug clearance, preexisting electroencephalogram (EEG) alterations, and general physical illness, probably plays an important role in facilitation and may explain those case reports of seizures or even status epilepticus triggered by low or therapeutic dosages of a given drug. Concomitant treatment with additional drugs acting on the central nervous system and/or altering drug plasma concentrations is another aggravating factor (Pisani et al., 1999, 2002). Most antipsychotics are substrates and inhibitors of cytochrome P450 isoenzymes, which can cause interactions with a wide variety of other drugs and even food components (Lee et al., 2003). Interactions can cause either an increase, or a decrease in the plasma concentrations of antipsychotics and of antiepileptic medication.

9.3   CLINICAL AND LABORATORY FEATURES

Drug-induced seizures fall into the category of "conditions with epileptic seizures that do not require a diagnosis of epilepsy" (Engel, 2001). With respect to their pathogenesis, drug-induced seizures are classified as "provoked," "situation-related," "occasional," "acute symptomatic," or "reactive" seizures (Bast and Carmant, 2013; Fröscher, 2004). These seizures occur only when there is an acute trigger such as drug intake (Commission on Classification and Terminology of the International League Against Epilepsy, 1989). Only exceptionally do they pass over to classic epilepsy. The clinical appearance of drug-induced seizures (and other provoked seizures) is identical to seizures in "chronic" epilepsy (Fröscher, 2004). Seizures associated with medication are typically generalized seizures (in more than 90% of cases), although focal seizures may be observed (Bast and Carmant, 2013; Meyer and Fröscher, 2004). Generalized seizures are subdivided into the categories tonic−clonic, myoclonic, clonic, tonic, atonic, and absences. Focal seizures should be described according to their manifestations (Berg et al., 2010; Berg and Cross, 2012).

Case reports on drug-induced "seizures" often describe only "seizures" without a more precise description and appropriate classification; as a rule, these reports concern generalized tonic−clonic seizures. In case of seizures induced by antipsychotic drugs, besides generalized tonic−clonic seizures, the following clinical types of seizures have been described: generalized myoclonic seizures, absences (one case), "probable" complex focal seizures, "suspected" simple focal seizures, and "astatic" seizures (Gouzoulis-Mayfrank et al., 1994; Pacia and Devinsky, 1994; Silvestri et al., 1998; Wong and Delva, 2007). Astatic seizures are seizures of short duration leading to falls, but do not represent a distinct type of seizure from the current perspective and can be categorized among one of the other aforementioned categories. Generalized myoclonic seizures were predominantly observed in patients treated with clozapine. The myoclonic jerks were similar to the myoclonic jerks of juvenile myoclonic epilepsy and were accompanied by spike-wave-activity in the EEG (Gouzoulis-Mayfrank et al., 1994). Clozapine-related myoclonic jerks may precede a generalized tonic−clonic seizure (Pacia and Devinsky, 1994).

Although most drug-induced seizures are self-limiting and do not result in permanent sequelae, as many as 15% of these seizures (especially those related to overdose) may present as status epilepticus (Garcia and Alldredge, 1994).

9.3.1   Diagnostic Relevance of the EEG

Most psychotropic agents, particularly antipsychotics and antidepressants, reduce the proportion of basal activity in the EEG, while the proportion of theta- and, to a less extent, delta-waves increases. In a study of 293 patients treated by an antipsychotic, an abnormal EEG was found in 19% (Centorrino et al., 2002). However, this finding was also obtained in 13% of those 30 patients of the sample who received no medication, pointing to the abovementioned assumption that individuals with mental disorders seem to have an increased liability to subtle signs of brain dysfunction, manifesting themselves in such unspecific EEG alterations. Among patients treated with antipsychotics, EEG abnormalities were most frequently found with clozapine (47%), followed by olanzapine (39%), risperidone (28%), typical antipsychotics (14% on average, highest under fluphenazine) and, lastly, quetiapine (0%). This reflects the ranking in the liability to cause seizures as mentioned above. Severe EEG abnormalities such as spikes and spike wave complexes were found among 3% of patients treated with antipsychotics, but none of the drug-naïve patients (Centorrino et al., 2002). A study on 81 patients treated by a single antipsychotic reported similar results (Amann et al., 2003): EEG abnormalities were found in 35.1% with olanzapine, in 22.8% with haloperidol, and in 4.6% with quetiapine, which was comparable to a healthy control group. More specific epileptic activity was found in only four patients with olanzapine. Patients given clozapine were not included in this study. Amisulpride seems to cause EEG abnormalities similar to olanzapine in frequency, but with significantly less occurrence of epileptic activity (Pogarell et al., 2004).

Most EEG abnormalities are observed during therapy with clozapine. Such abnormalities and associations with the incidence of seizures have been observed in several studies. In a prospective study of 50 patients treated by clozapine, EEG decelerations were more frequent and more pronounced at serum concentrations over 300 μg mL^{-1} than at lower concentrations. Out of three patients who developed seizures, one had higher serum concentrations, the two others had lower serum concentrations, but a history of seizures (Freudenreich et al., 1997). In a further study of 50 patients treated with clozapine, abnormal EEGs were found in 62%, predominantly with unspecific decelerations. A linear association was found between dosage and EEG alterations. Also in this sample, seizures occurred in only two out of 50 patients (Chung et al., 2002).

A question of high clinical importance is the correlation between nonspecific and specific EEG abnormalities on the one hand, and the occurrence of seizures on the other. A strong association of nonspecific EEG abnormalities such as spikes and sharp waves with the occurrence of seizures has been suggested for clozapine (Welch et al., 1994). Typical epileptic activity in the EEG (spikes, sharp waves, spike wave complexes) nearly exclusively occurs in patients with a history of epilepsy and a history of such EEG abnormalities (Pisani et al., 2002). EEG records in a time span of one or more days either before, or after occasional seizures under treatment with antipsychotics or other psychotropic agents typically show either only unspecific, or no abnormalities. EEG records are frequently performed after the occurrence of seizures and even sometimes routinely under therapy with antipsychotics, but actually have little predictive value and little impact on clinical decisions. Among patients with additional risk factors for seizures such as comorbid epilepsy, specific activity in EEG records can indicate an increased risk for seizures (Pisani et al., 2002). The available evidence on the association of EEG and seizures does not allow the conclusion that a single EEG record either before the beginning of treatment with antipsychotics, or under some other type of treatment as a control would increase either drug safety, or the doctor's safety in terms of forensic investigation of the treatment offered. The weak association between EEG records and seizures is not really surprising, taking into account that EEG records are time-limited records of the head surface, thus capturing an incidental sample of potential epileptic activity limited to a small window of time and space. Even in patients with epilepsy interictal EEG records can be completely inconspicuous, while on the other hand in patients with epilepsy and frequent interictal epileptic activity reliable prediction of seizure activity is again not possible (Gil-Nagel and Abou-Khalil, 2012).

9.3.2 Differential Diagnosis

The typical clinical picture of tonic—clonic seizures with loss of consciousness is highly characteristic and gives little occasion for misinterpretation. However, a symptom which is difficult to interpret is nocturnal enuresis under treatment with clozapine. Theoretically, it could be the consequence of an unobserved tonic—clonic seizure during sleep. However, nocturnal enuresis has been recognized as a rather frequent side effect of SGAs, notably clozapine, and occurs in up to one-fifth of patients treated with clozapine (Harrison-Woolrych et al., 2011). The underlying mechanisms are protean and not completely understood. Deep sleep is considered as the major reason, while epileptic seizures are not considered as a common cause for nocturnal enuresis, particularly in the absence of any other evidence of occurrence of a seizure (Barnes et al., 2012; Sagy et al., 2014).

The incidence of myoclonic or astatic seizures described in the literature gives rise to difficulties in differential diagnosis. However, according to our own experience, any type of seizure other than tonic—clonic seizure is very rare. Myocloni, which themselves are not necessarily epileptic in their nature, might be confused with tics or mannerisms. Astatic seizures could be confused with falls and sudden loss of consciousness for any other reason. Stuttering induced by myocloni, which has also been described under clozapine (Wong and Delva, 2007), could be confused with extrapyramidal side effects, with formal thought disorder and with speech disorder of another origin. Complex focal seizures are uncommon under therapy with antipsychotics, being caused by a local focus of brain tissue which is not a typical feature of psychotic disorders. If complex focal seizures occur, they could be confused with catatonic symptoms such as mannerisms and "dreamy states" of psychotic origin.

In clinical units specializing in epilepsy, the most challenging differential diagnosis is between tonic−clonic seizures and nonepileptic (psychogenic) seizures (Widdess-Walsh et al., 2012). Nonepileptic seizures, sometimes closely resembling true epileptic seizures, are viewed as a kind of dissociative symptom, occurring predominantly in patients with other dissociative disorders, personality disorders, mental retardation, or a history of childhood sexual abuse (Direk et al., 2012; Magaudda et al., 2011; Myers et al., 2013). Among people with psychotic disorders, such nonepileptic seizures are very uncommon. However, it is conceivable that patients with dissociative disorders and nonepileptic seizures could receive antipsychotics as an off-label treatment for one or other reason, which could give rise to problems of differential diagnosis.

Retrospective evidence that a tonic−clonic seizure has occurred relies on measuring blood creatine kinase (CK) activity. CK activity is increased after seizures due to strong muscular activity. According to a recent meta-analysis, the specificity of elevated blood CK activity in differentiating epileptic from nonepileptic seizures is very high, but the sensitivity is low (Brigo et al., 2014). Seizure activity does not necessarily lead to elevation of CK activity in seizures of short duration. Therefore normal CK blood data do not exclude the occurrence of an epileptic seizure. With respect to the claimed high specificity, none of the studies reviewed in the meta-analysis included individuals with psychotic disorders. Elevation of blood CK is frequent in patients with psychotic disorders for many reasons, among others catatonic muscular activity and increased physical activity in general. Thus determining blood CK activity is of little value in the differential diagnosis of seizures and nonepileptic phenomena in patients treated with antipsychotics.

9.3.3 Complications and Significant Sequelae

The occurrence of seizures has adverse consequences, most of which are the same as for patients with epilepsy. First, the occurrence of seizures in patients treated with clozapine limits the use of the drug and can prevent an increase in dosage that may be desirable for therapeutic reasons. Second, seizures impose possible life-threatening risks such as accidents or falls. Third, prolonged seizures themselves and accidents with head injury can lead to additional brain damage, and thus, in the worst case, can progress from occasional seizures to post-traumatic epilepsy. Fourth, adverse consequences for the quality of life are inability to drive a vehicle and the need to take additional antiepileptic drugs with additional side effects if there have been repeated seizures. Lastly, the possible occurrence of status epilepticus represents a life-threatening complication. Occurrence of a status epilepticus with a fatal outcome has been described in a case where a comprehensive post-mortem analysis could not detect any other possible reason except for monotherapy with olanzapine carried out for 5 months in the usual therapeutic dosages (Wyderski et al., 1999). However, doubt remains in such cases whether the regular intake of drugs can really be considered as the relevant causal factor for the occurrence of occasional seizures, or if it is only a coincidence.

If therapy with antiepileptics is necessary, the spectrum of side effects of the selected drug has to be taken into consideration. Side effects can add and reinforce themselves mutually. Hematologic, cardiogenic, psychiatric, and metabolic side effects are of particular importance. Carbamazepine can cause neutropenia or agranulocytosis and must not be combined with antipsychotics with an increased risk for these complications, notably clozapine. Also combination with olanzapine should be avoided for the same reason. Valproic acid may induce thrombocytopenia and disturbances of coagulation. Under coadministration of antiepileptics and antipsychotics (and other psychotropic drugs, as well as antibiotics and hormones), QT_C intervals can increase, imposing a risk of cardiac arrhythmias up to torsades de pointes (Feldman and Gidal, 2013). The risk is higher with amisulpride and sertindole than with other antipsychotics (Leucht et al., 2013). ECG controls therefore are required particularly when new combinations are started.

Any antiepileptic drug can cause psychiatric side effects like tiredness, depression, irritability, and aggressiveness, albeit to a different extent. Psychotic symptoms only exceptionally occur as side effects of antiepileptic drugs. Weight gain particularly is a problem with valproic acid, gabapentin, and pregabalin. Lamotrigine mostly is not a good choice if an antiepileptic is necessary as an add-on because of the very slow titration required due to the risk of allergic rash. Coadministration of various drugs can lead to interactions of different kinds. Enzyme induction leading to lower serum concentrations and loss of efficacy is possible as well as inhibition of P450 enzymes leading to higher serum concentrations and features of toxicity, both mechanisms can refer to both types of drugs. Therefore, drug monitoring by control of serum concentrations is recommended, particularly if dosages and drugs are changed.

9.3.4 Risk Stratification for Death or Permanent Disability

Exceptionally a single tonic—clonic seizure or status epilepticus can be fatal. The above-mentioned patient of Wyderski et al. (1999) died (despite successful treatment of the status epilepticus) from secondary rhabdomyolysis and disseminated intravascular coagulation. Patients at risk are predominantly those with overdoses or intoxications, abrupt withdrawal, those given clozapine, under treatment with multiple psychotropic agents, with rapid increases or abrupt changes of dose, and with an increased liability to seizures for other reasons, for example, comorbid epilepsy, a history of occasional seizures or alcohol or benzodiazepine withdrawal syndrome, brain injury, cerebral arteriosclerosis, and CNS-infections (Lee et al., 2003).

9.4   PREVENTION AND MANAGEMENT

Recommendations for the clinical management of seizures in patients given antipsychotics can be outlined according to the evidence described above. Generally, the situation with a first seizure (Table 9.1) should be distinguished from the situation with reoccurrence of seizures (Table 9.2).

Considering the slightly increased liability of individuals with psychotic disorders of developing seizures and the increased risk of seizures with the most effective antipsychotic drugs, seizures cannot be prevented completely. Since seizures are relatively rare and (except for status epilepticus, which is rare) only exceptionally life-threatening, prophylactic administration of antiepileptics is not justified without a history of seizures. If there is a history of

---

TABLE 9.1 Management Guidelines After a First Epileptic Seizure in Patients Treated With Antipsychotic Drugs

- Check whether drugs with a known increased risk for seizures can be responsible (among antipsychotics: clozapine, olanzapine, chlorpromazine, if still in use)
- Check whether changes of concomitant pharmacologically active substances have taken place, for example, smoking cessation, add-on of drugs with enzyme-inhibiting properties
- If causation by an antipsychotic agent seems possible, measure serum concentration
- Taking into account dosage, serum concentration, and efficacy, is dose reduction possible?
- In case of clozapine or olanzapine (or chlorpromazine), consider switching to a different antipsychotic
- Alternatively, in case of treatment with clozapine and occurrence of a seizure, consider reducing the dosage and supplementing with a second antipsychotic, for example, risperidone or amisulpride
- If neither switching to a different agent, nor reduction of dosage seems advisable (which is sometimes the case under high dosage-treatment with clozapine due to therapy resistance with other antipsychotics), add an antiepileptic drug such as valproic acid or lamotrigine (Williams and Park, 2015)
- But consider that lamotrigine mostly is not helpful in such situations because the required slow titration takes too much time until efficacy is achieved
- Don't combine clozapine and olanzapine with carbamazepine because of similar possible deleterious effects on white blood cells
- If an antiepileptic is prescribed in addition, carry out ECG (QT_C interval) and take into account drug interactions. Adapt dosages after measuring plasma concentrations if necessary
- If no clear reason is obvious such as drug intake, sleep deprivation, or alcohol withdrawal, exclude other origin by brain scan
- Examine EEG record in order to exclude preexisting epileptic disposition (spikes or spike-wave complexes)
- But don't draw clinical consequences from EEG abnormalities without clinical symptoms
- Inform patient that she/he should not drive a motor vehicle for a defined period (according to national guidelines)

TABLE 9.2 Management After Reoccurrence of Epileptic Seizures in Patients Treated With Antipsychotic Drugs

- Check whether typical and avoidable triggers can be detected (clozapine, sleep deprivation, alcohol, and alcohol withdrawal)
- Check whether changes of concomitant pharmacologically active substances have taken place, for example, smoking cessation, add-on of drugs with enzyme-inhibiting properties
- If such triggers cannot be avoided, administer valproic acid as add-on. Take into account side effect of weight gain, probably in addition to similar side effects from prescribed antipsychotics. Carry out ECG (QT_C interval) and take into account drug interactions. Adapt dosages after measuring serum concentrations if necessary
- EEG records are not helpful to determine the efficacy of the therapeutic regimen
- However, EEG decelerations (compared to previous EEG records) can indicate overdosage
- Make clinical decisions dependent on occurrence of subsequent seizures, not on EEG records

seizures in typical trigger situations, the situation should be avoided if possible and patients should be encouraged to get enough sleep and to avoid alcohol. If the patient develops alcohol withdrawal syndrome after all, prophylactic administration of antiepileptics with rapid dose titration is justified for some days until termination of the withdrawal syndrome. Only in the case of repeated seizures and the impossibility to avoid triggers or giving drugs, prophylactic antiepileptic medication is justified. In the management of antipsychotic drug therapy, those agents with the highest risk (clozapine, olanzapine) should be avoided, if possible, in individuals with a history of seizures. Generally, caution is recommended with high doses, rapid changes of dose, and use of multiple psychotropic drugs.

ACKNOWLEDGMENT

We thank Dr. Hartmut Baier for valuable hints and references.

REFERENCES

Acri, A.A., Henretig, F.M., 1998. Effects of risperidone in overdose. Am. J. Emerg. Med. 16, 498–501.

Alper, K., Schwartz, K.A., Kolts, R.L., Khan, A., 2007. Seizure incidence in psychopharmacological clinical trials: an analysis of Food and Drug Administration (FDA) Summary Basis of Approval Reports. Biol. Psychiatry 62, 345–354.

Amann, B.L., Pogarall, O., Mergl, R., Juckel, G., Grunze, H., Mulert, C., et al., 2003. EEG abnormalities associated with antipsychotics: a comparison of quetiapine, olanzapine, haloperidol and healthy subjects. Hum. Psychopharmacol. 18, 641–646.

Anton-Stephens, D., 1954. Preliminary observations on the psychiatric use of chlorpromazine. J. Ment. Sci. 100, 543–557.

Barnes, T., Drake, M.J., Paton, C., 2012. Nocturnal enuresis with antipsychotic medication. Br. J. Psychiatry 200, 7−9.

Bast, T., Carmant, L., 2013. Febrile and other occasional seizures. In: Dulac, O., Lassonde, M., Sarnat, H.B. (Eds.), Handbook of Clinical Neurology, vol. 111 (3rd series). Elsevier, Edinburgh, pp. 477−491.

Berg, A., Cross, J.H., 2012. Classification of epilepsies and seizures: historical perspective and future directions. In: Stefan, H., Theodore, W.H. (Eds.), Handbook of Clinical Neurology, vol. 107 (3rd series), Epilepsy, Part I. Elsevier, Edinburgh, pp. 99−111.

Berg, A.T., Berkovic, S.F., Brodie, M.J., Buchhalter, J., Cross, J.H., van Emde Boas, W., et al., 2010. Revised terminology and concepts for organization of seizures and epilepsies: report of the ILAE Commission on Classification and Terminology. Epilepsia 51, 676−685.

Bianchi, A., Viaggi, S., Chiossi, E., 2003. Family study of epilepsy in first degree relatives: data from the Italian Episcreen Study. Seizure 12, 203−210.

Brigo, F., Igwe, S.C., Erro, R., Bongiovanni, L.G., Marangi, A., Nardone, R., et al., 2015. Postictal serum creatine kinase for the differential diagnosis of epileptic seizures and psychogenic non-epileptic seizures: a systematic review. J. Neurol. 262 (2), 251−257.

Cavalleri, G.L., Weale, M.E., Shianna, K.V., Singh, R., Lynch, J.M., Grinton, B., et al., 2007. Multicentre search for genetic susceptibility loci in sporadic epilepsy syndrome and seizure types: a case-control study. Lancet Neurol. 6, 1970−1980.

Centorrino, F., Price, B.H., Tuttle, M.I., Bahk, W.M., Hennen, J., Albert, M.J., et al., 2002. EEG abnormalities during treatment with typical and atypical antipsychotics. Am. J. Psychiatry 159, 109−115.

Chung, S.J., Jeong, S.H., Ahn, Y.M., Kang, U.G., Koo, Y.J., Ha, J.H., et al., 2002. A retrospective study of clozapine and electroencephalographic abnormalities in schizophrenic patients. Prog. Neuropsychopharmacol. Biol. Psychiatry 26, 139−144.

Commission on Classification and Terminology of the International League Against Epilepsy, 1989. Proposal for revised classification of epilepsies and epileptic syndromes. Epilepsia 30, 389−399.

Cormac, I., Brown, A., Creasey, S., Ferriter, M., Huckstep, B., 2010. A retrospective evaluation of the impact of total smoking cessation on psychiatric inpatients taking clozapine. Acta Psychiatr. Scand. 121, 393−397.

Devinsky, O., Honigfeld, G., Patin, J., 1991. Clozapine-related seizures. Neurology 41, 369−371.

Direk, N., Kulaksizoglu, I.B., Alpay, K., Gurses, C., 2012. Using personality disorders to distinguish between patients with psychogenic nonepileptic seizures and those with epileptic seizures. Epilepsy Behav. 23, 138−141.

Engel Jr., J., 2001. ILAE commission report. A proposed diagnostic scheme for people with epileptic seizures and with epilepsy. Report of the ILAE task force on classification and terminology. Epilepsia 46, 796−803.

Eyer, F., Pfab, R., Felgenhauser, N., Strubel, T., Saugel, B., Zilker, T., 2011. Clinical and analytical features of severe suicidal quetiapine overdoses—retrospective cohort study. Clin. Toxicol. 49, 846−853.

Feldman, A.E., Gidal, B.E., 2013. QTc prolongation by antiepileptic drugs and the risk of torsade de pointes in patients with epilepsy. Epilepsy Behav. 26, 421−426. Available from: http://dx.doi.org/10.1016/j.yebeh.2012.09.021.

Fisher, R.S., van Emde Boas, W., Blume, W., Elger, C., Genton, P., Lee, P., et al., 2005. Epileptic seizures and epilepsy: definition proposed by the International League Against Epilepsy (ILAE) and the International Bureau for Epilepsy (IBE). Epilepsia 46, 470−472.

Fisher, R.S., Acevedo, C., Arzimanoglou, A., Bogacz, A., Cross, J.H., Elger, C.E., et al., 2014. A practical clinical definition of epilepsy. Epilepsia 55, 475−482.

Freudenreich, O., Richard, D., McEvoy, W., 1997. Clozapine-induced electroencephalogram changes as a function of clozapine serum levels. Biol. Psychiatry 42, 132−137.

Fröscher, W., 2004. Akute symptomatische Epilepsien und Gelegenheitsanfälle des Erwachsenenalters. In: Fröscher, W., Vassella, F., Hufnagel, A. (Eds.), Die Epilepsien, 2. Aufl. Schattauer, Stuttgart, New York, pp. 220−223.

Garcia, P.A., Alldredge, B.K., 1994. Drug-induced seizures. Neurol. Clin. 12, 85−99.

Gelisse, P., Samuelian, J.C., Genton, P., 1999. Is schizophrenia a risk factor for epilepsy or acute symptomatic seizures? Epilepsia 40, 1566−1571.

Gil-Nagel, A., Abou-Khalil, B., 2012. Electroencephalography and video-electroencephalography. In: Stefan, H., Theodore, W.H. (Eds.), Handbook of Clinical Neurology, vol. 107 (3rd series), Epilepsy, Part I. Elsevier, Edinburgh, pp. 323−345.

Gonzalez-Heydrich, J., Pandina, G.J., Fleisher, C.A., Hsin, O., Raches, D., Bourgeois, B.F., et al., 2004. No seizure exacerbation from risperidone in youth with comorbid epilepsy and psychiatric disorders: a case series. J. Child Adolesc. Psychopharmacol. 14, 295−310.

Gouzoulis-Mayfrank, E., Kasper, J., Grunze, H., 1994. Generalisierte epileptische Anfälle unter Behandlung mit Clozapin. Nervenarzt 65, 792−794.

Grover, S., Hazari, N., Chakrabarti, S., Avasthi, A., 2015. Association of clozapine with seizures: a brief report involving 222 patients prescribed clozapine. East Asian Arch. Psychiatry 25, 73−78.

Harrison-Woolrych, N., Skegg, K., Ashton, J., Herbison, P., Skegg, D.C., 2011. Nocturnal enuresis in patients taking clozapine, risperidone, olanzapine and quetiapine. A comparative cohort study. Br. J. Psychiatry 199, 140−144.

Hori, M., Suzuki, T., Sasaki, M., Shiraishi, H., Koizumi, J., 1992. Convulsive seizures in schizophrenic patients induced by zotepine administration. Jpn. J. Psychiatry Neurol. 46, 161−167.

Hyde, T.M., Weinberger, D.R., 1997. Seizures and schizophrenia. Schizophr. Bull. 23, 611−622.

Isbister, G.K., Balit, C.R., Macleod, D., Duffull, S.B., 2010. Amisulpride overdose is frequently associated with QT prolongation and torsades de pointes. J. Clin. Psychopharmacol. 30, 391−395.

Itil, T.M., Soldatos, C., 1980. Epileptogenic side effects of psychotropic drugs. Practical recommendations. JAMA 26, 1460−1463.

Ko, D.Y., Benbadis, S.R., 2014. Epilepsy and Seizures—Pathophysiology. Updated November 18, 2014. Retrieved from: <http://emedicine.medscape.com/article/1184846-overview# aw2aab6b2b4/>.

Kumlien, E., Lundberg, P.O., 2009. Seizure risk associated with neuroactive drugs: data from the WHO adverse drug reactions database. Seizure 19, 69−73.

Landowski, J., Cubala, W.J., 2007. Psychotropic drugs in epilepsy: effect on seizure threshold. A clinical perspective. Epileptologia 15, 49−56.

Lee, K.C., Finley, P.R., Alldredge, B.K., 2003. Risk of seizures associated with psychotropic medications: emphasis on new drugs and new findings. Expert Opin. Drug Saf. 2, 233−247.

Lertxundi, U., Hernandez, R., Medrano, J., Domingo-Echaburu, S., García, M., Aguirre, C., 2013. Antipsychotics and seizures: higher risk with atypicals? Seizure 22, 141−143. Available from: http://dx.doi.org/10.1016/j.seizure.2012.10.009.

Leucht, S., Cipriani, A., Spineli, L., Mavridis, D., Örey, D., Richter, F., et al., 2013. Comparative efficacy and tolerability of 15 antipsychotic drugs in schizophrenia: a multiple-treatments meta-analysis. Lancet 382, 951−962. Available from: http://dx.doi.org/10.1016/S0140-6736(13)60733-3.

Magaudda, A., Gugliotta, S.C., Tallarico, R., Buccheri, T., Alfa, R., Laganà, A., 2011. Identification of three distinct groups of patients with both epilepsy and psychogenic nonepileptic seizures. Epilepsy Behav. 22, 318−323.

Maher, A.R., Maglione, M., Bagley, S., Suttorp, M., Hu, J.H., Ewing, B., et al., 2011. Efficacy and comparative effectiveness of atypical antipsychotic medications for off-label uses in adults: a systematic review and meta-analysis. JAMA 306, 1359−1369. Available from: http://dx.doi.org/10.1001/jama.2011.1360.

Meyer, A., Fröscher, W., 2004. Anfallssteigernde Medikamente und Drogen. In: Fröscher, W., Vassella, F., Hufnagel, A. (Eds.), Die Epilepsien, 2. Aufl. Schattauer, Stuttgart, New York, pp. 523−541.

Myers, L., Perrine, K., Lancman, M., Fleming, M., Lancman, M., 2013. Psychological trauma in patients with psychogenic nonepileptic seizures: trauma characteristics and those who develop PTSD. Epilepsy Behav. 28, 121−126.

Neligan, A., Hauser, W.A., Sander, W.A., 2012. The epidemiology of the epilepsies. In: Stefan, H., Theodore, W.H. (Eds.), Handbook of Clinical Neurology, vol. 107 (3rd series), Epilepsy, Part I. Elsevier, Edinburgh, pp. 113−133.

Ngugi, A.K., Kariuki, S.M., Bottomley, C., Kleinschmidt, I., Sander, J.W., Newton, C.R., 2011. Incidence of epilepsy. A systematic review and meta-analysis. Neurology 77, 1005−1012. Available from: http://dx.doi.org/10.1212/WNL.0b013e31822cfc90.

Ottman, R., 1997. Family studies. In: Engel, J., Pedley, T.A. (Eds.), Epilepsy: A Comprehensive Text Book. Lippincott Raven, Philadelphia, PA, pp. 177−183.

Pacia, S., Devinsky, O., 1994. Clozapine-related seizures. Neurology 44, 2247−2249.

Pisani, F., Spina, E., Oteri, G., 1999. Antidepressant drugs and seizure susceptibility: from in vitro data to clinical practice. Epilepsia 40 (Suppl. 10), S48−S56.

Pisani, F., Oteri, G., Costa, C., Di Raimondo, G., Di Perri, R., 2002. Effects of psychotropic drugs on seizure threshold. Drug Safety 25, 91−110.

Pogarell, O., Juckel, G., Mulert, C., Amann, B., Möller, H.J., Hegerl, U., 2004. EEG abnormalities under treatment with atypical antipsychotics: effects of olanzapine and amisulpride as compared to haloperidol. Pharmacopsychiatry 37, 303−304.

Sagy, R., Weizman, A., Katz, N., 2014. Pharmacological and behavioral management of some often-overlooked clozapine-induced side effects. Int. J. Clin. Psychopharmacol. 29, 313−317.

Seneviratne, U., Cook, M., D'Souza, W., 2014. Focal abnormalities in idiopathic generalized epilepsy: a critical review of the literature. Epilepsia 55, 1157−1169.

Silvestri, R.C., Bromfield, E.B., Koshbin, S., 1998. Clozapine-induced seizures and EEG abnormalities in ambulatory psychiatric patients. Ann. Pharmacother. 32, 1147−1151.

Steinlein, O.K., Mulley, J.C., Propping, P., Wallace, R.H., Phillips, H.A., Sutherland, G.R., et al., 1995. A missense mutation in the neuronal nicotinic acetylcholine receptor alpha 4 subunit is associated with autosomal dominant nocturnal frontal lobe epilepsy. Nat. Genet. 11, 201−203.

Swinkels, W.A., Kuyk, J., van Dyck, R., Spinhoven, P., 2005. Psychiatric comorbidity in epilepsy. Epilepsy Behav. 7, 37–50.

Welch, J., Manschreck, T., Redmond, D., 1994. Clozapine-induced seizures and EEG changes. J. Neuropsychiatr. Clin. Neurosci. 6, 250–256.

Widdess-Walsh, P., Mostacci, B., Tinuper, P., Devinsky, O., 2012. Psychogenic nonepileptic seizures. In: Stefan, H., Theodore, W.H. (Eds.), Handbook of Clinical Neurology, vol. 107 (3rd series), Epilepsy, Part I. Elsevier, Edinburgh, pp. 277–295.

Williams, A.M., Park, S.H., 2015. Seizure associated with clozapine: incidence, etiology, and management. CNS Drugs 29, 101–111.

Wong, J., Delva, N., 2007. Clozapine-induced seizures: recognition and treatment. Can. J. Psychiatry 52, 457–463.

Wyderski, R.J., Starrett, W.G., Abou-Saif, A., 1999. Fatal status epilepticus associated with olanzapine. Ann. Psychopharmacother. 33, 787–789.

Chapter 10

Neuroleptic Malignant Syndrome

Julie Langan Martin and Daniel J. Martin
University of Glasgow, Glasgow, United Kingdom

10.1 EPIDEMIOLOGY

Although neuroleptic malignant syndrome (NMS) is a relatively uncommon consequence of medications which act on the central dopaminergic system, due to the large number of people treated with these medications, clinicians must remain vigilant to its possibility. Estimates of incidence vary from 0.167 cases/1000 people (Neppe, 1984) to 32.6 cases/1000 (Argyriou et al., 2012). A meta-analysis in 2007 yielded an overall estimate of 0.991 cases/1000 people (Gurrera et al., 2007). Retrospective reporting of the incidence of NMS has also been done by many in this field and it too has yielded inconsistent results. In particular Pope and colleagues (1986) reported an incidence of 1.4% of definite or suspected NMS at a hospital in Belmont, TN, USA while Gelenberg and colleagues (1988) reported a lower incidence rate of just 0.07%.

Throughout the world, estimates of incidence of NMS vary. In China, one psychiatric unit reported a rate of 0.12% over 6 years (Deng et al., 1990). While in Russia, an incidence rate of 0.02% over 10 years was reported (Spivak et al., 1991). In Australia, cases of NMS from clozapine administration were reviewed and a rate of 0.08−0.16% of new cases was estimated for an 8-month period (Sachdev et al., 1995). Trends in rates of cases of NMS have also been investigated, with some suggestion that new cases of NMS are declining. This is possibly due to increased pharmacovigilance (Keck et al., 1991) or due to the increased prescribing of atypical antipsychotics (Su et al., 2014). While there is a plausible mechanistic rationale for a reduction in NMS related to atypical antipsychotics, the evidence of a

Life-Threatening Effects of Antipsychotic Drugs. DOI: http://dx.doi.org/10.1016/B978-0-12-803376-0.00010-1
© 2016 Elsevier Inc. All rights reserved.

true reduction in rates of NMS is inconclusive (Rittmannsberger, 2002). As psychotropic prescribing has become more common (Rittmannsberger, 2002) within both primary and secondary care, clinicians need to remain aware and vigilant of this potentially fatal condition.

10.1.1 Genetic Vulnerability

Cases series have suggested that there is a familial clustering of NMS and therefore an underlying genetic vulnerability to this condition. Given the important role of the D2 receptor in the etiology of NMS, much research has focused on polymorphisms for this receptor. Three potential polymorphisms have been identified: TaqI A, -141C Ins/Del, and Ser311Cys (Kishida et al., 2004). Other genetic vulnerability lies in polymorphisms for the CYP2D6 isozyme, which is involved in the hepatic metabolism of many psychotropic medications. More than 40 different polymorphisms in the allele which affects the enzymatic activity of CYP2D6 have been identified. The resulting phenotypes of the CYP2D6 polymorphisms led to individuals being classified as extensive, poor, or ultrarapid metabolizers (Bertilsson et al., 2002). Some studies have suggested that the prevalence of *5 alleles in the group of patients with NMS was higher than that in the controls of individuals who have had NMS (Zivković et al., 2010) although more detailed work in this area is required.

10.1.2 Risk Factors

Although at times NMS is considered to be idiosyncratic and unpredictable, a number of risk factors have been identified.

10.1.2.1 Demographic Factors

Major demographic risk factors include: male sex (Tsai et al., 2003) and medical comorbidity. Variables relating to the individuals overall health and resilience are also important. The presence of an organic brain syndrome or previous brain injury (Pelonero et al., 1998), or poorly-controlled antipsychotic-induced extrapyramidal side effects have also been found to increase the risk of NMS. Males under 40 are often considered to be at greater risk of NMS but it is unclear if this is a reflection of increased use of antipsychotics within this population. It should also be noted that this patient group are also exposed to increased rates of risk factors for NMS including parenteral medication and physical restraint, further complicating the association. Postpartum women may also be at slightly elevated risk (Alexander et al., 1998). Advancing age, malnutrition, agitation, physical exhaustion, biochemical and metabolic abnormalities, such as hyponatremia, thyrotoxicosis, and iron deficiency (Rosebush and Mazurek, 1991), along with psychiatric and medical comorbidity, such as Parkinson's disease (Takubo et al., 2003), can also have an important influence on risk of developing NMS (Caroff and Mann, 1993). Alcohol or other psychoactive substance misuse (Itoh et al., 1977) is also associated with increased risk of NMS.

10.1.2.2   Genetic Liability

It is also well recognized that a prior history of NMS or a personal history or family history of catatonia is a risk factor for NMS (Otani et al., 1991a,b). Within the literature there are reports of identical twins, a mother, and two of her daughters all having suffered an episode of NMS (Otani et al., 1991a,b), increasing the possibility of a genetic basis for the condition, albeit within case reports. This likely represents the underlying genetic predisposition which is as yet not fully understood although this may be linked to a genetically-induced reduction in the function of the dopamine D2 receptor (Mihara et al., 2003).

10.1.2.3   Environmental Factors

Dehydration (Keek et al., 1989), physical restraint, and high external temperature have all been cited in the literature as environmental risk factors for NMS. These risk factors themselves may be increased in situations where individuals are mentally unwell, distressed, or living in difficult situations.

10.1.2.4   Pharmacological Factors

While NMS can occur at any time during the course of drug treatment, it occurs more frequently during the initial phase of drug treatment or after a dose change. More recently rapid alteration and in particular escalation of antipsychotic dose has emerged an important risk factor for the development of NMS (Caroff and Mann, 1993), with most cases occurring shortly after initial exposure (Pelonero et al., 1998). NMS is less likely to occur in patients who have been stable on their dose of antipsychotic medication for a long time or who have good long-term compliance (Berman, 2011; Sachdev et al., 1997). However, it is important to note that NMS has been reported to occur at all standard doses and in all routes of administration.

Higher total doses of antipsychotic drugs, along with parenteral routes of administration—intramuscular (Viejo et al., 2003; Tse et al., 2015) or rarely intravenous—are also associated with increased risk of NMS. It is also thought that typical (or "first-generation") drugs are associated with higher risk of NMS compared to atypical or "second-generation" antipsychotic drugs (Buckley and Hutchinson, 1995). The common rationale for this is related to the higher dopamine D2 affinity of typical antipsychotics, which have a lower binding dissociation constant from the reception. Antipsychotic polypharmacy and the concomitant use of medications which predispose to NMS (such as lithium and carbamazepine) (Pajonk et al., 2006) also increase the risk of NMS.

Rate of dose escalation of antipsychotic medication has been recognized as a risk factor for NMS (Baker et al., 2003). Although it is recognized that rate of patient titration onto a therapeutic dose is often multifactorial, with factors, such as age, comorbid physical health problems, previous antipsychotic exposure, history of side effects, severity of illness, and the need for a rapid clinical response, being important considerations, individual clinician preference and experience also plays a role. While there are titration schedules available for certain medications, most notably quetiapine (BNF 63, 2012) and clozapine, guidance is not available for all medications. In clinical practice there are occasions where antipsychotic dose is escalated more quickly than would be seen routinely and caution should be undertaken where "rapid dose escalation" occurs (Langan et al., 2012).

10.2 PATHOBIOLOGY

Historically NMS was considered to be a condition affecting only people with psychotic disorders prescribed antipsychotic medications, however, with the increased use of antipsychotics "off-label" NMS has been reported in individuals with Parkinson's disease, delirium, encephalitis, and dementia (Tse et al., 2015). An increasing issue to be considered by healthcare professionals is the possibility of "over the counter" or online purchases of antipsychotic medication. Due to the sedative effects, increased availability, and the possible stigma associated with mental health problems, increasing numbers of patients worldwide are using medications which affect the central dopamine system without appropriate supervision from healthcare professionals. Thus when taking a drug history it is important to ask about: over the counter medications, herbal remedies, online medications and "legal highs" (new psychoactive substances). Other medications such as the tricyclic antidepressants amoxapine (Madakasira, 1989) and amitriptyline (Janati et al., 2012), the mood stabilizers lithium (Gill et al., 2003) and carbamazepine (Sharma et al., 2013) and phenelzine (Heyland and Sauve, 1991) have all been reported to cause NMS. This is thought to be a result of their dopamine blocking properties. In addition to psychotropic medication there have also been cases of NMS associated with other agents with antidopaminergic activity such as the antiemetic metoclopramide (Friedman et al., 1987; Patterson, 1988), promethazine, tetrabenazine, droperidol, and diatrizoate.

10.2.1 Dopamine Receptor Blockade Hypothesis

A marked and sudden reduction in central dopaminergic activity resulting from D_2 receptor blockade within the nigrostriatal, hypothalamic, mesolimbic, and mesocortical pathways may help to explain some of the clinical features of NMS, such as rigidity, hyperthermia, and altered mental state (Bhanushali and Tuite, 2004; Strawn et al., 2007). The general consensus that the risk of NMS is higher in conditions associated with antipsychotic sensitivity—such as learning disability (Viejo et al., 2003) and dementia with Lewy bodies (Kobayashi et al., 2006)—also provides evidence for this pathophysiological mechanism. Dopamine neurotransmission is important in thermoregulation and antagonism of dopamine receptor-mediated signaling by antipsychotics in the thermoregulatory center can potentially lead to a dysregulation of thermoregulation (Henderson and Wooten, 1981). Sudden blockade of the postsynaptic receptor, a sudden reduction in postsynaptic receptor stimulation, or a lack of neurotransmitter will all lead to a lack of dopaminergic signaling in the thermoregulatory system subsequently leading to hyperthermia, which is one of the classical features of NMS.

Disrupted dopamine receptor-mediated signaling as a mechanism of NMS is also supported by a number of factors including the observation that antipsychotic medication is the primary agent in most cases of NMS and the observation that NMS can also be induced by the abrupt withdrawal of dopamine agonists (e.g., in Parkinson's Disease). Even though the NMS can occur at any point during the course of treatment with implicated agents, it is thought to occur more frequently during both the initial period of treatment or after change in the dose of a drug affecting the central dopamine system. Given this, it is unsurprising that higher doses of antipsychotic drugs have been correlated with a greater risk of developing NMS. Similarly, parenteral routes of administration (such as intramuscular or intravenous) have also been associated with increased incidence of the NMS. In relation to the type of medication affecting the central dopamine system, typical (conventional or first generation) antipsychotics are also associated with a higher risk for development of NMS compared to atypical or second-generation antipsychotics. This is often explained by the higher dopamine D2 receptor affinity of typical antipsychotics, which often have a lower binding dissociation constant from the receptor.

The occurrence of NMS in individuals treated with catecholamine depleting drugs also provides further evidence for disrupted dopaminergic signaling being a possible mechanism underlying NMS (Haggerty et al., 1987). Altered dopamine neurotransmission in the basal ganglia, which is important for regulating muscle tone and motor coordination, may explain the rigidity, increased muscle tone, and tremor reported in NMS. Furthermore it is possible that the increased muscular tone as a secondary symptom of NMS can lead to a further increased body temperature.

10.2.2   Sympathoadrenal Hyperactivity

D2 receptor antagonism does not fully explain all the signs and symptoms of NMS. In particular the occurrence of NMS with medications with low D_2 affinity has led to the proposal that sympathoadrenal hyperactivity resulting from the removal of tonic inhibition within the sympathetic nervous system may play an important role in NMS (Gurrera, 1999). This is supported by the frequent occurrence of autonomic symptoms in NMS, as well as demonstrated changes in urine and plasma catecholamine levels.

10.2.3 Musculoskeletal Fiber Toxicity Hypothesis

Similarities with malignant hyperthermia have led to theories that a defect in calcium regulatory proteins within sympathetic neurons may be a key factor which triggers the onset of NMS (Gurrera, 2002). Release of calcium from the sarcoplasmic reticulum of muscle cells has been shown to be increased with antipsychotic usage (Adnet et al., 2000) and it may be that this could lead to the rigidity, muscle breakdown, and hyperthermia seen in NMS. The therapeutic effect of dantrolene in treating NMS also supports this theory. Malignant hyperthermia is a rare condition characterized by high body temperature after the administration of halogenate anesthetics. Individuals who develop this condition have a characteristic in vitro musculoskeletal contractile response to halothane and caffeine. Similar results are noted when biopsied muscular fibers of individuals with NMS are challenged to halothane or caffeine (Gurrera, 2002). This laboratory finding supports this hypothesis.

10.2.4 Neuroimmunological Hypothesis

A neuroimmunological hypothesis for NMS has also been postulated by a number of researchers (Anglin et al., 2010). NMS is known to be associated with a reduction in serum iron levels, which is a key feature of the immunological driven acute phase response (Rosebush and Mazurek, 1991). It is hypothesized that the acute phase response in NMS may occur due to autoantibody production, heat stress, muscle breakdown, and psychological stress. There is also strong evidence to suggest that iron is essential for the normal functioning of the dopamine D2 receptor (Kato et al., 2007) and that the reduction in serum iron levels that occurs may result in a decreased number of functional D2 receptors in the brain.

10.3 CLINICAL AND LABORATORY FEATURES

The diagnosis of NMS is largely based on clinical history and the presence of specific clinical signs (Table 10.1). NMS can be quite variable in its clinical manifestations and all four classical features may not be present leading to diagnostic difficulty and delay. The fever seen in NMS is characteristically high and without major fluctuations. Therapeutic response to conventional antipyretic drugs (such as paracetamol) may also be poor. Muscular rigidity is classically generalized and symmetrical, although it may vary from a mild increase in tone to extreme generalized rigidity. Opisthotonus and oculogyric crises may occur and nystagmus, dysphagia, or dysarthria

TABLE 10.1 The Classic NMS Tetrad

- Fever
- Rigidity
- Altered mental state, and
- Autonomic instability

TABLE 10.2 Biochemical Abnormalities in NMS

- Raised creatinine kinase at times >600 UI L^{-1}
- High white cell count (in particular a leukocytosis)
- Reduced glomerular filtration rate
- Raise inflammatory markers (such as C-reactive protein and Erythrocyte Sedimentation Rate), and
- Low serum iron

may occur again due to increased muscular tone. Delirium is also often present and is characterized with typical fluctuations in levels of orientation, consciousness, and psychomotor agitation. Autonomic instability is a common feature and may present with labile blood pressure, unstable heart rate and extreme diaphoresis. Urinary incontinence along with sialorrhea may also occur. Although there is significant heterogeneity in presentations of NMS, authors have suggested that the clinical course typically begins with muscle rigidity followed by a fever within hours of onset and mental status changes that can range from mild drowsiness, agitation, or confusion to a severe delirium or coma.

There is no specific diagnostic test for NMS and biochemical abnormalities can be variable and far-ranging (Table 10.2). Electromyography and muscle biopsy yield nonspecific results with minimal capacity to rule in or rule out NMS and may be indicated depending on the clinical picture. In general, muscle biopsy should be considered when there is a significant suspicion of an alternative diagnosis. Neuroimaging, electroencephalography (EEG), and lumbar puncture may also be required.

When considering the possibility of NMS, many clinicians place significant emphasis on the levels of creatinine kinase. Although this laboratory marker is very important in the diagnosis of the condition, there are several potential pitfalls when considering it in an unwell patient. Firstly, in episodes of NMS, CK levels are usually >6000−1000 UI L^{-1}. Several other conditions including physical restraint or the intramuscular injection of medication increase levels of CK, albeit more modestly (usually below 600 UI L^{-1}). The further and ongoing monitoring of CK levels in a patient with suspected NMS is vital, as one would expect levels to decline over time in a patient recovering from the condition. Measurements of liver, kidney, electrolyte, and fluid base balance should also be sought as part of a comprehensive medical work up. Although less likely to yield positive results, if possible an EEG could also be considered to rule out seizure activity if this investigation is available and practical to perform on the patient. Furthermore, EEG tracings typically show generalized slowing in cases of NMS. Similarly, lumbar puncture is an important part of the work-up in a patient presenting with symptoms suggestive of NMS in order to help rule out infections of the central nervous system.

Given the heterogeneity and lack of consistent biological markers, there are a number of diagnostic criteria currently used to aid diagnosis, which include the DSM IV criteria (DSM-IV-TR, 2000), Pope's criteria (Pope et al., 1986), Levenson's criteria (Levenson, 1985), and Adityanjee's criteria (Adityanjee et al., 1988) (Table 10.3).

10.3.1 Differential Diagnosis

Many conditions can mimic the presentation of NMS, and a high level of clinician suspicion, vigilance, and expertise is required in order to diagnose and initiate treatment of NMS promptly. The main differential diagnoses for NMS include: bacterial or viral meningitis and other CNS infections; toxic or metabolic encephalopathies; serotonin syndrome (SS); severe dehydration; heat stroke; drug toxicities; cholinergic reactions; drug overdose or withdrawal; lethal catatonia; vasculitis (including primary CNS vasculitis); malignant hyperthermia; heavy metal poisoning (e.g., with thallium or arsenic); intermittent acute porphyria; thyroid storm; and febrile syndromes occurring in patients with neuroleptic-induced parkinsonism. Clinical heterogeneity creates diagnostic uncertainty and it is imperative that any underlying source of infection in particular is excluded. Consequentially patients may need extensive investigations with serial blood and urine cultures, chest X-rays, neuroimaging, and CSF analysis being obtained before underlying infections can confidently be excluded.

10.3.1.1 NMS and SS

SS is a life-threatening adverse reaction caused by serotonergic antidepressants and neuroleptics. It is thought to occur due to increased serotonin activity in the central nervous system and its clinical presentation overlaps substantially with NMS (Table 10.4). Given the autonomic, neuromuscular, and mental state changes that occur in SS, distinction between the two syndromes (NMS and SS) can be challenging (Dosi et al., 2014). While SS is classically associated with myoclonus and hyperreflexia, NMS is classically associated with severe muscle rigidity. Gastrointestinal features, such as diarrhea, nausea, and vomiting, which are more commonly reported in SS, are quite unusual in NMS. CK, which is classically elevated in NMS, may

TABLE 10.3 Diagnostic Criteria for Neuroleptic Malignant Syndrome

DSM IV Research Criteria for Neuroleptic Malignant Syndrome	Pope's Criteria (All 3 Major Criteria Required) Retrospective: 2 of 3 With Additional Criteria	Levenson Criteria (All 3 Major Symptoms, or 2 Major and 4 Minor)	Adityanjee Criteria (All 4 Major and at Least 2 From the Autonomic Dysfunction Category)
A. Development of severe muscle rigidity and elevated temperature associated with the use of neuroleptic medication B. Two (or more) of the following: • diaphoresis, • dysphagia, • tremor, • incontinence, • changes in level of consciousness (ranging from confusion to coma), • mutism, • tachycardia, • elevated or labile blood pressure, • leukocytosis • Laboratory evidence of muscle injury (e.g., elevated creatinine kinase) C. The symptoms in criteria A and B are not due to another substance, neurological or general medical condition D. The symptoms in A and B are no better accounted for by a mental disorder	*Major Criteria:* A. **Hyperthermia** (>37.5°C) B. **Severe EPS** (2 or more) of: • Lead pipe rigidity • Cog wheeling • Sialorrhea • Oculogyric crisis • Retrocollis • Opisthotonus • Trismus • Dysphagia • Choreiform movements • Dyskinetic movements • Festinating gait • Flexor-extensor posturing C. **Autonomic dysfunction** (2 or more) of: • Hypertension ≥ 20 mmHg rise in diastolic BP • Tachycardia ≥ 30 above baseline • Tachypnea ≥ 25 • Diaphoresis • Incontinence *Retrospective Criteria:* A. **Clouded consciousness** B. **Leukocytosis >15,000** C. **CPK > 300 U L^{-1}**	*Major Criteria:* A. **Fever** B. **Muscle rigidity** C. **Elevated CPK** *Minor Criteria:* A. **Tachycardia** B. **Abnormal BP** C. **Tachypnea** D. **Altered consciousness** E. **Diaphoresis** F. **Leukocytosis**	*Major Features:* A. **Altered sensorium (except agitation) documented by 2 different observers,** B. **Muscle rigidity,** C. **Hyperthermia >39°C oral** D. **Autonomic dysfunction** • Tachycardia (>90 bpm) • Tachypnea (>25 min^{-1}) • BP fluctuation of at least 30 mmHg systolic or 15 mmHg diastolic • Diaphoresis • Incontinence *Supportive Features:* CPK elevation Leukocytosis

CPK, creatinine phosphokinase; EPS, extrapyramidal symptoms; BP, blood pressure.

TABLE 10.4 Clinical Features of Serotonin Syndrome

- *Neuromuscular abnormalities*: tremor, myoclonus, clonus, muscular rigidity, and hyperreflexia,
- *Mental state changes*: anxiety, agitation, and hypomania, and
- *Autonomic hyperactivity*: fever, diaphoresis, and tachycardia.

also be elevated in SS. This may enhance diagnostic confusion. SS tends to resolve within a few days of discontinuation of the likely offending drug(s) while NMS takes a longer time to resolve (often 9−14 days).

Published case reports highlight the difficulties encountered when attempting to differentiate between the two conditions. In one case, a 62-year-old male patient had been treated with imipramine and lithium carbonate. He developed symptoms of hyperthermia, myoclonus, tremor, tachycardia, mental status changes, diaphoresis, and mild muscle rigidity following an increase in his imipramine dose. Despite the pharmacological and clinical features being more consistent with SS, the clinical picture evolved and included grossly elevated creatinine kinase and severe muscle rigidity as well as myoclonus and hyperreflexia. The patient had also been prescribed metoclopramide, a dopamine antagonist. Following admission to a general medical unit he was found to satisfy criteria for both SS and the NMS. The final diagnosis was most likely initial SS followed by the development of NMS. Although unusual, this case underlines the possibility of cooccurring and indeed related episodes of the two conditions. This consideration has direct relevance to common prescribing patterns. Due to widened availability of drugs, the increasing recognition of diagnostic uncertainty in psychiatry and the increasing number of indications for different psychotropic medication, it is not uncommon for antidepressants or mood stabilizers to be prescribed alongside antipsychotic medication. As a result, it is important to keep an open mind as to the possibility of, or comorbidity of, both SS and the NMS.

10.3.1.2 Catatonia and NMS

A debated issue is whether NMS should be thought of as an extreme form of catatonia. Those who argue that NMS is an individual entity support the view that NMS is caused primarily by dopamine receptor blockade. Conversely, authors Taylor and Fink are among the many scholars who argue that NMS is a form of malignant catatonia. This argument is strengthened by the knowledge and observation that NMS often presents with the clinical features of a catatonic syndrome but also includes the presence of severe autonomic nervous system dysregulation. NMS also responds very well to the same treatments as catatonic syndrome including electroconvulsive therapy (ECT). Furthermore, there are documented presentations

TABLE 10.5 Clinical Presentation of Catatonia

- Agitation
- Catalepsy: prolonged maintenance of a fixed body posture
- Echolalia: immediate and involuntary repetition of words
- Echopraxia: involuntary mimicking of movements of others
- Grimacing
- Mannerism: a distinctive behavioral trait
- Mutism
- Negativism
- Posturing
- Stereotypy
- Stupor
- Waxy flexibility

consistent with NMS prior to the development of antipsychotic medications. Catatonia was first described in 1874 by Kahlbaum and consists of affective, behavioral, and motor symptoms (Table 10.5).

Stauder (1934) coined the term "lethal catatonia," when reporting a case series of individuals with catatonia who presented with autonomic disturbance and who had a high fatality rate. Other authors have referred to this as "pernicious" or "malignant" catatonia (Gabris and Muller, 1983; Philbrick and Rummans, 1994). Given the autonomic features present it is largely indistinguishable from NMS (although when Stauder first reported this, it was in the preantipsychotic era). Given the overlap between the two conditions, some researchers have hypothesized that NMS and malignant catatonia are on a continuum and that NMS is an iatrogenic, drug-induced form of malignant catatonia (Fricchione et al., 2000).

10.3.2   Complications and Significant Sequelae

There is evidence to suggest that in some individuals when the offending pharmacological agent is stopped, NMS will resolve in 7–10 days (Caroff, 1980). However, in some the clinical course is much more severe and is life-threatening: this largely depends on the severity of the illness and resultant medical complications. It is noteworthy that prompt recognition and action can significantly improve prognosis of NMS. In cases of delayed diagnosis and treatment, the illness can last for several weeks and there is an increased risk of patients being left with residual catatonic symptoms or parkinsonism as well as longer lasting cardiopulmonary effects.

Potential complications include: seizures, renal failure, cognitive impairment, and residual catatonic states. Some individuals have also been reported to develop compartment syndrome after an episode of NMS. In cases where death occurs as a result of NMS, it is often due to cardiac arrhythmias, disseminated intravascular coagulation, cardiac failure, respiratory failure, or renal failure.

10.3.3   Risk of Recurrence

Given that many individuals who develop NMS have a major mental illness (schizophrenia or bipolar disorder) future antipsychotic treatment may be required. Rechallenging with antipsychotics after an episode of NMS has occurred, but is not always safe. McCarthy (1988) reported a fatal case of NMS after a milder episode 3 months previously and others have reported recurrence of NMS when using similarly potent antipsychotics (Gonzalez-Blanco et al., 2013). Therefore consideration to the use of other treatments such as lithium or ECT should be given. If reintroduction of antipsychotics is required, it should occur with the utmost caution and with close monitoring most likely as an inpatient.

10.3.4   Risk Stratification for Death or Permanent Disability

NMS characteristically runs a fluctuating course and is known to be heterogenic with some having a mild illness while others have a severe life-threatening one. Illness severity is difficult to predict and to date there are no risk stratification tools available. Although creatinine phosphokinase (CPK) is typically raised in NMS, it may also be elevated for other reasons for example, due to muscular injuries or after exertion (Sahoo et al., 2014). Moreover CPK is not a particularly specific test, as individuals who are treated with antipsychotics who become pyrexial may have an elevated CPK for other reasons (Adnet et al., 2000).

10.4   PREVENTION AND MANAGEMENT

Prompt cessation of the offending medication is of paramount importance in NMS. There is very little purpose in continuing the treatment with medications suspected of causing the condition, even to obtain laboratory measurements such as CPK to confirm the diagnosis. Elevated CPK is likely to remain for several days following the cessation of medication and in any case, further administration of the medication may worsen the clinical picture.

Initial treatment is largely supportive and rehydration and electrolyte management is often required. Although not confirmed through systematic research, keeping the patient in a comfortable ambient temperature not higher than $21-23°C$ may enable better heat dissipation. Other physical measures to control temperature, including the use of wet cold cataplasms, have again not been fully evaluated, but are both low-cost and low-risk interventions. In cases of severe autonomic instability, admission and treatment in the Intensive Care

Unit may be required. For individuals with severe hypotension, inotropic support may be required. For individuals with a reduced conscious level, mechanical ventilation may also be required. As is the case in any situation involving reduced conscious level, the risk of aspiration pneumonia should be considered and addressed accordingly as this is a major source of mortality within patients suffering from NMS. Simple measures include placing the patient in a semirecumbent position (45 degrees) and keeping physical restraint to a minimum, although this in itself may not be possible. A rarer, although not insignificant risk is that of reversible dilated cardiomyopathy—a baseline chest X-ray and echocardiograph as well as an ECG should all be considered and clinical vigilance maintained to this possibility.

Antipyretics can be used to treat the elevated temperature, although there are reports of decreased efficacy in NMS. Due to initial diagnostic uncertainty, antibiotics and/or antivirals are often prescribed (especially if encephalitis had been suspected). It is also important to ensure adequate oxygenation of the patient. It is also important to consider investigating and correcting any possible electrolyte imbalance or acid—base disturbance. It has been suggested that maintaining a slightly alkalotic pH benefits the excretion of myoglobinuric detritus, which itself can be supported by the administration of loop diuretics.

Specific treatments for NMS can at times be controversial as evidence is often empirical or based on case reports. However some pharmacological interventions are thought to reduce the mortality in NMS (Table 10.6). Electroconvulsive treatment has been used successfully as a treatment for NMS and is usually considered after failure to respond to one of the above treatment options. A case review by Trollor and Sachdev (1999) found that ECT was effective even after drug treatment had failed and that a few treatments were

---

TABLE 10.6 Pharmacological Therapy for NMS

- *Benzodiazepines*: this is based on the premise that NMS is a form of catatonia. Successful use of lorazepam to treat NMS has been reported (Davis et al., 2000)
- *Dantrolene*: a hydantoin derivate which causes muscle relaxation by inhibiting calcium release by the endoplasmic reticulum, and consequently decreases intracellular calcium availability. As a result it can be beneficial with regards the musculoskeletal toxicity seen in neuroleptic malignant syndrome. It has been used to successfully treat cases of the condition (Kouparanis et al., 2015)
- *Bromocriptine*: a dopamine agonist and has been shown to reduce rigidity and pyrexia and has been used successfully in the treatment of NMS (Yang et al., 2014). It is important to monitor for adverse side effects such as nausea, vomiting, or deterioration in mental status
- *Amantadine*: a weak antagonist at the NDMA-like glutamate receptor and increases dopamine release and reduces reuptake. It has also been reported to be effective in the treatment of NMS (Woo et al., 1986)

necessary before response was apparent. The therapeutic effect of ECT may be due to increased sensitivity to dopamine receptors (Wielosz, 1981), however, it is largely unclear as treatment response is not predictable on the basis of age, gender, psychiatric diagnosis, or any particular feature of NMS including catatonia.

A series of case studies have indicated that the fastest resolution of NMS resulted from bromocriptine followed by dantrolene administration. Both drugs resulted in a remission of NMS significantly quicker than supportive treatment alone. There are also some reports which support the use of both drugs at the same time (Rosenberg and Green, 1989).

An important aspect of the management of NMS is the subsequent management of patients who have suffered an episode of the condition who require ongoing treatment with medications which affect the central dopaminergic system. In many instances patients who have recovered from an episode of NMS require ongoing treatment with centrally acting dopaminergic drugs. This introduces a significant management challenge as a previous episode of NMS is a known risk factor for a further episode. Although there is no well-established approach to this, in general clinicians should attempt to minimize other risk factors, use low potency dopamine antagonists, avoid the use (where possible) of parenteral routes of administration, and perhaps consider the use of ECT. Furthermore, given the challenges faced by many patients with chronic mental illness with regards communication and in some cases cognition, careful consideration should be given to developing a system of medication alert, such as a sticker on their case notes or an electronic alert on their system, if they have previously suffered an episode of NMS.

REFERENCES

Adityanjee, Singh, S., Singh, G., Ong, S., 1988. Spectrum concept of neuroleptic malignant syndrome. Br. J. Psychiatry 153, 107–111.

Adnet, P., Lestavel, P., Krivosic-Horber, R., 2000. Neuroleptic malignant syndrome. Br. J. Anaesth. 85, 129–135.

Alexander, P.J., Thomas, R.M., Das, A., 1998. Is risk of neuroleptic malignant syndrome increased in the postpartum period? J. Clin. Psychiatry 59, 254–255.

Anglin, R.E., Rosebush, P.I., Mazurek, M.F., 2010. Neuroleptic malignant syndrome: a neuroimmunologic hypothesis. CMAJ 182 (18), E834–E838.

Argyriou, A.A., Drakoulgona, O., Karanasios, P., Kouliasa, L., Leonidou, L., Giannakopoulou, F., et al., 2012. Lithium induced fatal neuroleptic malignant syndrome in a patient not being concomitantly treated with commonly offending agents. J. Pain Symptom Manage. 44 (6), e4–e6.

Baker, R.W., Kinon, B.J., Maguire, G.A., Liu, H., Hill, A.L., 2003. Effectiveness of rapid initial dose escalation of up to forty milligrams per day of oral olanzapine in acute agitation. J. Clin. Psychopharmacol. 23, 342–348.

Berman, B.D., 2011. Neuroleptic malignant syndrome: a review for neurohospitalists. Neurohospitalist 1, 41–47.

Bertilsson, L., Dahl, M.L., Dalen, P., Al-Shurbaji, A., 2002. Molecular genetics of CYP2D6: clinical relevance with focus on psychotropic drugs. Br. J. Clin. Pharmacol. 53, 111–122.

Bhanushali, M.J., Tuite, P.J., 2004. The evaluation and management of patients with Neuroleptic malignant syndrome. Neurologic Clin. 22, 389–441.

BNF 63, March 2012. 4.2.1 Antipsychotic Drugs 235. <http://www.medicinescomplete.com/mc/bnf/current/PHP2284-quetiapine.htm/>.

Buckley, P.F., Hutchinson, M., 1995. Neuroleptic malignant syndrome. J. Neurol. Neurosurg. Psychiatry 58, 271–273.

Caroff, S.N., 1980. The neuroleptic malignant syndrome. J. Clin. Psychiatry 41 (3), 79–83.

Caroff, S.N., Mann, S.C., 1993. Neuroleptic malignant syndrome. Med. Clin. North Am. 77 (1), 185–202.

Davis, J.M., Caroff, S.N., Mann, S.C., 2000. Treatment of neuroleptic malignant syndrome. Psychiatr. Ann. 30 (5), 325–331.

Deng, M.Z., Chen, G.Q., Phillips, M.R., 1990. Neurolpetic Malignant Syndrome in 12 of 9,792 Chinese inpatients exposed to neuroleptics: a prospective study. Am. J. Psychiatry 147 (9), 1149–1155.

Dosi, R., Ambaliya, A., Joshi, H., Patell, R., 2014. Serotonin syndrome versus neuroleptic malignant syndrome: a challenging clinical quandary. BMJ Case Rep. Available from: http://dx.doi.org/10.1136/bcr-2014-204154.

DSM-IV-TR, 2000. Medication-induced movement disorders: neuroleptic malignant syndrome. Diagnostic and Statistical Manual of Mental Disorders. American Psychiatric Association, Washington, DC, pp. 795–798.

Fricchione, G., Mann, S., Caroff, S., 2000. Catatonia, lethal catatonia and neuroleptic malignant syndrome. Psychiatr. Ann. 30 (5), 347–355.

Friedman, L.S., Weinrauch, L.A., D'Elia, J.A., 1987. Metoclopramide induced neuroleptic malignant syndrome. Arch. Intern. Med. 147, 1495–1497.

Gabris, G., Müller, C., 1983. So-called pernicious catatonia. Encéphale 9, 365–385.

Gelenberg, A.J., Bellinghausen, B., Wojcik, J.D., Falk, W.E., Sachs, G.S., 1988. A prospective survey of neuroleptic malignant syndrome in a short term psychiatric hospital. Am. J. Psychiatry 154 (4), 517–518.

Gill, J., Singh, H., Nugent, K., 2003. Acute lithium intoxication and neuroleptic malignant syndrome. Pharmacotherapy 23, 811–815.

González-Blanco, L., García-Prada, H., Santamarina, S., Jiménez-Treviño, L., Bobes, J., 2013. Recurrence of neuroleptic malignant syndrome. Actas Esp. Psiquiatr. 41 (5), 314–318, Epub September 1, 2013.

Gurrera, R.J., 1999. Sympathoadrenalhyoactivity and the aetiology of neuroleptic malignant syndrome. Am. J. Psychiatry 156, 169–180.

Gurrera, R.J., 2002. Is neuroleptic malignant syndrome a neurogenic form of malignant hyperthermia? Clin. Neuropharmacol. 25, 183–193.

Gurrera, R.J., Simpson, J.C., Tsuang, M.T., 2007. Meta-analytic evidence of systemic bias in estimates of neuroleptic malignant syndrome incidence. Compr. Psychiatry 48 (2), 205–211.

Haggerty Jr., J.J., Bentsen, B.S., Gillette, G.M., 1987. Neuroleptic malignant syndrome superimposed on tardive dyskinesia. Br. J. Psychiatry 150, 104–105.

Henderson, V.M., Wooten, G.F., 1981. Neuroleptic malignant syndrome: a pathogenic role for dopamine receptor blockade? Neurology 31 (2), 132–137.

Heyland, D., Sauve, M., 1991. Neuroleptic malignant syndrome without the use of neuroleptics. Can. Med. Ass. J. 145, 817–819.

Itoh, H., Ohtuska, N., Ogita, K., 1977. Malignant neuroleptic syndrome: its present status in Japan and clinical problems. Folia Psychiatr. Neurol. Jpn. 31, 565−576.

Janati, A.B., Alghasab, N., Osman, A., 2012. Neuroleptic malignant syndrome caused by a combination of carbamazepine and amitriptyline. Case Rep. Neurol. Med.183252.

Kato, D., Kawanishi, C., Kishida, I., et al., 2007. Effects of CYP2D6 polymorphisms on neuroleptic malignant syndrome. Eur. J. Clin. Pharmacol. 63, 991−996.

Keck Jr, P.E., Pope Jr, H.G., McElroy, S.E., 1991. Declining frequency of neuroleptic malignant syndrome in a hospital population. Am. J. Psychiatry 148 (7), 880−882.

Keek, P.E., Pope, H.G., Cohen, B.M., McElroy, S.L., Nierenberg, A.A., 1989. Risk factors for neuroleptic malignant syndrome. Arch. Gen. Psychiatry 46, 914−9198.

Kishida, I., Kawanishi, C., Furuno, T., Kato, D., Ishigami, T., Kosaka, K., 2004. Association in Japanese patients between neuroleptic malignant syndrome and functional polymorphisms of the dopamine D(2) receptor gene. Mol. Psychiatry 9 (3), 293−298.

Kobayashi, A., Kawanishi, C., Matsumura, T., Kato, D., Furukawa, R., Kishida, I., et al., 2006. Quetiapine induced neuroleptic malignant syndrome in dementia with Lewy bodies: a case report. Prog. Neuropsychopharmacol. Biol. Psychiatry 30, 1170−1172.

Kouparanis, A., Bozikas, A., Spilioti, M., Tziomalos, K., 2015. Neuroleptic malignant syndrome in a patient on long-term olanzapine treatment at a stable dose: successful treatment with dantrolene. Brain Inj. 29 (5), 658−660. Available from: http://dx.doi.org/ 10.3109/ 02699052.2014.1002002/. Epub January 27, 2015.

Langan, J., Martin, D., Shahajan, P., Smith, D., 2012. Antipsychotic dose escalation as a trigger for Neuroleptic Malignant Syndrome (NMS): literature review and case series report. BMC Psychiatry 12, 214, ISSN: 1471-244X. Available from: http://dx.doi.org/10.1186/1471-244X-12-214/.

Levenson, J.L., 1985. Neuroleptic malignant syndrome. Am. J. Psychiatry 142 (10), 1137−1145.

Madakasira, S., 1989. Amoxapine induced neuroleptic malignant syndrome. Drug Intelligence Clin. Pharm. 23, 50−61.

McCarthy, A., 1988. Fatal recurrence of neuroleptic malignant syndrome. Br. J. Psychiatry 152, 558−559.

Mihara, K., Kondo, T., Suzuki, A., Yasui-Furukori, N., Ono, S., Sano, A., et al., 2003. Relationship between functional dopamine D2 and D3 receptors gene polymorphisms and neuroleptic malignant syndrome. Am. J. Med. Genet. B. Neuropsychiatr. Genet. 117B (1), 57−60.

Neppe, V.M., 1984. The neuroleptic malignant syndrome, a priority system. South Afr. Med. J. 65 (13), 523−525.

Otani, K., Horiuchi, M., Kondo, T., Kanedo, S., Fuskushima, Y., 1991a. Is the predisposition to neuroleptic malignant syndrome genetically transmitted? Br. J. Psychiatry 158, 850−853.

Otani, K., Kaneko, S., Fukushima, Y., Chiba, K., Ishizaki, T., 1991b. NMS and genetic drug oxidation. Br. J. Psychiatry 159 (4), 595−596. Available from: http://dx.doi.org/10.1192/bjp.159.4.595.

Pajonk, F.-G.B., Schwertner, A.K., Seelig, M.A., 2006. Rapid dose titration of quetiapine for the treatment of acute schizophrenia and acute mania: a case series. J. Psychopharmacol. 20, 119−124.

Patterson, J.F., 1988. Neuroleptic malignant syndrome associated with Metoclopramide. South Med. J. 81, 674−675.

Pelonero, A.L., Levebson, J.L., Pandurangi, A.K., 1998. Neuroleptic malignant syndrome; a review. Psychiatr. Serv 49, 1163−1172.

Philbrick, K.L., Rummans, T.A., 1994. Malignant catatonia. J. Neuropsychiatr. Clin. Neurosci. 6, 1−13.

Pope Jr, H.G., Keck Jr, P.E., McElroy, S.L., 1986. Frequency and presentation of neuroleptic malignant syndrome in a large psychiatric hospital. Am. J. Psychiatry 143 (10), 1227−1233.

Rittmannsberger, H., 2002. The use of drug monotherapy in psychiatric inpatient treatment. Prog. Neuropsychopharmacol. Biol. Psychiatry. 26, 547−551.

Rosebush, P.I., Mazurek, M.F., 1991. Serum iron and neuroleptic malignant syndrome. Lancet 2013, 149−151.

Rosenberg, M.R., Green, M., 1989. Neuroleptic malignant syndrome. Review of response to therapy. Arch. Intern. Med. 149, 1927.

Sachdev, P., Kruk, J., Kneebone, M., Kissane, D., 1995. Clozapine induced neuroleptic malignant syndrome: review and report of new cases. J. Clin. Psychopharmacol. 15 (5), 365−371.

Sachdev, P., Mason, C., Hadzi-Pavlovic, D., 1997. Case control study of neuroleptic malignant syndrome. Am. J. Psychiatry 154, 1156−1158.

Sahoo, M.K., Agarwal, S., Biswas, H., 2014. Catatonia versus neuroleptic malignant syndrome: the diagnostic dilemma and treatment. Ind. Psychiatry J. 23 (2), 163−165. Available from: http://dx.doi.org/10.4103/0972-6748.151703.

Sharma, B., Sannegowda, R.B., Gandhi, P., Dubey, P., Panagariya, A., 2013. Combination of Steven-Johnson syndrome and neuroleptic malignant syndrome following carbamazepine therapy: a rare occurrence. BMJ Case Rep. June 11, 2013. pii:bcr2013008908. Available from: http://dx.doi.org/10.1136/bcr-2013-008908/.

Spivak, B., Maline, D.I., Kozyrev, V.N., Mester, R., Neduva, S.A., Ravilov, R.S., et al., 1991. Frequency of neuroleptic malignant syndrome in a large psychiatric hospital in Moscow. Eur. Psychiatry. 147, 880−882.

Stauder, K.H., 1934. Die tödliche Katatonie. Arch. Psychiatr. Nervenkr. 102, 614−634.

Strawn, J.R., Keck, P.E., Caroff, S.N., 2007. Neuroleptic malignant syndrome. Am. J. Psychiatry 164, 870−876.

Su, Y.P., Chang, C.K., Hayes, R.D., Harrison, S., Lee, W., Broadbent, M., et al., 2014. Retrospective chart review on exposure to psychotropic medications associated with neuroleptic malignant syndrome. Acta Psychiatr. Scand. 130 (1), 52−60. Available from: http://dx.doi.org/10.1111/acps.12222/. Epub November 15, 2013.

Takubo, H., Harada, T., Hashimoto, T., Inaba, Y., Kanazawa, I., Kuno, S., et al., 2003. A collaborative study on the malignant syndrome in Parkinson's disease and related disorders. Parkinson. Relat. Disord. 9 (Suppl. 1), S31−S41.

Trollor, J.N., Sachdev, P.S., 1999. Electroconvulsive treatment of neuroleptic malignant syndrome: a review and report of cases. Aust. N. Z. J. Psychiatry 33 (5), 650−659.

Tsai, H.C., Kuo, P.H., Yang, P.C., 2003. Fever, consciousness disturbance, and muscle rigidity in a 68-year-old man with depressive disorder. Chest 124 (4), 1598−1601.

Tse, L., Barr, A.M., Scarapicchia, V., Vila-Rodriguez, F.V., 2015. Neuroleptic malignant syndrome: a review from a clinically oriented perspective. Curr. Neuropharmacol. 13, 395−406.

Viejo, L.F., Morales, V., Punal, P., Perez, J.L., Sancho, R.A., 2003. Risk factors in neuroleptic malignant syndrome a case control study. Acta Psychiatri. Scand. 107, 45−49.

Wielosz, M., 1981. Increased sensitivity to dopaminergic agonists after repeated electroconvulsive shock (ECS) in rats. Neuropharmacology. 20 (10), 941−945.

Woo, J., Teoh, R., Vallance-Owen, J., 1986. Neuroleptic malignant syndrome successfully treated with amantidine. Postgrad. Med. J. 62, 809–810.

Yang, Y., Guo, Y., Zhang, A., 2014. Neuroleptic malignant syndrome in a patient treated with lithium carbonate and haloperidol. Shanghai Arch Psychiatry 26 (6), 368–370. Available from: http://dx.doi.org/10.11919/j.issn.1002-0829.214099.

Zivković, M., Mihaljević-Peles, A., Sagud, M., Silić, A., Mihanović, M., 2010. The role of CYP2D6 and TaqI A polymorphisms in malignant neuroleptic syndrome: two case reports with three episodes. Psychiatr. Danub. 22 (1), 112–116.

Chapter 11

Heat Stroke and Rhabdomyolysis

Kathlyn J. Ronaldson
Monash University, Melbourne, VIC, Australia

11.1 HEAT STROKE

11.1.1 Definition

Heat stroke is defined as a core body temperature of more than 40°C with central nervous system impairment, such as loss of consciousness, convulsions, and delirium, in the context of high ambient temperature (Martin-Latry et al., 2007) (Box 11.1).

11.1.2 Epidemiology

Many studies have found the risk of heat stroke is increased with mental illness and/or with use of antipsychotics (Kim et al., 2014; Nordon et al., 2009; Semenza et al., 1996; Bouchama et al., 2007; Martin-Latry et al., 2007). However, the incidence with specified climatic conditions, exposure, and drug use is uncertain, even in broad terms. A Finnish study by Tacke and Venalainen (1987) conducted among healthy psychiatric inpatients on stable medication and enjoying a sauna for 10 minutes at 64°C found no difference in body temperature postsauna between these patients and the control group of psychiatric nurses. As sauna use was a regular occurrence at this psychiatric facility, the authors also checked the past 20 years' experience and found seven convulsive seizures (six had prediagnosed epilepsy) and two episodes of loss of consciousness. The latter two cases were considered to be heat stroke and one of these patients died of aspiration of vomitus. This study suggests that heat stroke is rare following a sauna, but does not address the situation of a psychiatric patient in poor health spending a

Life-Threatening Effects of Antipsychotic Drugs. DOI: http://dx.doi.org/10.1016/B978-0-12-803376-0.00011-3
© 2016 Elsevier Inc. All rights reserved.

BOX 11.1 Heat Stroke

- Heat stroke is defined as body temperature $\geq 40°C$ with central nervous system involvement (loss of consciousness, confusion, seizure) in the context of high ambient temperature.
- The risk of heat stroke is increased in those with mental illness and with antipsychotic use.
- Antipsychotics suppress the hypothalamus resulting in reduced peripheral vasodilation and sweat generation.
- The mainstays of treatment are cooling, and support of ventilation and circulation, but additional measures may be required if multiorgan dysfunction develops.
- Preventive strategies include staying in a room with air-conditioning, keeping out of the sun, taking cool showers, drinking chilled drinks, and limiting exertion.

number of hours in a temperature above 35°C, or enduring several consecutive days when the temperature does not fall below 22°C.

In a meta-analysis of six case-control studies of heat-related deaths in the context of high ambient temperature, Bouchama et al. (2007) found that mental illness (odds ratio (OR) 3.61; 95% confidence interval (CI) 1.3−9.8) and taking psychotropic medication (OR 1.9; 95% CI 1.3−2.8) increased the risk of dying. A more recent study conducted in 2012 in South Korea (Kim et al., 2014) observed that neuropsychiatric disorders were more common among patients with heat stroke than among a group with mild heat-related illness (adjusted OR 7.69; 95% CI 4.06−14.54).

Nordon et al. (2009) conducted a study of deaths among persons aged 70−100 years during the French heat wave of Aug. 2003. In this elderly group, antipsychotic use increased the risk of death (adjusted OR 2.09; 95% CI 1.89−2.35). More specifically, phenothiazines (1.24; 1.06−1.46), olanzapine, clozapine or loxapine (1.76; 1.09−2.84), and benzamide (amisulpride) (2.25; 1.78−2.85) were associated with an increased risk of dying, as was use of tricyclic antidepressants and serotonin reuptake inhibitors. However, antipsychotic and antidepressant use among an elderly population may be more common among the more frail.

None of these studies permit calculation of either incidence of heat stroke or death from heat stroke among psychiatric patients, but they do provide evidence that this group of patients are at elevated risk. The epidemiological evidence is supported by the known mechanism of action of antipsychotic medication (see Pathophysiology) and by the observation that psychiatric patients with heat stroke typically are anhidrotic (without sweat) despite a very high body temperature (Tacke and Venalainen, 1987).

Most of the published cases of heat stroke with antipsychotic medication have occurred with phenothiazines (Zelman and Guillan, 1970; Sarnquist and

Larson, 1973; Ellis, 1976; Forester, 1978; Mann and Boger, 1978; Cooper, 1979; Bark, 1982; Stadnyk and Glezos, 1983; Tyndel and Labonte, 1983; Surmont et al., 1984; Lazarus, 1985, 1989; Koizumi et al., 1996; Kwok and Chan, 2005), but other first-generation antipsychotics including haloperidol (Bark, 1982; Surmont et al., 1984), pimozide (Fijnheer et al., 1995), and zuclopenthixol (Fijnheer et al., 1995; Kwok and Chan, 2005; Kao and Kelly, 2007) have also been implicated. Of the second-generation agents, one published case report involves clozapine (Kerwin et al., 2004) and another quetiapine with zuclopenthixol and benztropine (Kao and Kelly, 2007). The Australian Therapeutic Goods Administration has received one report involving amisulpride, clozapine, and venlafaxine (Hill, R. Personal Communication, Jul. 6, 2015). In some cases no exertion was involved (Ellis 1976; Bark, 1982), some were engaged in activities requiring mild exertion, albeit at 40°C in one case (Cooper 1979; Stadnyk and Glezos, 1983; Tyndel and Labonte, 1983), and others carried out activities such as builder's laborer (Kerwin et al., 2004), car cleaning (Kwok and Chan, 2005), returning shopping trolleys (Hill, R. Personal Communication, Jul. 6, 2015), and roofing a building (Kao and Kelly, 2007) despite the heat. In addition, two cases occurred following mountain climbing at 31−32°C (Koizumi et al., 1996).

While the case report data gives limited support for an association with second-generation antipsychotics, the epidemiological study by Nordon et al. (2009) suggests olanzapine, clozapine, loxapine, and amisulpride may increase the risk of heat stroke at least in elderly patients. With the expected increase in the frequency of hot temperatures associated with global warming, an increase in the risk of heat stroke among all members of the population and especially psychiatric patients can be expected unless suitable precautions are taken by all.

11.1.3   Pathobiology

Antipsychotics influence the hypothalamus, the body's center for thermoregulation (Kerwin et al., 2004; Mann and Boger, 1978; Cusack et al., 2011; Hajat et al., 2010). Consequently, peripheral vasodilation and sweat generation are reduced. Sweat generation and cooling from evaporation are particularly important when the ambient temperature rises above normal body temperature. The different antipsychotics will differ in their effect on thermoregulation and there may be a dose-relationship (Nordon et al., 2009), but these factors have been given little attention (Hajat et al., 2010). Concomitant benzatropine (benztropine), antiparkinsonian drugs, tricyclic antidepressants, and serotonin reuptake inhibitors have a synergistic or additive effect (Lazarus, 1985, 1989; Hajat et al., 2010; Sarnquist and Larson, 1973; Fijnheer et al., 1995).

Schizophrenia itself, and other indications for antipsychotic medication, may also be associated with an elevated risk of heat stroke (Semenza et al., 1996; Bouchama et al., 2007; Kim et al., 2014) by behavioral and physiological mechanisms (Kim et al., 2014). The physiological mechanism involves impairment of the vascular function of conducting heat away from the core to the periphery. The behavioral mechanism follows from reduced mobility and awareness and increased dependence resulting in neglect of precautions, including moving to a cool location, wearing cool clothing, and increasing fluid intake.

11.1.4 Clinical and Laboratory Features

As previously mentioned, heat stroke involves high core body temperature ($>40°C$) and central nervous system impairment, such as coma, seizure, and delirium. In addition, psychiatric patients will typically have hot dry skin, as a result of suppression of the sweating response. Further, tachycardia and tachypnea are the norm and many patients have hypotension (Kerwin et al., 2004). Laboratory investigation on admission may reveal respiratory alkalosis, hypophosphatemia, hypokalemia, leukocytosis, electrolyte disturbance, acidosis, and raised creatine kinase (CK; Kerwin et al., 2004).

11.1.5 Differential Diagnosis

A difficulty with neuroleptic facilitated heat stroke is that often the patient is found unconscious and is unable to give a history. A comatose patient may have overdosed, suffered trauma, or have some medical condition leading to coma. Key to the diagnosis of heat stroke is the patient's body temperature. The ambient temperature may also be an indicator, but heat stroke may occur with over- or sustained exertion at relatively moderate temperatures. The features of heat stroke are similar to those with neuroleptic malignant syndrome (NMS), but it can be distinguished from this condition by the absence of muscular rigidity and sweating (see Chapter 10, Neuroleptic Malignant Syndrome). In addition, NMS seldom leads to a body temperature of more than $40°C$ (Kerwin et al., 2004; Kwok and Chan, 2005).

11.1.6 Complications and Significant Sequelae

Complications are common with heat stroke and death is said to be the outcome in about 50% of cases (Martin-Latry et al., 2007). The complications include multiorgan dysfunction, including encephalopathy, rhabdomyolysis, acute renal failure, adult respiratory distress syndrome, myocardial injury, hepatocellular injury, intestinal ischemia or infarction, pancreatic injury, and disseminated intravascular coagulopathy with thrombocytopenia (Kerwin et al., 2004). Aspiration of vomitus is a further complication which typically results in death following pneumonia (Lazarus, 1985). Death may occur within a few hours of admission (Ellis, 1976; Bark, 1982; Stadnyk and Glezos, 1983; Kao and Kelly, 2007) or it may occur after a prolonged illness (Sarnquist and Larson, 1973; Bark, 1982; Surmont et al., 1984). Completeness of recovery is not often described, but Mann and Boger (1978) report persisting refractory anemia, and Kerwin et al. (2004) report mental slowness and muscle necrosis in a patient who no longer had any sign of psychotic illness.

11.1.7 Risk Stratification for Death or Permanent Disability

Varghese et al. (2005) reported a 71% mortality among heat stroke patients in southern India, but they noted that with improved awareness among medical staff, mortality fell to 50%, indicating the importance of prompt and aggressive treatment. The mean time to admission after development of pyrexia in this study was more than 3 days.

11.1.8 Management

Support of ventilation and circulation as well as prevention of aspiration in the comatose patient are fundamental to treatment of heat stroke (Sarnquist and Larson, 1973). Cooling is essential, but care should be taken to avoid surface cooling occurring so quickly as to induce shivering and trigger peripheral vasoconstriction to retain heat in the core (Cusack et al., 2011; Stadnyk and Glezos, 1983). Cooling using ice packs, cold baths, fanning with cool air, and peritoneal lavage with chilled (26°C) dialysate (Stadnyk and Glezos, 1983) have all been employed. Recently, a case report described aggressive cooling using a specially designed intravascular balloon-catheter system (Hamaya et al., 2015). Dehydration may not be an issue, due to the absence of sweating, and excessive fluid administration should be avoided. Acidosis, if present, should be corrected. Treatment to prevent seizures may be required and diazepam has been used for this purpose.

In some cases, heat stroke has been treated with dantrolene (Kerwin et al., 2004). It is indicated for malignant hyperthermia associated with anesthetics, but not for heat stroke, for which there is no evidence base. If shock develops, vasoconstrictors should be avoided as vasodilation is a mechanism for heat loss. Dialysis will be required if renal failure develops.

11.1.9 Prevention

A meta-analysis of epidemiological studies found that the most effective preventive measure against death in a heat wave is working air-conditioning in the home (OR 0.23; 95% CI 0.1−0.6) (Bouchama et al., 2007). In particular, for those with psychiatric illness, the risk of dying was reduced for those who were institutionalized (1.1; 1.0−1.2) compared with those who were not (4.8; 3.0−7.6; $p < 0.001$ for comparison). However, proposing removal of all psychiatric patients to institutions or requiring all to have functional air-conditioning is not practicable. Prevention requires health carers to educate patients about measures to take to prevent heat stroke and to monitor them, especially those unable to care for themselves (Cusack et al., 2011). Wearing cool, loose clothing, visiting places with air-conditioning, having frequent cool showers, drinking chilled drinks, staying out of the sun, and limiting exertion are all measures that can be taken (Hajat et al., 2010). Use of electric fans in a hot room is not recommended (Bouchama et al., 2007). The onset of heat stroke in psychiatric patients has been said to be abrupt (Kwok and Chan, 2005), but it is likely that monitoring body temperature in hot weather would give an early warning and signal a need to upgrade the preventive measures should the body temperature rise to 38°C or more.

11.2   RHABDOMYOLYSIS

11.2.1   Definition

Rhabdomyolysis is the breakdown of skeletal muscle tissue (Zutt et al., 2014). The intracellular components are released into the circulation leading to a rise in serum CK. Three factors may result in the condition becoming life-threatening: myoglobin precipitation in the glomerular filtrate leading to acute renal failure; electrolyte disturbance causing cardiac arrhythmias; and disseminated intravascular coagulation producing multiple organ damage (Parekh et al., 2012) (Box 11.2).

11.2.2   Epidemiology

Rhabdomyolysis has many causes including alcohol and drug abuse, prescribed medication (particularly statins), severe infection, intramuscular injection, electrolyte disturbance, hyperthermia, NMS, extreme physical exertion, status epilepticus, multiple injury, crush injury, extensive third degree burns, prolonged immobility, and polydipsia (Parekh et al., 2012; Zutt et al., 2014). Psychosis may also be associated with rises in CK by as much as 30-fold above normal in the absence of other risk factors (Meltzer, 2000).

Several studies have reviewed serum CK concentrations in patients taking antipsychotics with a view to assessing frequency and causality (Reznik et al., 2000; Scelsa et al., 1996; Melkersson, 2006). Scelsa et al. (1996) found serial measurements of CK among 37 patients treated with clozapine and monitored weekly for a mean of 8.2 months showed wide fluctuations and 78% of patients had a value above the normal range at some point. Three patients had extreme CK elevations ($>20,000 \, U \, L^{-1}$) without myoglobinuria or recorded muscle weakness or pain. All three recovered rapidly on withdrawal of clozapine. One patient tolerated rechallenge with clozapine at a lower dose with only mild increases in CK.

A study conducted using VigiBase data (WHO Collaborating Centre for International Drug Monitoring) found that rhabdomyolysis was reported more frequently with antipsychotics than would be expected for a random event and that olanzapine was the most frequently implicated (Star et al., 2012).

11.2.3 Pathobiology

The causal pathway for raised CK with antipsychotics is unclear and the cause may not be the antipsychotic but some aspect(s) of the patient's underlying condition.

11.2.4 Clinical and Laboratory Features

Many of the published cases of raised CK were identified from a routine test (Perlov et al., 2005; Oulis et al., 2007; Shuster, 2000; Boot and de Haan, 2000). Symptoms have included myalgia and weakness (Ceri et al., 2011), falling (Rosebraugh et al., 2001), and difficulty walking (Dickmann and Dickmann, 2010). Psychiatric patients may not volunteer that they have muscle symptoms. In addition, to the muscle symptoms, tachycardia and pyrexia are sometimes (Strawn et al., 2008; Klein et al., 2006; Eiser et al., 1982; Strachan et al., 2007) but not always (Marti-Bonmati et al., 2003; Marinella, 1997) present. Overt myoglobinuria has been reported in very few; even those with CK in excess of $10,000 \, U \, L^{-1}$ are unlikely to display this sign (Strawn et al., 2008; Meltzer et al., 1996; Perlov et al., 2005).

Mild rises in liver enzymes are the norm. Although renal dysfunction is a cause for major concern with rhabdomyolysis, raised creatinine is reported in very few cases (Eiser et al., 1982), but rises may not develop until several days after the initial elevation of CK (Yang and McNeely, 2002).

11.2.5 Differential Diagnosis

NMS is a potential competing diagnosis (see Chapter 10, Neuroleptic Malignant Syndrome). It is characterized by muscle rigidity, altered mental status, pyrexia, tachycardia, unstable blood pressure, renal failure, and elevated CK concentration (Meltzer et al., 1996). Only the first two features are not associated with rhabdomyolysis, when rhabdomyolysis is the primary condition. The absence of muscle rigidity is usually taken as a reason to exclude NMS in the presence of markedly raised CK (Perlov et al., 2005; Yang and McNeely, 2002). Altered mental status is not uncommon in psychiatric patients, and is likely to occur following overdose or seizure. The differential diagnosis should include a review for other potential primary or contributing causes.

BOX 11.2 Rhabdomyolysis
- Rhabdomyolysis is breakdown of skeletal muscle tissue, leading to a rise in creatine kinase (CK).
- Substantial rises in CK may occur in psychiatric patients without identified cause.
- Many cases of substantial rises in CK have apparently occurred without symptoms and have been identified by routine testing.
- Mild and moderate cases may resolve without antipsychotic withdrawal or other intervention.
- Severe cases are very rare and there may not be a causal relationship between antipsychotic use and clinically significant rises in CK.

11.2.6   Complications and Significant Sequelae

Very few published cases of rhabdomyolysis with therapeutic use of antipsychotics have experienced the complication of renal failure, as mentioned earlier. Only one published case was fatal and only one report describes residual impairment (Eiser et al., 1982). The evidence indicates that complications are rare, even in cases involving overdose (Waring et al., 2006).

11.2.7   Management

It may be possible to avoid withdrawal of antipsychotic medication following a mild or moderate rise in CK. Careful history taking for other possible contributors and repeat CK determination within a day or 2 may resolve the concern and prevent psychiatry relapse. In more severe cases, or if CK does not fall with a repeat determination despite addressing other possible causes, withdrawal of all medication may be sufficient to facilitate recovery. However, those with renal impairment, serum myoglobin, myoglobinuria, or very high CK ($>5000 \text{ U L}^{-1}$) should receive intravenous hydration with isotonic saline to reduce the risk of renal failure. Serial creatinine determinations are recommended for early detection of renal dysfunction.

11.2.8   Conclusion

While it appears that extreme, life-threatening rises in CK with antipsychotic treatment are rare, the evidence points to substantial rises in CK not being uncommon among patients with psychiatric diagnoses. These rises may be associated with the illness, rather than the treatment, and the mechanism is unknown.

REFERENCES

Heat Stroke

Bark, N.M., 1982. Heatstroke in psychiatric patients: two cases and a review. J. Clin. Psychiatry 43, 377–380.

Bouchama, A., Dehbi, M., Mohamed, G., et al., 2007. Prognostic factors in heat wave related deaths: a meta-analysis. Arch. Intern. Med. 167, 2170–2176.

Cooper, R.A., 1979. Heat and neuroleptics: a deadly combination. Am. J. Psychiatry 136, 466–467.

Cusack, L., de Crespigny, C., Athanasos, P., 2011. Heatwaves and their impact on people with alcohol, drug and mental health conditions: a discussion paper on clinical practice considerations. J. Adv. Nurs. 67, 915–922.

Ellis, F., 1976. Heat wave deaths and drugs affecting temperature regulation. Br. Med. J. 2, 474.

Fijnheer, R., van de Ven, P.J., Erkelens, D.W., 1995. [Psychiatric drugs as risk factor in fatal heat stroke] [Dutch]. Ned. Tijdschr. Geneeskd. 139, 1391–1393.

Forester, D., 1978. Fatal drug-induced heat stroke. J. Am. Coll. Emerg. Phys. 7, 243–244.

Hajat, S., O'Connor, M., Kosatsky, T., 2010. Health effects of hot weather: from awareness of risk factors to effective health protection. Lancet 375, 856–863.

Hamaya, H., Hifumi, T., Kawakita, K., et al., 2015. Successful management of heat stroke associated with multiple-organ dysfunction by active intravascular cooling. Am. J. Emerg. Med. 33 (124), e125–e127.

Kao, R.L., Kelly, L.M., 2007. Fatal exertional heat stroke in a patient receiving zuclopenthixol, quetiapine and benztropine. Can. J. Clin. Pharmacol. 14, e322–e325.

Kerwin, R.W., Osborne, S., Sainz-Fuertes, R., 2004. Heat stroke in schizophrenia during clozapine treatment: rapid recognition and management. J. Psychopharmacol. 18, 121–123.

Kim, S.H., Jo, S.N., Myung, H.N., et al., 2014. The effect of pre-existing medical conditions on heat stroke during hot weather in South Korea. Environ. Res. 133, 246–252.

Koizumi, T., Nomura, H., Kobayashi, T., et al., 1996. Fatal rhabdomyolysis during mountaineering. J. Sports Med. Phys. Fitness 36, 72–74.

Kwok, J.S., Chan, T.Y., 2005. Recurrent heat-related illnesses during antipsychotic treatment. Ann. Pharmacother. 39, 1940–1942.

Lazarus, A., 1985. Heatstroke in a chronic schizophrenic patient treated with high-potency neuroleptics. Gen. Hosp. Psychiatry 7, 361–363.

Lazarus, A., 1989. Differentiating neuroleptic-related heatstroke from neuroleptic malignant syndrome. Psychosomatics 30, 454–456.

Mann, S.C., Boger, W.P., 1978. Psychotropic drugs, summer heat and humidity, and hyperpyrexia: a danger restated. Am. J. Psychiatry 135, 1097–1100.

Martin-Latry, K., Goumy, M.P., Latry, P., et al., 2007. Psychotropic drugs use and risk of heat-related hospitalisation. Eur. Psychiatry 22, 335–338.

Nordon, C., Martin-Latry, K., de Roquefeuil, L., et al., 2009. Risk of death related to psychotropic drug use in older people during the European 2003 heatwave: a population-based case-control study. Am. J. Geriatr. Psychiatry 17, 1059–1067.

Sarnquist, F., Larson Jr., C.P., 1973. Drug-induced heat stroke. Anesthesiology 39, 348–350.

Semenza, J.C., Rubin, C.H., Falter, K.H., et al., 1996. Heat-related deaths during the July 1995 heat wave in Chicago. N. Engl. J. Med. 335, 84–90.

Stadnyk, A.N., Glezos, J.D., 1983. Drug-induced heat stroke. Can. Med. Assoc. J. 128, 957–959.

Surmont, D.W., Colardyn, F., De Reuck, J., 1984. Fatal complications of neuroleptic drugs. A clinico-pathological study of three cases. Acta Neurol. Belg. 84, 75–83.

Tacke, U., Venalainen, E., 1987. Heat stress and neuroleptic drugs. J. Neurol. Neurosurg. Psychiatry 50, 937−938.

Tyndel, F., Labonte, R., 1983. Drug-facilitated heat stroke. Can. Med. Assoc. J. 129, 680−682.

Varghese, G.M., John, G., Thomas, K., et al., 2005. Predictors of multi-organ dysfunction in heatstroke. Emerg. Med. J. 22, 185−187.

Zelman, S., Guillan, R., 1970. Heat stroke in phenothiazine-treated patients: a report of three fatalities. Am. J. Psychiatry 126, 1787−1790.

Rhabdomyolysis

Boot, E., de Haan, L., 2000. Massive increase in serum creatine kinase during olanzapine and quetiapine treatment, not during treatment with clozapine. Psychopharmacology 150, 347−348.

Ceri, M., Unverdi, S., Altay, M., et al., 2011. Comment on: low-dose quetiapine-induced severe rhabdomyolysis. Ren. Fail. 33, 463−464.

Dickmann, J.R., Dickmann, L.M., 2010. An uncommonly recognized cause of rhabdomyolysis after quetiapine intoxication. Am. J. Emerg. Med. 28 (1060), e1061−e1062.

Eiser, A.R., Neff, M.S., Slifkin, R.F., 1982. Acute myoglobinuric renal failure. A consequence of the neuroleptic malignant syndrome. Arch. Intern. Med. 142, 601−603.

Klein, J.P., Fiedler, U., Appel, H., et al., 2006. Massive creatine kinase elevations with quetiapine: report of two cases. Pharmacopsychiatry 39, 39−40.

Marinella, M.A., 1997. Rhabdomyolysis associated with haloperidol without evidence of NMS. Ann. Pharmacother. 31, 927−928.

Marti-Bonmati, E., San Valero-Carcelen, E., Ortega-Garcia, M.P., et al., 2003. Olanzapine elevation of serum creatine kinase. J. Clin. Psychiatry 64, 483−484.

Melkersson, K., 2006. Serum creatine kinase levels in chronic psychosis patients—a comparison between atypical and conventional antipsychotics. Prog. Neuropsychopharmacol. Biol. Psychiatry 30, 1277−1282.

Meltzer, H.Y., 2000. Massive serum creatine kinase increases with atypical antipsychotic drugs: what is the mechanism and the message? Psychopharmacology 150, 349−350.

Meltzer, H.Y., Cola, P.A., Parsa, M., 1996. Marked elevations of serum creatine kinase activity associated with antipsychotic drug treatment. Neuropsychopharmacology 15, 395−405.

Oulis, P., Koulouris, G.C., Konstantakopoulos, G., et al., 2007. Marked elevation of creatine kinase with sertindole: a case report. Pharmacopsychiatry 40, 295−296.

Parekh, R., Care, D.A., Tainter, C.R., 2012. Rhabdomyolysis: advances in diagnosis and treatment. Emerg. Med. Pract. 14, 1−15.

Perlov, E., Tebartz van Elst, L., Czygan, M., et al., 2005. Serum creatine kinase elevation as a possible complication of therapy with olanzapine. Naunyn Schmiedebergs Arch. Pharmacol. 372, 168−169.

Reznik, I., Volchek, L., Mester, R., et al., 2000. Myotoxicity and neurotoxicity during clozapine treatment. Clin. Neuropharmacol. 23, 276−280.

Rosebraugh, C.J., Flockhart, D.A., Yasuda, S.U., et al., 2001. Olanzapine-induced rhabdomyolysis. Ann. Pharmacother. 35, 1020−1023.

Scelsa, S.N.M., Simpson, D.M.M., McQuistion, H.L.M., et al., 1996. Clozapine-induced myotoxicity in patients with chronic psychotic disorders. Neurology 47, 1518−1523.

Shuster, J., 2000. Olanzapine and rhabdomyolysis. Nursing 30, 87.

Star, K., Iessa, N., Almandil, N.B., et al., 2012. Rhabdomyolysis reported for children and adolescents treated with antipsychotic medicines: a case series analysis. J. Child Adolesc. Psychopharmacol. 22, 440−451.

Strachan, P., Prisco, D., Multz, A.S., 2007. Recurrent rhabdomyolysis associated with polydipsia-induced hyponatremia—a case report and review of the literature. Gen. Hosp. Psychiatry 29, 172–174.

Strawn, J.R., Adler, C.M., Strakowski, S.M., et al., 2008. Hyperthermia and rhabdomyolysis in an adolescent treated with topiramate and olanzapine. J. Child Adolesc. Psychopharmacol. 18, 116–118.

Waring, W.S., Wrate, J., Bateman, D.N., 2006. Olanzapine overdose is associated with acute muscle toxicity. Hum. Exp. Toxicol. 25, 735–740.

Yang, S.H., McNeely, M.J., 2002. Rhabdomyolysis, pancreatitis, and hyperglycemia with ziprasidone. Am. J. Psychiatry 159, 1435.

Zutt, R., van der Kooi, A.J., Linthorst, G.E., et al., 2014. Rhabdomyolysis: review of the literature. Neuromuscul. Disord. 24, 651–659.

Part V

Metabolic Complications of Antipsychotic Drug Treatment

Chapter 12

Type 2 Diabetes Mellitus

Davy Vancampfort[1], Richard I.G. Holt[2], Brendon Stubbs[3,4],
Marc De Hert[1], Katherine Samaras[5] and Alex J. Mitchell[6]
[1]University Psychiatric Center University of Leuven, Kortenberg, Belgium,
[2]University of Southampton, Southampton, United Kingdom, [3]King's College London,
London, United Kingdom, [4]Maudsley NHS Foundation Trust, London, United Kingdom,
[5]Garvan Institute of Medical Research, Sydney, NSW, Australia, [6]University of Leicester,
Leicester, United Kingdom

12.1 EPIDEMIOLOGY

Diabetes mellitus is a metabolic disorder characterized by hyperglycemia (American Diabetes Association, 2010). Several pathogenic processes are involved in the development of diabetes mellitus. These range from autoimmune destruction of the β-cells of the pancreas with consequent insulin deficiency to abnormalities that result in resistance to insulin action (American Diabetes Association, 2010). The basis of the abnormalities in carbohydrate, fat, and protein metabolism in diabetes is the deficient action of insulin on target tissues. The vast majority of cases of diabetes fall into two broad etio-pathogenetic categories. In one category, type 1 diabetes, the cause is an absolute deficiency of insulin secretion (American Diabetes Association, 2014). Individuals at increased risk of developing this type of diabetes can often be identified by serological evidence of an autoimmune pathologic process occurring in the pancreatic islets and by genetic markers. In the other, much more prevalent category, type 2 diabetes mellitus (T2DM), deficient insulin action results from a heterogeneous combination of inadequate insulin secretion and diminished tissue responses to insulin (insulin resistance) at one or more points in the complex pathways of hormone action (American Diabetes Association, 2010). Chronic hyperglycemia in turn is associated with long-term damage, dysfunction, and failure of various organs, especially the eyes, kidneys, nerves, heart, and blood vessels (American Diabetes Association, 2010). In T2DM, a degree of hyperglycemia sufficient to cause

Life-Threatening Effects of Antipsychotic Drugs. DOI: http://dx.doi.org/10.1016/B978-0-12-803376-0.00012-5
© 2016 Elsevier Inc. All rights reserved.

pathologic and functional changes in various target tissues, but without the classical triad of diabetes symptoms, thirst, polydipsia, and polyuria, may be present for a long period of time before it is detected. In this chapter, as there is no evidence of an increase in type 1 diabetes in people receiving antipsychotics, we will focus on T2DM.

Obtaining precise T2DM prevalence rates in people taking antipsychotics is challenging because of the high level of undiagnosed T2DM in this population (Holt and Mitchell, 2014; Samaras et al., 2014). For example, up to 70% of diabetes cases in people with severe mental illness are estimated to be undiagnosed, which is in contrast to the rate of around 25−30% in the general population (Taylor et al., 2005). Nevertheless, the best estimate from the literature is that approximately 10% of people with severe mental illness also have T2DM. For instance, in a meta-analysis including 26 studies and encompassing 145,744 individuals with schizophrenia, the overall pooled prevalence of T2DM was 9.7% (95% confidence interval (CI) = 6.7−13.1%) (Stubbs et al., 2015). Another recent meta-analysis including 19 studies ($n = 18,053$) showed that the overall prevalence of T2DM was 9.4% (95% CI = 6.5−12.7%) in people with bipolar disorder (Vancampfort et al., 2015a). Third, a meta-analysis including 15 studies in clearly defined major depression disorder ($n = 14,049$) showed an overall prevalence of T2DM of 8.6% (95% CI = 6.4−11.0%) (Vancampfort et al., 2015a). The literature is also consistent in demonstrating that people with severe mental illness have a two to three times increased risk for T2DM (Stubbs et al., 2015; Vancampfort et al., 2013a, 2015a,b).

12.1.1 The Increased Risk of T2DM in People With Severe Mental Illness

Knowledge about factors that are associated with T2DM can help identify persons at greatest risk. There is evidence that lifestyle and environmental factors, biological effects of the mental illness, antipsychotic medication use, and genetic vulnerability all contribute to the increased risk for T2DM in people with severe mental illness.

12.1.1.1 Lifestyle and Environmental Factors

People with severe mental illness are more likely than the general population to be sedentary (Vancampfort et al., 2012), smoke (Dickerson et al., 2013), and have diets that are rich in saturated fats and refined sugars while avoiding fruit and vegetables (Bly et al., 2014), all of which are known risk factors for T2DM (American Diabetes Association, 2014). For instance, a study of 501,161 US veterans found that compared with the general population, those with schizophrenia or bipolar disorder were more likely to smoke (odds ratio (OR) = 1.69, 95% CI = 1.63−1.75 and OR = 1.18, 95%

CI = 1.13−1.24, respectively) and less likely to be physically active (OR = 0.92, 95% CI = 0.89−0.95 and OR = 0.94, 95% CI = 0.90−0.98, respectively) (Chwastiak et al., 2011). In the same way, a poor-quality neighborhood environment and poverty might predispose people with severe mental illness to T2DM as dietary and physical activity choices might be adversely affected by poor physical and social environments (Soundy et al., 2014; Vancampfort et al., 2013b, 2014a).

12.1.1.2 Biological Effects of the Mental Illness

A number of inflammatory and neuroendocrine changes occur in people with severe mental illness (Manu et al., 2014), which tend to increase insulin resistance and thus predispose to T2DM (Mitchell and Dinan, 2010). In addition, an emerging body of evidence shows that alterations in the immune system, especially those related to inflammation, are associated with an increased risk of schizophrenia, suggesting that chronic inflammation might be a precursor to both conditions (Fineberg and Ellman, 2013). More specifically, severe mental illness seems to be associated with hypothalamic−pituitary−adrenal axis dysfunctions (Bradley and Dinan, 2010) and increased basal cortisol secretion (especially in the early stages of the disease), an abnormal diurnal rhythm, and a blunted cortisol response to psychological stressors.

12.1.1.3 Antipsychotic Medication Use

Antipsychotic drugs have a propensity to induce weight gain (Bak et al., 2014) as well as other metabolic abnormalities (Rummel-Kluge et al., 2010), thereby increasing the patient's risk of obesity, T2DM, and cardiovascular diseases (Mitchell et al., 2013a,b; Vancampfort et al., 2013b, 2014c). The risk of diabetes related adverse events differs for individual agents. Olanzapine and clozapine, and to a lesser extent quetiapine, are associated with the highest risk for T2DM (Rummel-Kluge et al., 2010; De Hert et al., 2012) (Table 12.1).

12.1.1.4 Genetic Vulnerability

Molecular inference and genome-wide association studies point out that schizophrenia shares substantial polygenetic components with T2DM (Lin and Shuldiner, 2010). An estimated 11% and 14% of putative risk genes for T2DM and schizophrenia, respectively, might account for risk of developing the other condition (Lin and Shuldiner, 2010). It has been recently suggested that serine/threonine kinase, protein kinase B (PKB), also known as AKT, could be one of the important shared components and may play a pivotal role to link both of the pathogenetic processes (Liu et al., 2013). Polymorphisms in the gene that encodes tyrosine hydroxylase might also have an important role in the development of T2DM in people with severe

TABLE 12.1 Risk for Antipsychotic-Induced Weight Gain and Hyperglycemia

Antipsychotic Drug	Associated Risk of Weight Gain	Associated Risk of Glucose Metabolism Abnormalities
Chlorpromazine	Substantial	High (limited data)
Fluphenazine	Neutral/low	Low (limited data)
Haloperidol	Neutral/low	Low
Molindone	Neutral	Low (limited data)
Perphenazine	Neutral/low	Low
Pimozide	Neutral/low	Low (limited data)
Thioridazine	Intermediate	High (limited data)
Amisulpride	Neutral/low	Mild
Aripiprazole	Neutral/low	Low
Asenapine	Neutral/low	Low (limited data)
Clozapine	Substantial	High
Iloperidone	Intermediate	Mild (limited data)
Lurasidone	Neutral/low	Low (limited data)
Olanzapine	Substantial	High
Paliperidone	Intermediate	Mild
Quetiapine	Intermediate	Moderate
Risperidone	Intermediate	Mild
Sertindole	Intermediate	Mild
Ziprasidone	Neutral/low	Low
Zotepine	Intermediate	Not reported

Source: Permission obtained from Nature Publishing Group © De Hert, M., Detraux, J., van Winkel, R., Yu, W., Correll, C.U., 2012 Metabolic and cardiovascular adverse effects associated with antipsychotic drugs. Nat. Rev. Endocrinol. 8, 114–126. Available from: http://dx.doi.org/10.1038/nrendo.2011.15.

mental illness (Chiba et al., 2000). A further example is the TCF7L2 gene (which encodes a transcription factor involved in Wnt/β-catenin signaling), which has a role in pancreatic β-cell function and is a susceptibility gene for T2DM (Lin and Shuldiner, 2010). The Wnt signaling pathway also has a role in the development of the central nervous system and abnormalities in the Wnt signaling pathway have been associated with schizophrenia (Alkelai et al., 2012).

12.1.1.5 Gene—Environment Interactions

As well as directly affecting an individual's risk of developing T2DM, genetic variations might explain some of the diversity in the response to exposure to various environmental factors, such as the degree of weight gain following antipsychotic treatment. Among the most consistent findings from studies of the genetic influence on antipsychotic-induced weight gain are serotonin 2C receptors (HTR2C) and leptin promoter gene variants, with more recent studies implicating methylenetetrahydrofolate reductase (MTHFR) and melanocortin receptor 4 (MC4R) genes. There is also evidence, although less frequently reported, for the histamine H1 receptor gene (HRH1), brain-derived neurotrophic factor (BDNF), neuropeptide Y (NPY), cannabinoid receptor type 1 (CNR1), ghrelin/obestatin prepropeptide (GHRL), fat mass- and obesity-associated, alpha-ketoglutarate-dependent dioxygenase (FTO), and adenosine monophosphate-activated protein kinase (AMPK) genes (Kao and Müller, 2013). Some methodological limitations pertinent to genome-wide association studies should, however, be considered when interpreting the current evidence. Published studies vary in their methodologies with respect to study designs, sample sizes, ethnicities, type of antipsychotic, covariates, comedication, statistical measures, and in their study design (cross-sectional vs prospective cohort study), which may account for differences in the results. In addition, although weight represents a reliable and universal measure, some studies used kilogram weight change and others used percentage weight change (correcting for baseline weight) or body mass index (BMI) changes, while other studies used the metabolic syndrome as the outcome variable (Kao and Müller, 2013).

12.2 PATHOBIOLOGY

The current evidence shows that antipsychotic medication use is an important risk factor for developing T2DM in people with severe mental illness. T2DM might develop rapidly after treatment initiation. In one case series, more than half of patients who developed T2DM did so within 3 months of the initiation of treatment (Jin et al., 2002). However, T2DM is more likely to develop gradually following many years of treatment (Holt and Peveler, 2006). Based on these findings, and as can be seen in Fig. 12.1, there is a consensus that hyperglycemia in people taking antipsychotics develops in two distinct patterns; first, there is gradually worsening glucose metabolism, akin to T2DM, whereby increasing insulin resistance, particularly as a result of weight gain, overcomes the capacity of the pancreatic β-cells to increase secretion. The second occurs more acutely with a more rapid and marked β-cells decline and may present with diabetic ketoacidosis (DKA). These reports of DKA, albeit uncommon, argue against the position that glucose dysregulation associated with antipsychotic use is related to weight gain

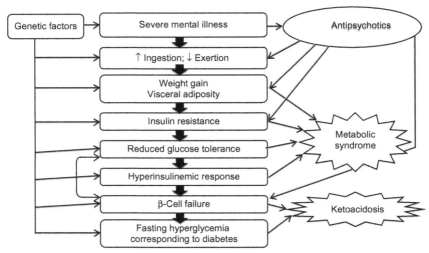

FIGURE 12.1   Pathways for antipsychotic drug-induced metabolic abnormalities. *Permission obtained from Elsevier © Scheen, A.J., van Winkel, R., De Hert, M., 2008. Traitements neuroleptiques et troubles metaboliques. Méd. Maladies Métaboliq., 2, 593–599.*

alone (Guenette et al., 2013a). While excessive adiposity represents a significant risk factor for T2DM, this is not the case with DKA, which is caused by marked insulin deficiency. DKA has been reported soon after the initiation of antipsychotic treatment and in individuals who experience no significant changes in weight. These cases emphasize that weight gain cannot be used as the sole proxy for concerns regarding possible glucose abnormalities following antipsychotic medication use. The occurrence of DKA also raises questions from a mechanistic standpoint; it remains unclear whether antipsychotic agents impact insulin and glucose metabolism via a single mechanism or multiple distinct mechanisms (i.e., one through antipsychotic-induced weight gain and other more direct effects on insulin secretion which may be more acute in nature).

Although the exact mechanisms underlying antipsychotic-induced altered glucose regulation remain poorly understood, it has been proposed that a heterogeneous receptor-binding pharmacology, which differentiates antipsychotic agents from each other, may be implicated. Antipsychotic binding to dopaminergic, serotonergic, adrenergic, and cholinergic sites is understood to influence receptors and transporters in essential body tissues implicated in glucose metabolism. One hypothesis is that antipsychotic drugs contribute to weight gain and associated hyperglycemia via effects mediated by binding to the serotonergic receptors 5-HT_{1a} and 5-HT_{2c} (Guenette et al., 2013b). Stimulation of 5-HT_{1a} is associated with an increase in food intake whereas stimulation of 5-HT_{2c} is related to a decrease in food intake. Antagonism of the 5-HT$_{2c}$ receptor can, in turn, lead to an increase in food intake. In particular clozapine and olanzapine are potent 5-HT$_{2c}$ antagonists. The fact that aripiprazole and ziprasidone have only a weak association with metabolic dysregulation, despite their high affinities for 5-HT$_{2c}$ receptors, could be explained by other receptor-specific mechanisms that potentially counterbalance inhibition of the 5-HT$_{2c}$ receptors. For example, aripiprazole is a partial agonist of 5-HT$_{1a}$ receptors.

Blockade of the dopamine D2 receptors is another potential mechanism involved (Hahn et al., 2011). Prolonged D2 blockade with antipsychotics may predispose to depletion of insulin granule stores. Moreover, synergistic effects between the blockade of D2 receptors and 5-HT$_{1a}$ or 5-HT$_{2c}$ receptors might have a key role in triggering a cascade of events that lead to increased energy intake, weight gain, and hyperglycemia (Correll et al., 2009). Third, the affinity of antipsychotic agents for M3 receptors also seems relevant for the glucose homeostasis, perhaps because M3 receptors on pancreatic β cells, control cholinergic-dependent insulin release (Weston-Green et al., 2013). Some antipsychotic drugs, such as clozapine and olanzapine, might impair both cholinergic-dependent and glucose-dependent insulin secretion from pancreatic β cells. Among antipsychotic agents a high affinity for the M3 receptor, as is seen with clozapine and olanzapine, seems to be the best predictor of a propensity to promote glucose dysregulation and T2DM (Starrenburg and Bogers, 2009; Weston-Green et al., 2013). In addition, to these pharmacological mechanisms, there is also unpublished evidence from in vitro experiments that clozapine and haloperidol, but not aripiprazole, may reduce β-cell viability (Bowen et al., 2012). It is clear that antipsychotics act on the metabolism in a variety of ways. However, much remains unclear and difficult to comprehend, and further research into these mechanisms is needed. Step by step, more data are emerging to help unravel the puzzle.

12.3 CLINICAL AND LABORATORY FEATURES

In the United States, T2DM accounts for more than 90% of all cases of diabetes in adults (American Diabetes Association, 2010). Many people with T2DM are asymptomatic and hyperglycemia is noted on routine laboratory evaluation, prompting further testing. Classic symptoms of hyperglycemia include polyuria, polydipsia, weight loss, sometimes with polyphagia, and blurred vision (American Diabetes Association, 2010). Diabetes is diagnosed based on plasma glucose criteria, either the fasting plasma glucose (FPG), random plasma glucose (RPG) or the 2-hour plasma glucose (2-h PG) value after a 75-g oral glucose tolerance test (OGTT) (American Diabetes Association, 2014). While once considered the gold standard, the OGTT is used less commonly now because the FPG and RPG tests are easier and faster to perform, more convenient and acceptable to patients, and less expensive. FPG has greater sensitivity than RPG but this must be balanced against the inconvenience of fasting. More recently, an International Expert Committee (2009) added glycated hemoglobin (HbA$_{1c}$) (threshold $\geq 6.5\%$, 48 mmol mol^{-1}) as a third option to diagnose diabetes. Epidemiological data show a similar relationship of HbA$_{1c}$ with the risk of retinopathy as seen with FPG and 2-h PG (Cheng et al., 2009). HbA$_{1c}$ has several advantages to the FPG and OGTT, including greater convenience (fasting not required), possibly greater preanalytical stability, and less day-to-day perturbations during stress and illness. These advantages must be balanced by greater cost and the incomplete correlation between HbA$_{1c}$ and average glucose in certain individuals (Bonora and Tuomilehto, 2011). In particular, a single measurement of HbA$_{1c}$ levels has a low positive predictive value; however, this measurement can be used as part of a screening algorithm with repeat testing, or combined with other tests. Measuring HbA$_{1c}$ levels might also give a false negative result if the concentration of glucose is rising rapidly, which can happen shortly after treatment initiation.

As with most diagnostic tests, a test result should be repeated when feasible to rule out laboratory error unless there is a clear clinical diagnosis (e.g., a patient in a hyperglycemic crisis or presenting with classic symptoms of hyperglycemia and a RPG ≥ 200 mg dL^{-1}) (American Diabetes Association, 2014). It is preferable that the same test be repeated for confirmation, since there will be a greater likelihood of concurrence (American Diabetes Association, 2014) because each of the tests identifies a slightly different population, at least in the early stages of diabetes. If a patient has discordant results on two different tests, then the test result that is above the diagnostic cut point should be repeated (American Diabetes Association, 2014). The diagnosis may then be made on the basis of the confirmed test. For example, if a patient meets the diabetes criterion of the HbA$_{1c}$ (two results $\geq 6.5\%$, 48 mmol mol^{-1}) but not the FPG (<126 mg dL^{-1} or 7.0 mmol L^{-1}), or vice versa, that person should be considered to have diabetes (American Diabetes Association, 2014) (Table 12.2).

12.3.1 Categories of Increased Risk for Diabetes (Prediabetes)

Expert Committee on the Diagnosis and Classification of Diabetes Mellitus (1997) recognized a group of individuals whose glucose levels did not meet the criteria for diabetes, but were too high to be considered normal. "Prediabetes" is defined as having FPG levels ≥ 100 mg dL^{-1} (5.6 mmol L^{-1}) but <126 mg dL^{-1} (7.0 mmol L^{-1}) and/or 2-hour OGTT values of ≥ 140 mg dL^{-1} (7.8 mmol L^{-1}) but <200 mg dL^{-1} (11.1 mmol L^{-1}). In the absence of pregnancy, impaired fasting glucose (IFG) and impaired glucose tolerance (IGT) are not clinical entities in their own right but should rather be considered to be indicative of impaired glucose regulation and risk factors for future T2DM as

TABLE 12.2 Diagnostic Criteria for the Diagnosis of Diabetes (American Diabetes Association, 2014)

$HbA_{1c} \geq 6.5\%$ (48 mmol mol^{-1})

OR

Fasting plasma glucose $\geq$ 126 mg dL^{-1} (7.0 mmol L^{-1}). Fasting is defined as no caloric intake for at least 8 h[a]

OR

Two-hour plasma glucose $\geq$ 200 mg dL^{-1} (11.1 mmol L^{-1}) during an oral glucose tolerance test. The test should be performed using a glucose load containing the equivalent of 75 g anhydrous glucose dissolved in water[a]

OR

In a patient with classic symptoms of hyperglycemia or hyperglycemic crisis, a random plasma glucose $\geq$ 200 mg dL^{-1} (11.1 mmol L^{-1})

[a]In the absence of unequivocal hyperglycemia, result should be confirmed by repeat testing.
Source: Permission obtained from American Diabetes Association © American Diabetes Association, 2014. Standards of medical care in diabetes—2014. Diabetes Care, 37 (Suppl. 1), S14—S80. Available from: http://dx.doi.org/10.2337/dc14-S014.

well as cardiovascular disease. IFG and IGT are associated as well with the metabolic syndrome, which includes obesity (especially abdominal or visceral obesity), dyslipidemia of the high-triglyceride and/or low-HDL type, and hypertension (Alberti et al., 2009).

12.3.1.1   At-Risk Groups

Children and adolescents taking antipsychotics are at heightened risk of metabolic effects compared with their peers. In clinical trials, the absolute weight gain in drug-naïve patients given antipsychotics was three- to fourfold greater than in patients switching antipsychotics drugs (Alvarez-Jiménez et al., 2008). In another study (Bobo et al., 2013), children and young people treated with an antipsychotic had a threefold increase in risk of diabetes compared with propensity score matched controls who had recently commenced other psychotropic medication. A similar strong association was also found in a systematic review (Galling and Correll, 2015). Olanzapine and quetiapine caused significant increases in total cholesterol, triglycerides, and low-density lipoprotein cholesterol in children and adolescents treated for a median of 11 weeks (Correll et al., 2009). Compared with age-matched patients not taking antipsychotics, with data in the same drug-claims database, one study (Hammerman et al., 2008) reported an OR of 8.9 (95% CI = 7.0−11.3) in those aged <24 years compared with an OR of 4.2 (95% CI = 3.8−4.5) for those aged 25−44 years, an OR of 1.9 (95% CI = 1.8−2.1) for those 45−54 years old, an OR of 1.3 (95% CI = 1.2−1.4) for those aged 55−64 years for T2DM. A reason might be that the low background risk for T2DM at a young age makes the diabetogenic effect of the antipsychotic drugs noticeable, whereas at an older age, the effects of the biological and behavioral risk factors becomes more pronounced than those of the antipsychotic drugs (Holt and Mitchell, 2014).

12.3.1.2 Differential Diagnosis

The differential diagnosis for T2DM is limited and most importantly includes type 1 diabetes as this requires urgent treatment with insulin. Clinicians should consider type 1 diabetes when patients are younger than 40 years of age, have a history of ketoacidosis, or are of low or normal weight (American Diabetes Association, 2010).

12.3.1.3 Complications, Significant Sequelae, and Risk Stratification for Death or Permanent Disability

Long-term complications of diabetes can be divided into microvascular and macrovascular. Microvascular complications include: (1) retinopathy with potential loss of vision; (2) nephropathy leading to renal failure; (3) peripheral neuropathy with risk of foot ulcers, amputations, and Charcot joints; and (4) autonomic neuropathy causing gastrointestinal, genitourinary, and cardiovascular symptoms and sexual dysfunction (American Diabetes Association, 2010). People with diabetes are known to have a double increased incidence of atherosclerotic cardiovascular, peripheral arterial, and cerebrovascular disease (Sarwar et al., 2010).

In people with severe mental illness, the consequences of T2DM appear to be much more profound than the general population, with higher rates of acute metabolic disturbance, microvascular and macrovascular complications and deaths related to T2DM (Becker and Hux, 2011). In a recent Danish study (Ribe et al., 2014) involving 4.7 million participants, the overall age- and calendar-period adjusted mortality ratios for those with severe mental illness and T2DM ($n = 1083$) were 4.14 (95% CI = 3.81−4.51) for men and 3.13 (95% CI = 2.88−3.40) for women, compared with those with neither illness. The cumulative risks of death following the diagnosis of T2DM were substantial for people with severe mental illness; 15.0% (95% CI = 12.4−17.6%) of those aged <50 years died within 7 years of diagnosis, with the risk rising to 30.7% (95% CI = 27.8−33.4%) for those aged 50−69 years and to 63.8% (95% CI = 58.9−68.2%) for those aged ≥70 years. Of deaths from physical causes, 33.4% were attributed to T2DM and 14% of deaths from physical causes were attributed to the interaction between T2DM and severe mental illness.

There are several proposed reasons for the increased risk of T2DM morbidity and premature mortality including psychiatric symptoms (e.g., depression) and cognitive deficits that lead to lower adherence to hypoglycemic drugs, poorer diabetes self-management through glucose self-monitoring and follow-up (Ciechanowski et al., 2003; Dickerson et al., 2005), and low compliance with lifestyle measures including diet, physical activity, smoking and alcohol restrictions, and general physical health care (De Hert et al., 2011a).

12.4 PREVENTION AND MANAGEMENT

People with severe mental illness are at greatly elevated risk of T2DM and so additional preventative measures must be undertaken. To this end, the Healthy Active Lives (HeAL) statement from the International Physical Health in Youth Stream Working Group has advocated positive discrimination in young people with severe mental illness during their first episode in order to improve the care of these individuals and reduce the inequality of care (HeAL; www.iphys.org.au) (Curtis et al., 2012). The HeAL declaration states that any young person developing psychosis should expect their risks for future physical health complications (particularly obesity, premature cardiovascular disease, and diabetes), when assessed 2 years after initial diagnosis, to be equivalent to their peers from a similar background who have not experienced psychosis.

12.4.1 Screening for T2DM in People Taking Antipsychotics

Despite clear guidance and demonstration of its potential benefits, routine glucose screening has not been translated into clinical practice and is suboptimal (Mitchell et al., 2012), particularly in children and adolescents initiating antipsychotic treatment (Raebel et al., 2014). For example, only 11% of children and adolescents in a large US cohort ($n = 16,304$) had glucose assessed between 90 days before and 3 days after starting an antipsychotic. Expanding the time frame to include the 30 days after starting only increased the proportion to 15%. Importantly, this US study included 6 years (2006−11) subsequent to the publication of guidelines and product labeling recommending metabolic screening before initiating antipsychotic treatment. The low rates of glucose screening might reflect both patient and professional barriers. People with severe mental illness might be less likely than other groups to take opportunities for health screening (Lord et al., 2010). Professional barriers to screening within mental health settings include lack of clarity about whose responsibility screening is, lack of understanding about what should be measured and when, lack of confidence in interpreting results and lack of access to necessary equipment (Barnes et al., 2007; De Hert et al., 2011a).

The high rates of undiagnosed T2DM have led to recommendations that all people under psychotropic treatment, regardless of their specific psychotropic treatment, should be offered regular screening for T2DM and for other cardiovascular risk factors. The European Psychiatric Association supported by the European Association for the Study of Diabetes and the European Society of Cardiology (De Hert et al., 2009) proposed guidelines for screening and monitoring. The World Psychiatric Association also reviewed the evidence for the association between severe mental illness and physical illnesses and proposed recommendations both on the individual level and a systems level to achieve somatic health care on a par with that of the general population (De Hert et al., 2011a,b). Although the details of the various international guidelines differ to varying degrees, screening is recommended before the start or change of treatment, several weeks after treatment initiation (to identify the minority of patients who develop diabetes mellitus rapidly after antipsychotic initiation) and annually thereafter. It is particularly important to establish baseline diabetes and cardiovascular risk at initial presentation so that any subsequent change during treatment can be monitored. The medical history and examination should, at a minimum, include: (1) history of previous cardiovascular diseases, T2DM or other related diseases; (2) family history of premature cardiovascular diseases, T2DM, or other related diseases; (3) smoking habits; (4) weight and height in order to calculate the BMI and waist circumference; (5) fasting blood glucose and/or HbA_{1c}; and (6) blood pressure (measured twice and average taken) (overview: see Table 12.3). It is recommended that fasting blood glucose and/or HbA_{1c} measurements should also be taken before the first prescription of psychotropic medication (De Hert et al., 2009, 2011a). The frequency of testing will depend on the patient's medical history and the prevalence of baseline risk factors.

TABLE 12.3 Monitoring Guidelines of the European Psychiatric Association Supported by the European Association for the Study of Diabetes and the European Society of Cardiology

Ask	Measure	Decide
Personal/family history: • Diabetes • Hypertension • Coronary heart disease • Smoking • Diet • Physical activity	• Height • Weight • Waist circumference • Blood pressure • Fasting glucose and/or HbA_{1c} • Fasting lipids	• Behavioral treatments (e.g., obesity, prediabetes) • Smoking cessation • Referral (intern/extern) • Switch medications

Source: Permission obtained from Elsevier © De Hert, M. Dekker, J.M., Wood, D., Kahl, K.G., Holt, R.I., Möller, H.J., 2009. Cardiovascular disease and diabetes in people with severe mental illness position statement from the European Psychiatric Association (EPA), supported by the European Association for the Study of Diabetes (EASD) and the European Society of Cardiology (ESC). Eur. Psychiatry, 24, 412–424. Available from: http://dx.doi.org/10.1016/j.eurpsy.2009.01.005.

12.4.2   Screening in People With Normal Baseline Tests

For patients with normal baseline tests, it is recommended that measurements are repeated between 6 and 12 weeks after initiation of treatment and at least annually thereafter (De Hert et al., 2009, 2011a). During the initial phase, it is important to measure weight weekly to identify those individuals who gain weight rapidly with psychotropic treatment. The annual examination should also include measurement of cardiovascular diseases risk factors, urinary albumin excretion and serum creatinine, an eye examination, ideally including fundus photography, and foot examination to diagnose early signs of complications (De Hert et al., 2009, 2011a).

12.4.3   Screening in People With Risk Factors

Those who have significant risk factors for T2DM (family history, $BMI \geq 25 \ kg \ m^{-2}$, abdominal obesity, gestational diabetes, minority ethnicity) should have their FPG concentration or HbA_{1c} monitored at the same time points as other patients starting medication (baseline, between week 6 and 12), but thereafter they need to be checked more frequently (approximately every 3−6 months) (De Hert et al., 2009, 2011a). People who gain 7% or more of their baseline weight should also have their FPG concentration or HbA_{1c} value monitored more frequently (De Hert et al., 2009, 2011a).

In people with (pre-)diabetes starting antipsychotic treatment, special attention should be given to DKA (De Hert et al., 2009, 2011a). The signs and symptoms often develop quickly, sometimes within 24 hours (Guenette et al., 2013a). Polyuria, polydipsia, and weight loss may be present for several days before the development, and vomiting and abdominal pain are frequently the presenting symptoms. Physical examination reveals signs of dehydration, including loss of skin turgor, dry mucous membranes, tachycardia, and hypotension. Mental status can vary from full alertness to profound lethargy. Most patients are normothermic or even hypothermic at presentation. Acetone on breath may also be present on admission, particularly in patients with severe metabolic acidosis. When fatal DKA occurs, it usually occurs in the setting of a physiologic stressor (e.g., intercurrent infection, pancreatitis, myocardial infarction, or surgery) (Umpierrez and Kitabchi, 2003). By contrast, in drug-induced DKA, the precipitating factors are less clear. For example, no physiologic stressors were identified by history or autopsy in a clinical report of 17 deaths due to DKA in psychiatric patients treated with second-generation antipsychotic medications (Ely et al., 2013).

12.4.4   Lifestyle Modification

Studies over the last 20 years have shown conclusively that lifestyle-modification programs reduce the risk of diabetes in the general population (Norris et al., 2008). These programs are based on weight loss with a goal to normalize body weight; reduction in dietary fat intake; reduction in saturated fat intake; increase in dietary fiber; and increase in physical activity/exercise to at least 30 minutes a day, 5 days per week.

Although no diabetes prevention studies have been performed in people with severe mental illness, lifestyle-modification programs are the basis for recent efforts to assist individuals with serious mental illnesses in improving health and reducing cardiometabolic risks (Rosenbaum et al., 2014; Vancampfort and Faulkner, 2014). These programs apply behavioral approaches to weight loss and management, including education and behavioral self-management skills. A meta-analysis (Caemmerer et al., 2012) reported that compared with controls, patients following such lifestyle interventions experienced significant decreases in waist circumference (weighted mean difference, WMD $= -3.58$ cm, CI: -5.51, -1.66, $p = 0.03$), percent body fat (WMD $= -2.82\%$, CI: -5.35, -0.30, $p = 0.03$), fasting glucose (WMD $= -5.79$ mg dL^{-1}, CI: -9.73, -1.86, $p = 0.004$), insulin (WMD $= -4.93$ μIU mL^{-1}, CI: -7.64, -2.23, $p = 0.0004$), total cholesterol (WMD $= -20.98$ mg dL^{-1}, CI: -33.78, -8.19; $p = 0.001$), low-density lipoprotein cholesterol (WMD $= -22.06$ mg dL^{-1}, CI: -37.80, -6.32, $p = 0.006$), and triglycerides (WMD $= -61.68$ mg dL^{-1}, CI: -92.77, -30.59, $p = 0.0001$), and less weight gain of $\geq 7\%$ (29.7% vs 61.3%; risk ratio (RR) $= -0.52$, CI: -0.35, -0.78, $p = 0.002$). Up to 12 months after the intervention ended (mean $= 3.6$ months), benefits endured regarding weight (WMD $= -3.48$ kg, CI: -6.37, -0.58, $p = 0.02$). Subgroup analyses showed the superiority of these nonpharmacological interventions over the control interventions irrespective of treatment duration, or whether the intervention was applied in an individual or group setting, whether it involved cognitive behavioral or nutritional interventions, or the trials were for prevention or treatment. However, weight and BMI were significantly improved only in outpatient trials ($p < 0.0001$), but not in inpatient or mixed samples ($p = 0.09 - 0.96$) (Caemmerer et al., 2012). Recently, Green et al. (2015) extend these findings by showing participants ($n = 104$) following a 6-month once weekly (2 hours) combined physical activity and diet counseling program (followed by 6 months maintenance intervention) were 2.39 times as likely as participants in the control group (care as usual) to have normal fasting glucose levels at 12 months. The participants in this trial (Green et al., 2015) particularly appreciated the self-determination approach. Evidence for the success of this approach in adopting and maintaining lifestyle changes in people taking antipsychotic medications is rapidly growing (Vancampfort et al., 2013c, 2014b). Unfortunately many with severe mental illness struggle to participate in self-help programs and need a more assisted approach to ensure uptake (Daumit et al., 2013).

12.4.5   Pharmacological Interventions

Metformin and orlistat reduce incident T2DM in the general population (Knowler et al., 2002; Chiasson et al., 2002; Ramachandran et al., 2006). While neither drug has been used to prevent T2DM in people with severe mental illness, attempts have been made to manage antipsychotic-induced weight gain with these drugs. Again there have been no pharmacological diabetes prevention trials in people with severe mental illness but a recent systematic review (Mizuno et al., 2014) reported that the mean difference in weight between patients treated with metformin and placebo was -3.17 kg (95% CI = -4.44 to -1.90 kg), either through attenuation of weight gain or promotion of weight loss in patients taking antipsychotics. Research is needed to assess whether metformin can prevent the occurrence of T2DM in this population as well. However, in light of the current evidence in the general population and the established safety profile and low cost of metformin, several international guidelines (De Hert et al., 2009; McIntyre et al., 2012) recommend that metformin can be considered in people treated with antipsychotics. These guidelines suggest that metformin could be particularly relevant when additional risk factors are present, such as a personal or family history of metabolic dysfunction or when lifestyle interventions have been unsuccessful.

In an RCT of orlistat in people prescribed either clozapine or olanzapine, a modest weight reduction was seen after 16 weeks in men but not in women (-2.39 ± 5.45 kg, $p = 0.023$). Prolonged (32 weeks) orlistat treatment yielded no additional benefits as compared to short (16 weeks) treatment (Tchoukhine et al., 2011). The NICE (2012) guidance on the prevention of diabetes mellitus in high-risk individuals suggests that orlistat might also be considered as an alternative to metformin when lifestyle interventions are not achieving improvements in metabolic factors. Holt and Mitchell (2014) recently recommended that orlistat should only be considered when metformin is contraindicated or poorly tolerated because of the difficulties in using orlistat because of its side effects and poor treatment persistence. Several other drugs have been tried in the management of weight gain associated with antipsychotics in a small number of trials involving small numbers of participants. Anticonvulsant medications such as topiramate and zonisamide have a modest effect on weight (Gierisch et al., 2014).

The therapeutic principles for T2DM in people taking antipsychotics are similar to those for managing the condition in the general population and should follow currently available treatment algorithms (Holt and Mitchell, 2014). The American Diabetes Association (2014) recommends that people with T2DM should be referred to an effective ongoing support program targeting weight loss of 7%. These patients should be advised to perform at least 150 minutes per week of moderate-intensity aerobic physical activity (50–70% of maximum heart rate), spread over at least 3 days per week with no more than 2 consecutive days without exercise. In the absence of contra-indications, they should be encouraged to perform resistance training at least twice per week. Furthermore, the American Diabetes Association (2014) states that there is not an ideal percentage of calories from carbohydrate, protein, and fat for all people with T2DM; therefore, macronutrient distribution should be based on individualized assessment of current eating patterns, preferences, and metabolic goals. A variety of eating patterns (combinations of different foods or food groups) are acceptable for the management of diabetes.

Carbohydrate intake from vegetables, fruits, whole grains, legumes, and dairy products should be advised over intake from other carbohydrate sources, especially those that contain added fats, sugars, or sodium (American Diabetes Association, 2014). People with T2DM should also consume at least the amount of fiber and whole grains recommended for the general public (at least 25 g of fiber each day). Those with T2DM and those at risk should limit or avoid intake of sugar-sweetened beverages (from any caloric sweetener including high-fructose corn syrup and sucrose) to reduce risk for weight gain and worsening of cardiometabolic risk. Evidence is inconclusive for an ideal amount of total fat intake for people with T2DM; therefore, goals should be individualized (American Diabetes Association, 2014). Fat quality appears to be far more important than quantity. In people with T2DM, a Mediterranean-style, monounsaturated fats-rich eating pattern may benefit glycemic control and CVD risk factors and can therefore be recommended as an effective alternative to a lower fat, higher-carbohydrate eating pattern. Lastly, as recommended for the general public, an increase in foods containing long-chain n-3 fatty acids (from fatty fish) and n-3 linolenic acid is recommended (American Diabetes Association, 2014).

Oral agents with a reduced likelihood of inducing weight gain or those that promote weight loss might have advantages given the high prevalence of obesity in people taking antipsychotic medication. Therapies based on the incretin effect, which include dipeptidyl peptidase 4 inhibitors and glucagon-like peptide 1 receptor agonists, or sodium–glucose cotransporter 2 inhibitors, are new classes of drugs that might have a particular role in people taking antipsychotics, as they are associated with either no change in weight or weight loss and a low risk of hypoglycemia (Larsen et al., 2014). Although the glucagon-like peptide 1 receptor agonists must be given by injection, once-weekly preparations, such as extended release exenatide or dulaglutide, that could be administered by mental health teams are now available. Managing impaired glucose regulation and T2DM involves lifestyle changes, regular monitoring, and taking regular medication (American Diabetes Association, 2014). Health-care professionals, both in primary care and in mental health teams, have a responsibility to ensure that people with severe mental illness are not disadvantaged with regards to the care they receive for T2DM. Despite an increase in the number of consultations people with severe mental illness have with health-care professionals, evidence is emerging to suggest that they receive inferior physical health care (Mitchell et al., 2009). They receive less education about T2DM, are less likely to be examined for retinopathy or diabetic foot complications and are less likely to be screened for HbA_{1c} levels and other cardiovascular risk factors than the general population. Some of these inequalities may result from clinicians' attitude to patients with mental illness (Welch et al., 2014).

When T2DM develops while receiving an antipsychotic, it is important to assess what role the treatment is likely to have had in the onset. Under some circumstances, it might be appropriate to switch to an alternative antipsychotic but this should be done with care and with due regard to the mental state of the patient (Holt and Mitchell, 2014). To date, three studies evaluated antipsychotic switching strategies with glycemic control measurements as secondary outcomes. In two studies, patients on olanzapine switched to either quetiapine (Deberdt et al., 2008) or orally disintegrating olanzapine (Karagianis et al., 2010), while in a third study (Stroup et al., 2011) patients on olanzapine, quetiapine, or risperidone switched to aripiprazole. However, none reported significant changes in HbA_{1c} indicating that more research is required before rigorous recommendations can be formulated.

12.5 CONCLUSION

The current evidence illustrates the multiple and complex mechanisms underlying the association between severe mental illness and T2DM. This interplay of lifestyle and environmental factors, disease, and treatment effects makes it difficult to determine which of the factors has precipitated the development of T2DM in an individual on psychotropic treatment. Overall, the evidence points to a causative link between specific antipsychotics and T2DM, but the magnitude of the risk remains uncertain and other risk factors for T2DM, such as obesity, poor diet, physical inactivity, and family history, might have a higher risk than psychotropic treatment per se. However, whereas antipsychotics might directly increase the risk of T2DM through several molecular pathways, most of the risk appears to be mediated through their effects on traditional risk factors, such as weight gain. We recommend that treating mental health professionals, general practitioners, and medical specialists should all be responsible for giving preventive and proactive lifestyle advice, implementing the necessary screening assessments following International standards, and orchestrating or conducting the appropriate timely treatment of clinically relevant, abnormal findings. In addition to these measures, improved health promotion strategies, programs focusing on lifestyle, exercise and diet, and changes to the built and social environment of those with mental illness are essential.

REFERENCES

Alberti, K.G., Eckel, R.H., Grundy, S.M., Zimmet, P.Z., Cleeman, J.I., Donato, K.A., et al., 2009. Harmonizing the metabolic syndrome: a joint interim statement of the International Diabetes Federation Task Force on Epidemiology and Prevention; National Heart, Lung, and Blood Institute; American Heart Association; World Heart Federation; International Atherosclerosis Society; and International Association for the Study of Obesity. Circulation 120 (16), 1640−1645. Available from: http://dx.doi.org/10.1161/CIRCULATIONAHA.109.192644.

Alkelai, A., Greenbaum, L., Lupoli, S., Kohn, Y., Sarner-Kanyas, K., Ben-Asher, E., et al., 2012. Association of the type 2 diabetes mellitus susceptibility gene, TCF7L2, with schizophrenia in an Arab-Israeli family sample. PLoS One 7 (1), e29228. Available from: http://dx.doi.org/10.1371/journal.pone.0029228.

Alvarez-Jiménez, M., González-Blanch, C., Crespo-Facorro, B., Hetrick, S., Rodríguez-Sánchez, J.M., Pérez-Iglesias, R., et al., 2008. Antipsychotic-induced weight gain in chronic and first-episode psychotic disorders: a systematic critical reappraisal. CNS Drugs 22, 547−562.

American Diabetes Association, 2010. Diagnosis and classification of diabetes mellitus. Diabetes Care 33 (Suppl. 1), S62−S69. Available from: http://dx.doi.org/10.2337/dc10-S062.

American Diabetes Association, 2014. Standards of medical care in diabetes—2014. Diabetes Care 37 (Suppl. 1), S14−S80. Available from: http://dx.doi.org/10.2337/dc14-S014.

Bak, M., Fransen, A., Janssen, J., van Os, J., Drukker, M., 2014. Almost all antipsychotics result in weight gain: a meta-analysis. PLoS One 9 (4), e94112. Available from: http://dx.doi.org/10.1371/journal.pone.0094112.

Barnes, T.R., Paton, C., Cavanagh, M.R., Hancock, E., Taylor, D.M., 2007. UK Prescribing observatory for mental health. A UK audit of screening for the metabolic side effects of antipsychotics in community patients. Schizophr. Bull. 33 (6), 1397−1403. Available from: http://dx.doi.org/10.1093/schbul/sbm038.

Becker, T., Hux, J., 2011. Risk of acute complications of diabetes among people with schizophrenia in Ontario, Canada. Diabetes Care 34, 398−402. Available from: http://dx.doi.org/10.2337/dc10-1139.

Bly, M.J., Taylor, S.F., Dalack, G., Pop-Busui, R., Burghardt, K.J., Evans, S.J., et al., 2014. Metabolic syndrome in bipolar disorder and schizophrenia: dietary and lifestyle factors compared to the general population. Bipolar Disord. 16 (3), 277−288. Available from: http://dx.doi.org/10.1111/bdi.12160.

Bobo, W.V., Cooper, W.O., Stein, C.M., Olfson, M., Graham, D., Daugherty, J., et al., 2013. Antipsychotics and the risk of type 2 diabetes mellitus in children and youth. JAMA Psychiatry 70 (10), 1067−1075. Available from: http://dx.doi.org/10.1001/jamapsychiatry.2013.2053.

Bonora, E., Tuomilehto, J., 2011. The pros and cons of diagnosing diabetes with A1C. Diabetes Care 34 (Suppl. 2), S184−S190. Available from: http://dx.doi.org/10.2337/dc11-s216.

Bowen, E., Holt, R., Harrison, M., 2012. β-cell specific effects of the antipsychotic drugs clozapine and haloperidol. Poster Presented at Diabetes UK Professional Conference, Glasgow.

Bradley, A.J., Dinan, T.G., 2010. A systematic review of hypothalamic-pituitary-adrenal axis function in schizophrenia: implications for mortality. J. Psychopharmacol. 24 (Suppl. 4), 91−118. Available from: http://dx.doi.org/10.1177/1359786810385491.

Caemmerer, J., Correll, C.U., Maayan, L., 2012. Acute and maintenance effects of non-pharmacologic interventions for antipsychotic associated weight gain and metabolic abnormalities: a meta-analytic comparison of randomized controlled trials. Schizophr. Res. 140 (1-3), 159−168. Available from: http://dx.doi.org/10.1016/j.schres.2012.03.017.

Cheng, Y.J., Gregg, E.W., Geiss, L.S., Imperatore, G., Williams, D.E., Zhang, X., et al., 2009. Association of A1C and fasting plasma glucose levels with diabetic retinopathy prevalence in the U.S. population: implications for diabetes diagnostic thresholds. Diabetes Care 32 (11), 2027−2032. Available from: http://dx.doi.org/10.2337/dc09-0440.

Ciechanowski, P.S., Katon, W.J., Russo, J.E., Hirsch, I.B., 2003. The relationship of depressive symptoms to symptom reporting, self-care and glucose control in diabetes. Gen. Hosp. Psychiatry 25 (4), 246−252. Available from: http://dx.doi.org/10.1016/S0163-8343(03)00055-0.

Chiasson, J.L., Josse, R.G., Gomis, R., Hanefeld, M., Karasik, A., Laakso, M., 2002. Acarbose for prevention of type 2 diabetes mellitus: the STOP-NIDDM randomised trial. Lancet 359, 2072−2077. Available from: http://dx.doi.org/10.1016/S0140-6736(02)08905-5.

Chiba, M., Suzuki, S., Hinokio, Y., Hirai, M., Satoh, Y., Tashiro, A., et al., 2000. Tyrosine hydroxylase gene microsatellite polymorphism associated with insulin resistance in depressive disorder. Metabolism 49, 1145−1149. Available from: http://dx.doi.org/10.1053/meta.2000.8611.

Chwastiak, L.A., Rosenheck, R.A., Kazis, L.E., 2011. Association of psychiatric illness and obesity, physical inactivity, and smoking among a national sample of veterans. Psychosomatics 52, 230−236. Available from: http://dx.doi.org/10.1016/j.psym.2010.12.009.

Correll, C.U., Manu, P., Olshanskiy, V., Napolitano, B., Kane, J.M., Malhotra, A.K., 2009. Cardiometabolic risk of second-generation antipsychotic medications during first-time use in children and adolescents. J. Am. Med. Assoc. 302, 1765−1773. Available from: http://dx.doi.org/10.1001/jama.2009.1549.

Curtis, J., Newall, H.D., Samaras, K., 2012. The heart of the matter: cardiometabolic care in youth with psychosis. Early Interv. Psychiatry 6, 347−353. Available from: http://dx.doi.org/10.1111/j.1751-7893.2011.00315.x.

Daumit, G.L., Dickerson, F.B., Wang, N.Y., Dalcin, A., Jerome, G.J., Anderson, C.A., et al., 2013. A behavioral weight-loss intervention in persons with serious mental illness. N. Engl. J. Med. 368 (17), 1594−1602. Available from: http://dx.doi.org/10.1056/NEJMoa1214530.

Deberdt, W., Lipkovich, I., Heinloth, A.N., Liu, L., Kollack-Walker, S., Edwards, S.E., et al., 2008. Double-blind, randomized trial comparing efficacy and safety of continuing olanzapine versus switching to quetiapine in overweight or obese patients with schizophrenia or schizoaffective disorder. Ther. Clin. Risk Manag. 4 (4), 713−720.

De Hert, M., Dekker, J.M., Wood, D., Kahl, K.G., Holt, R.I., Möller, H.J., 2009. Cardiovascular disease and diabetes in people with severe mental illness position statement from the European Psychiatric Association (EPA), supported by the European Association for the Study of Diabetes (EASD) and the European Society of Cardiology (ESC). Eur. Psychiatry 24, 412−424. Available from: http://dx.doi.org/10.1016/j.eurpsy.2009.01.005.

De Hert, M., Correll, C.U., Bobes, J., Correll, C.U., Bobes, J., Cetkovich-Bakmas, M., et al., 2011a. Physical illness in patients with severe mental disorders, I: prevalence, impact of medications and disparities in health care. World Psychiatry 10, 52−77.

De Hert, M., Cohen, D., Bobes, J., Cetkovich-Bakmas, M., Leucht, S., Ndetei, D.M., et al., 2011b. Physical illness in patients with severe mental disorders. II. Barriers to care, monitoring and treatment guidelines, plus recommendations at the system and individual level. World Psychiatry 10 (2), 138−151.

De Hert, M., Detraux, J., van Winkel, R., Yu, W., Correll, C.U., 2012. Metabolic and cardiovascular adverse effects associated with antipsychotic drugs. Nat. Rev. Endocrinol. 8, 114−126. Available from: http://dx.doi.org/10.1038/nrendo.2011.156.

Dickerson, F.B., Goldberg, R.W., Brown, C.H., Kreyenbuhl, J.A., Wohlheiter, K., Fang, L., et al., 2005. Diabetes knowledge among persons with serious mental illness and type 2 diabetes. Psychosomatics 46 (5), 418−424. Available from: http://dx.doi.org/10.1176/appi.psy.46.5.418.

Dickerson, F., Stallings, C.R., Origoni, A.E., Vaughan, C., Khushalani, S., Schroeder, J., et al., 2013. Cigarette smoking among persons with schizophrenia or bipolar disorder in routine clinical settings, 1999-2011. Psychiatr. Serv. 64 (1), 44−50. Available from: http://dx.doi.org/10.1176/appi.ps.201200143.

Ely, S.F., Neitzel, A.R., Gill, J.R., 2013. Fatal diabetic ketoacidosis and antipsychotic medication. J. Forensic Sci. 58 (2), 398−403. Available from: http://dx.doi.org/10.1111/1556-4029.12044.

Expert Committee on the Diagnosis and Classification of Diabetes Mellitus, 1997. Report of the Expert Committee on the Diagnosis and Classification of Diabetes Mellitus. Diabetes Care 20, 1183−1197.

Fineberg, A.M., Ellman, L.M., 2013. Inflammatory cytokines and neurological and neurocognitive alterations in the course of schizophrenia. Biol. Psychiatry 73, 951−966. Available from: http://dx.doi.org/10.1016/j.biopsych.2013.01.001.

Galling, B., Correll, C.U., 2015. Do antipsychotics increase diabetes risk in children and adolescents? Expert Opin. Drug Saf. 14 (2), 219−241. Available from: http://dx.doi.org/10.1517/14740338.2015.979150.

Gierisch, J.M., Nieuwsma, J.A., Bradford, D.W., Wilder, C.M., Mann-Wrobel, M.C., McBroom, A.J., et al., 2014. Pharmacologic and behavioral interventions to improve cardiovascular risk factors in adults with serious mental illness: a systematic review and meta-analysis. J. Clin. Psychiatry 75 (5), e424−e440. Available from: http://dx.doi.org/10.4088/JCP.13r08558.

Green, C.A., Yarborough, B.J., Leo, M.C., Yarborough, M.T., Stumbo, S.P., Janoff, S.L., et al., 2015. The STRIDE weight loss and lifestyle intervention for individuals taking antipsychotic medications: a randomized trial. Am. J. Psychiatry 172 (1), 71−81. Available from: http://dx.doi.org/10.1176/appi.ajp.2014.14020173.

Guenette, M.D., Hahn, M., Cohn, T.A., Teo, C., Remington, G.J., 2013a. Atypical antipsychotics and diabetic ketoacidosis: a review. Psychopharmacology 226 (1), 1−12. Available from: http://dx.doi.org/10.1007/s00213-013-2982-3.

Guenette, M.D., Giacca, A., Hahn, M., Teo, C., Lam, L., Chintoh, A., et al., 2013b. Atypical antipsychotics and effects of adrenergic and serotonergic receptor binding on insulin secretion in-vivo: an animal model. Schizophr. Res. 146 (1−3), 162−169. Available from: http://dx.doi.org/10.1016/j.schres.2013.02.023.

Hahn, M., Chintoh, A., Giacca, A., Xu, L., Lam, L., Mann, S., et al., 2011. Atypical antipsychotics and effects of muscarinic, serotonergic, dopaminergic and histaminergic receptor binding on insulin secretion in vivo: an animal model. Schizophr. Res. 131 (1−3), 90−95. Available from: http://dx.doi.org/10.1016/j.schres.2011.06.004.

Hammerman, A., Dreiher, J., Klang, S.H., Munitz, H., Cohen, A.D., Goldfracht, M., 2008. Antipsychotics and diabetes: an age-related association. Ann. Pharmacother. 42, 1316−1322. Available from: http://dx.doi.org/10.1345/aph.1L015.

Holt, R.I., Peveler, R.C., 2006. Antipsychotic drugs and diabetes—an application of the Austin Bradford Hill criteria. Diabetologia 49, 1467−1476.

Holt, R.I., Mitchell, A.J., 2014. Diabetes mellitus and severe mental illness: mechanisms and clinical implications. Nat. Rev. Endocrinol. Available from: http://dx.doi.org/10.1038/nrendo.2014.203.

International Expert Committee, 2009. International Expert Committee report on the role of the A1C assay in the diagnosis of diabetes. Diabetes Care 32, 1327–1334. Available from: http://dx.doi.org/10.2337/dc09-9033.

Jin, H., Meyer, J.M., Jeste, D.V., 2002. Phenomenology of and risk factors for new-onset diabetes mellitus and diabetic ketoacidosis associated with atypical antipsychotics: an analysis of 45 published cases. Ann. Clin. Psychiatry 14, 59–64.

Kao, A.C., Müller, D.J., 2013. Genetics of antipsychotic-induced weight gain: update and current perspectives. Pharmacogenomics 14 (16), 2067–2083. Available from: http://dx.doi.org/10.2217/pgs.13.207.

Karagianis, J., Landry, J., Hoffmann, V.P., Grossman, L., de Haan, L., Maguire, G., et al., 2010. An exploratory analysis of factors associated with weight change in a 16-week trial of oral vs. orally disintegrating olanzapine: the PLATYPUS study. Int. J. Clin. Pract. 64 (11), 1520–1529. Available from: http://dx.doi.org/10.1111/j.1742-1241.2010.02485.x.

Knowler, W.C., Barrett-Connor, E., Fowler, S.E., Hamman, R.F., Lachin, J.M., Walker, E.A., et al., 2002. Reduction in the incidence of type 2 diabetes with lifestyle intervention or metformin. N. Engl. J. Med. 346, 393–403. Available from: http://dx.doi.org/10.1056/NEJMoa012512.

Larsen, J.R., Vedtofte, L., Holst, J.J., Oturai, P., Kjær, A., Corell, C.U., et al., 2014. Does a GLP-1 receptor agonist change glucose tolerance in patients treated with antipsychotic medications? Design of a randomised, double-blinded, placebo-controlled clinical trial. BMJ Open 4, e004227. Available from: http://dx.doi.org/10.1136/bmjopen-2013-004227.

Lin, P.I., Shuldiner, A.R., 2010. Rethinking the genetic basis for comorbidity of schizophrenia and type 2 diabetes. Schizophr. Res. 123 (2–3), 234–243. Available from: http://dx.doi.org/10.1016/j.schres.2010.08.022.

Liu, Y., Li, Z., Zhang, M., Deng, Y., Yi, Z., Shi, T., 2013. Exploring the pathogenetic association between schizophrenia and type 2 diabetes mellitus diseases based on pathway analysis. BMC Med. Genom. 6 (Suppl. 1), 17. Available from: http://dx.doi.org/10.1186/1755-8794-6-S1-S17.

Lord, O., Malone, D., Mitchell, A.J., 2010. Receipt of preventive medical care and medical screening for patients with mental illness: a comparative analysis. Gen. Hosp. Psychiatry 32, 519–543. Available from: http://dx.doi.org/10.1016/j.genhosppsych.2010.04.004.

Manu, P., Correll, C.U., Wampers, M., Mitchell, A.J., Probst, M., Vancampfort, D., et al., 2014. Markers of inflammation in schizophrenia: association vs. causation. World Psychiatry 13 (2), 189–192. Available from: http://dx.doi.org/10.1002/wps.20117.

McIntyre, R.S., Alsuwaidan, M., Goldstein, B.I., Taylor, V.H., Schaffer, A., Beaulieu, S., et al., 2012. The Canadian Network for Mood and Anxiety Treatments (CANMAT) task force recommendations for the management of patients with mood disorders and comorbid metabolic disorders. Ann. Clin. Psychiatry 24, 69–81.

Mitchell, A.J., Dinan, T.G., 2010. Schizophrenia: a multisystem disease? J. Psychopharmacol. 24 (Suppl. 4), 5–7. Available from: http://dx.doi.org/10.1177/1359786810382059.

Mitchell, A.J., Malone, D., Doebbeling, C.C., 2009. Quality of medical care for people with and without comorbid mental illness and substance misuse: systematic review of comparative studies. Br. J. Psychiatry 194, 491–499.

Mitchell, A.J., Delaffon, V., Vancampfort, D., Correll, C.U., De Hert, M., 2012. Guideline concordant monitoring of metabolic risk in people treated with antipsychotic medication: systematic review and meta-analysis of screening practices. Psychol. Med. 42, 125–147. Available from: http://dx.doi.org/10.1017/S003329171100105X.

Mitchell, A.J., Vancampfort, D., Sweers, K., van Winkel, R., Yu, W., De Hert, M., 2013a. Prevalence of metabolic syndrome and metabolic abnormalities in schizophrenia and related disorders-a systematic review and meta-analysis. Schizophr. Bull. 39 (2), 306–318. Available from: http://dx.doi.org/10.1093/schbul/sbr148.

Mitchell, A.J., Vancampfort, D., De Herdt, A., Yu, W., De Hert, M., 2013b. Is the prevalence of metabolic syndrome and metabolic abnormalities increased in early schizophrenia? A comparative meta-analysis of first episode, untreated and treated patients. Schizophr. Bull. 39 (2), 295–305. Available from: http://dx.doi.org/10.1093/schbul/sbs082.

Mizuno, Y., Suzuki, T., Nakagawa, A., Yoshida, K., Mimura, M., Fleischhacker, W.W., et al., 2014. Pharmacological strategies to counteract antipsychotic-induced weight gain and metabolic adverse effects in schizophrenia: a systematic review and meta-analysis. Schizophr. Bull. 40, 1385–1403. Available from: http://dx.doi.org/10.1093/schbul/sbu030.

NICE, 2012. Preventing Type 2 Diabetes: Risk Identification and Interventions for Individuals at High Risk. <http://guidance.nice.org.uk/PH38>.

Norris, S.L., Kansagara, D., Bougatsos, C., Fu, R., U.S. Preventive Services Task Force, 2008. Screening adults for type 2 diabetes: a review of the evidence for the U.S. Preventive Services Task Force. Ann. Intern. Med. 148 (11), 855–868.

Raebel, M.A., Penfold, R., McMahon, A.W., Reichman, M., Shetterly, S., Goodrich, G., et al., 2014. Adherence to guidelines for glucose assessment in starting second-generation antipsychotics. Pediatrics 34 (5), e1308–e1314. Available from: http://dx.doi.org/10.1542/peds.2014-0828.

Ramachandran, A., Snehalatha, C., Mary, S., Mukesh, B., Bhaskar, A.D., Vijay, V., et al., 2006. The Indian Diabetes Prevention Programme shows that lifestyle modification and metformin prevent type 2 diabetes in Asian Indian subjects with impaired glucose tolerance (IDPP-1). Diabetologia 49 (2), 289–297.

Ribe, A.R., Laursen, T.M., Sandbaek, A., Charles, M., Nordentoft, M., Vestergaard, M., 2014. Long-term mortality of persons with severe mental illness and diabetes: a population-based cohort study in Denmark. Psychol. Med. 44, 3097–3107. Available from: http://dx.doi.org/10.1017/S0033291714000634.

Rosenbaum, S., Tiedemann, A., Sherrington, C., Curtis, J., Ward, P.B., 2014. Physical activity interventions for people with mental illness: a systematic review and meta-analysis. J. Clin. Psychiatry 75 (9), 964–974. Available from: http://dx.doi.org/10.4088/JCP.13r08765.

Rummel-Kluge, C., Komossa, K., Schwarz, S., Hunger, H., Schmid, F., Lobos, C.A., et al., 2010. Head-to-head comparisons of metabolic side effects of second generation antipsychotics in the treatment of schizophrenia: a systematic review and meta-analysis. Schizophr. Res. 123 (2–3), 225–233. Available from: http://dx.doi.org/10.1016/j.schres.2010.07.012.

Samaras, K., Correll, C.U., Mitchell, A.J., De Hert, M., HeAL Collaborators Healthy Active Lives for People With Severe Mental Illness, 2014. Diabetes risk potentially underestimated in youth and children receiving antipsychotics. JAMA Psychiatry 71 (2), 209–210. Available from: http://dx.doi.org/10.1001/jamapsychiatry.2013.4030.

Sarwar, N., Gao, P., Seshasai, S.R., Gobin, R., Kaptoge, S., Di Angelantonio, E., et al., 2010. Diabetes mellitus, fasting blood glucose concentration, and risk of vascular disease: a collaborative meta-analysis of 102 prospective studies. Lancet 375, 2215–2222. Available from: http://dx.doi.org/10.1016/S0140-6736(10)60484-9.

Soundy, A., Freeman, P., Stubbs, B., Probst, M., Vancampfort, D., 2014. The value of social support to encourage people with schizophrenia to engage in physical activity: an international insight from specialist mental health physiotherapists. J. Ment. Health 23 (5), 256–260. Available from: http://dx.doi.org/10.3109/09638237.2014.951481.

Starrenburg, F.C., Bogers, J.P., 2009. How can antipsychotics cause diabetes mellitus? Insights based on receptor-binding profiles, humoral factors and transporter proteins. Eur. Psychiatry 24 (3), 164−170. Available from: http://dx.doi.org/10.1016/j.eurpsy.2009.01.001.

Stroup, T.S., McEvoy, J.P., Ring, K.D., Hamer, R.H., LaVange, L.M., Swartz, M.S., et al., 2011. A randomized trial examining the effectiveness of switching from olanzapine, quetiapine, or risperidone to aripiprazole to reduce metabolic risk: comparison of antipsychotics for metabolic problems (CAMP). Am. J. Psychiatry 168 (9), 947−956. Available from: http://dx.doi.org/10.1176/appi.ajp.2011.10111609.

Stubbs, B., Vancampfort, D., De Hert, M., Mitchell, A.J., 2015. The prevalence and predictors of type 2 diabetes in people with schizophrenia: a systematic review and comparative meta-analysis. Acta Psychiatr. Scand. 132 (2), 144−157.

Taylor, D., Young, C., Mohamed, R., Paton, C., Walwyn, R., 2005. Undiagnosed impaired fasting glucose and diabetes mellitus amongst inpatients receiving antipsychotic drugs. J. Psychopharmacol. 19, 182−186. Available from: http://dx.doi.org/10.1177/0269881105049039.

Tchoukhine, E., Takala, P., Hakko, H., Raidma, M., Putkonen, H., Räsänen, P., et al., 2011. Orlistat in clozapine- or olanzapine-treated patients with overweight or obesity: a 16-week open-label extension phase and both phases of a randomized controlled trial. J. Clin. Psychiatry 72 (3), 326−330. Available from: http://dx.doi.org/10.4088/JCP.09m05283yel.

Umpierrez, G.E., Kitabchi, A.E., 2003. Diabetic ketoacidosis: risk factors and management strategies. Treat. Endocrinol. 2, 95−108.

Vancampfort, D., Faulkner, G., 2014. Physical activity and serious mental illness: a multidisciplinary call to action. Ment. Health Phys. Activity 7 (3), 153−154. Available from: http://dx.doi.org/10.1016/j.mhpa.2014.11.001.

Vancampfort, D., Probst, M., Knapen, J., Carraro, A., De Hert, M., 2012. Associations between sedentary behaviour and metabolic parameters in patients with schizophrenia. Psychiatry Res. 200 (2−3), 73−78. Available from: http://dx.doi.org/10.1016/j.psychres.2012.03.046.

Vancampfort, D., Wampers, M., Mitchell, A.J., Correll, C.U., De Herdt, A., Probst, M., et al., 2013a. A meta-analysis of cardio-metabolic abnormalities in drug naive, first-episode and multi-episode patients with schizophrenia versus general population controls. World Psychiatry 12, 240−250. Available from: http://dx.doi.org/10.1002/wps.20069.

Vancampfort, D., De Hert, M., De Herdt, A., Vanden Bosch, K., Soundy, A., Bernard, P.P., et al., 2013b. Associations between physical activity and the built environment in patients with schizophrenia: a multi-centre study. Gen. Hosp. Psychiatry 35 (6), 653−658. Available from: http://dx.doi.org/10.1016/j.genhosppsych.2013.07.004.

Vancampfort, D., De Hert, M., Vansteenkiste, M., De Herdt, A., Scheewe, T.W., Soundy, A., et al., 2013c. The importance of self-determined motivation towards physical activity in patients with schizophrenia. Psychiatry Res. 210 (3), 812−818. Available from: http://dx.doi.org/10.1016/j.psychres.2013.10.004, Epub 2013 Oct 18.

Vancampfort, D., De Hert, M., De Herdt, A., Soundy, A., Stubbs, B., Bernard, P., et al., 2014a. Associations between perceived neighbourhood environmental attributes and self-reported sitting time in patients with schizophrenia: a pilot study. Psychiatry Res. 215 (1), 33−38. Available from: http://dx.doi.org/10.1016/j.psychres.2013.11.011.

Vancampfort, D., Vansteenkiste, M., De Hert, M., De Herdt, A., Soundy, A., Stubbs, B., et al., 2014b. Self-determination and stage of readiness to change physical activity behaviour in schizophrenia. Ment. Health Phys. Activity 7 (3), 171−176. Available from: http://dx.doi.org/10.1016/j.mhpa.2014.06.003.

Vancampfort, D., Correll, C.U., Wampers, M., Sienaert, P., Mitchell, A.J., De Herdt, A., et al., 2014c. Metabolic syndrome and metabolic abnormalities in patients with major depressive disorder: a meta-analysis of prevalences and moderating variables. Psychol. Med. 44 (10), 2017–2028.

Vancampfort, D., Mitchell, A.J., De Hert, M., Sienaert, P., Probst, M., Buys, R., et al., 2015a. Prevalence and predictors of type 2 diabetes in people with bipolar disorder: a systematic review and meta-analysis. J. Clin. Psychiatry 76 (11), 1490–1499.

Vancampfort, D., Stubbs, B., De Hert, M., Sienaert, P., Probst, M., Buys, R., et al., 2015b. Type 2 diabetes in patients with major depressive disorder: a meta-analysis of prevalence estimates and predictors. Depress. Anxiety 32 (10), 763–773.

Welch, L.C., Litman, H.J., Borba, C.P., Vincenzi, B., Henderson, D.C., 2014. Does a physician's attitude toward a patient with mental illness affect clinical management of diabetes? Results from a mixed-method study. Health Serv. Res 50 (4), 998–1020. Available from: http://dx.doi.org/10.1111/1475-6773.12267.

Weston-Green, K., Huang, X.F., Deng, C., 2013. Second generation antipsychotic-induced type 2 diabetes: a role for the muscarinic M3 receptor. CNS Drugs 27 (12), 1069–1080. Available from: http://dx.doi.org/10.1007/s40263-013-0115-5.

Part VI

Other Life-Threatening Effects of Antipsychotic Drugs

Chapter 13

Interstitial Nephritis and Interstitial Lung Disease

Kathlyn J. Ronaldson
Monash University, Melbourne, VIC, Australia

13.1 INTERSTITIAL NEPHRITIS

13.1.1 Definition

Tubulointerstitial nephritis is primarily drug-induced, but other causes include infection and autoimmune disease (Beck and Salant, 2012). As the name indicates, the focus of the disorder is the tubules and interstitium with limited impact on glomeruli and renal vessels. Its clinical presentation and laboratory findings are varied but there is consistency in manifestations of acute or subacute kidney injury. Renal biopsy of drug-induced interstitial nephritis reveals interstitial inflammation with infiltration of leukocytes, particularly lymphocytes and monocytes, but also eosinophils (Beck and Salant, 2012; Perazella and Markowitz, 2010; Box 13.1).

13.1.2 Epidemiology

Evidence points to an association between interstitial nephritis and clozapine, and other antipsychotics are not implicated. This is illustrated by the data from the Australian Therapeutic Goods Administration (TGA) (2015) on interstitial nephritis and renal failure or acute kidney injury with a range of antipsychotic drugs as well as sodium valproate and lithium carbonate (Table 13.1). These latter medications are often used with antipsychotics, and feature in published cases with clozapine, as will be seen below. Renal failure and acute kidney injury have been included in the table because of the possibility that a case of interstitial nephritis has been recorded with one of these terms in the absence of biopsy data confirming the nature of the kidney injury. Of the antipsychotics, none besides clozapine had more than two

Life-Threatening Effects of Antipsychotic Drugs. DOI: http://dx.doi.org/10.1016/B978-0-12-803376-0.00013-7
© 2016 Elsevier Inc. All rights reserved.

BOX 13.1 Interstitial Nephritis

- Clozapine is the only antipsychotic implicated as a cause of interstitial nephritis.
- Interstitial nephritis with clozapine occurs very rarely and there is no evidence that it is being missed.
- Key features are raised C-reactive protein (>100 mg L^{-1}) and creatinine, often with fever.
- It may occur with myocarditis and possibly develops by the same or similar mechanism.
- It is unclear whether full recovery occurs in severe cases.
- Early detection: follow the monitoring guidelines for myocarditis (Fig. 2.4) and check renal function if cardiac findings are insufficient to explain the course of the illness.

TABLE 13.1 Reports to the Australian Therapeutic Goods Administration of Interstitial Nephritis and Renal Failure or Acute Kidney Injury (to February 21, 2015) (Therapeutic Goods Administration (TGA), 2015)

Drug	Total Reports	Acute Interstitial Nephritis	Renal Failure/ Acute Kidney Injury	Fatal
Clozapine	7817	12	55	6
Valproate	1459	5	9	4
Lithium	770	3	22	2
Olanzapine	1715	2	10	2
Quetiapine	937	0	4	0
Haloperidol	821	0	3	1
Chlorpromazine	622	1	2	2
Paliperidone	416	0	0	0
Risperidone	1484	1	5	0
Aripiprazole	316	1	2	0
Amisulpride	305	0	2	1

reports of interstitial nephritis, but sodium valproate and lithium carbonate had five and three reports, respectively, and for a total of three clozapine was a suspected agent.

There is one published case of interstitial nephritis attributable to quetiapine and olanzapine (He et al., 2013). The disorder developed following up titration of quetiapine to 200 mg day^{-1} and 4 years later again after increasing the dose of olanzapine from 10 mg to 20 mg daily. On the second occasion renal biopsy examination demonstrated chronic interstitial nephritis. This single case is not sufficient to demonstrate causality. In addition, acute renal failure with overdose of paliperidone has been described, but despite exhaustive screening no inflammatory markers were raised (Liang et al., 2012).

Hunter et al. (2009) report that of 26,000 suspected adverse reactions to clozapine reported to the United Kingdom Medicines and Healthcare products Regulatory Agency, 10 were of acute interstitial nephritis and 31 of acute renal failure. This is in line with the data from Australia (Table 13.1). These data, together with the small number of published cases (Table 13.2), suggest that interstitial nephritis may be a very rare adverse reaction of clozapine. Cases of chronic interstitial nephritis or end-stage renal failure attributable to clozapine might be indicative of interstitial nephritis being missed in the early weeks of clozapine therapy. The Australian database holds two reports of chronic kidney disease for which clozapine was a suspected contributing factor (TGA, 2015). In one case the patient had diabetes mellitus, suggesting a different causal pathway. Omitting to diagnose interstitial nephritis does not appear to be a significant matter.

The presence of a causal association between clozapine and interstitial nephritis is supported by the nature of the adverse effect (typically drug-induced), the time to onset (≤ 2 weeks in seven cases) and recovery on cessation of clozapine (Table 13.2). In addition, rechallenge in one case resulted in recurrence with a shorter time to onset, although neither the initial event nor the event occurring after rechallenge were confirmed by biopsy (Hunter et al., 2009). In seven cases the patient was taking valproic acid or a salt of it, which may indicate that this exposure increases the risk as it does for myocarditis, another hypersensitivity reaction (see Chapter 2, Myocarditis and Cardiomyopathy) (Table 13.2; Ronaldson et al., 2012). In each of these seven cases, the patient had been stabilized on valproate for some time, and the adverse event was characterized by sudden deterioration as a response to a newly introduced substance. Published cases with valproate suggest that interstitial nephritis with valproate may have a long time to onset (Fukuda et al., 1996; Watanabe et al., 2005), meaning a direct contribution from valproate is possible, but not as the primary cause. In addition, four cases were taking lithium carbonate, but the association with this substance is of greater rarity.

13.1.3 Pathobiology

Interstitial nephritis with clozapine is an idiosyncratic hypersensitivity reaction. The presence of raised inflammatory markers, C-reactive protein (CRP), and eosinophils, as well as the histological evidence from renal biopsy are indicative of an inflammatory process involving the immune system.

TABLE 13.2 Published Cases of Clozapine-Induced Interstitial Nephritis

Authors, Year	Age, Sex	Drugs	Dose (mg d^{-1})	Time to Onset	Comment Retime to Onset	Diagnostic Data	Other Results	Treatment	Outcome
Parekh et al. (2014)	54 M	Clozapine Sodium valproate	100	2.5 mo	Two previous episodes of febrile illness, including 1 at 2 mo with raised creatinine treated with prednisolone	Creatinine 5.1 mg dL^{-1}. U/S: enlarged kidneys Biopsy: tubulo-interstitial nephritis	Pyrexia, proteinuria 100 mg dL^{-1}; CRP 261 mg L^{-1}	Prednisolone 30 mg d^{-1}	Improved renal function; still in follow-up
Mohan et al. (2013)	53 F	Clozapine Sodium valproate	200	60 d	Clozapine ceased after 2 w due to febrile illness; recommenced by slow titration. 60 d counted from reinitiation	Creatinine 2.9 mg dL^{-1} Biopsy: AIN; scarring in 50% of cortical area	Pyrexia, tachycardia, urea 42 mg dL^{-1}. Hypotension, tachycardia, pyrexia	Prednisolone 25 mg d^{-1}	Recovered to renal parameters near baseline
Kanofsky et al. (2011)	28 M	Clozapine Divalproex Lithium Perphenazine Benzatropine Amoxicillin clavulanate	125	7 d		Creatinine 7.1 mg dL^{-1}; no biopsy	Pyrexia, proteinuria (3 +), total serum protein 5.6 g dL^{-1}, urea nitrogen 92 mg dL^{-1}. No eosinophilia	Prednisone and hydration	Recovered

Hunter et al. (2009)	57 F	Clozapine Lithium		c. 1 mo		Acute renal failure			5 d after stopping clozapine creatinine 1.2 mg dL^{-1}
		Clozapine Sodium valproate Olanzapine	25	3 d	Rechallenge 4 yr later	Creatinine 1.4 mg dL^{-1}. No biopsy	Pyrexia, tachycardia CRP 197 mg L^{-1}		
Siddiqui et al. (2008)	26 M	Clozapine Valproic acid Lithium Clonazepam	125	14 d		Creatinine 5.0 mg dL^{-1}; no biopsy. Echo: LVEF 40%	Pyrexia, tachycardia. Proteinuria (2+), eosinophils 0.8 × 10^9 L^{-1}	IV hydration, steroid, β-blocker	2 w after stopping clozapine. LVEF 50%, renal function improving
Au et al. (2004)	33 M	Clozapine Valproic acid Ziprasidone Gabapentin	100	14 d		Creatinine 9.7 mg dL^{-1}. U/S: glomerular nephritis	Pyrexia, vomiting, diarrhea. Eosinophils 2.5×10^9 L^{-1}, urea nitrogen 87 mg dL^{-1}	IV hydration	After 7 d creatinine 4.1 mg dL^{-1}.
Estébanez et al. (2002)	69 M	Clozapine Valproic acid Trihexyphenidyl		3 mo	Renal failure found when investigated for epilepsy	Creatinine 4.1 mg dL^{-1}. Biopsy: AIN	Signs of dehydration. No eosinophilia	Methylprednisolone IV 1 g d^{-1} for 3 d	Improvement followed clozapine withdrawal
Fraser and Jibani (2000)	49 M	Clozapine Diazepam prn	200	10 d	Clozapine for 10 d, ceased for 4 d for pyrexia, recommenced for 3 d	Creatinine 7.3 mg dL^{-1}. Biopsy: florid IN	Pyrexia, dehydration	Methylprednisolone IV 1 g d^{-1} for 3 d; then oral prednisolone	Dialysis independent 17 d after stopping clozapine

(Continued)

TABLE 13.2 (Continued)

Authors, Year	Age, Sex	Drugs	Dose (mg d⁻¹)	Time to Onset	Comment Retime to Onset	Diagnostic Data	Other Results	Treatment	Outcome
Southall and Fernando (2000)	24 F	Clozapine	300	11 d		Proteinuria 3 g L⁻¹. No biopsy.	Pyrexia, tachycardia, vomiting, Eosinophils 0.54×10^9 L⁻¹, CRP 58 mg L⁻¹		Urinary parameters normal 8 d after stopping clozapine
Elias et al. (1999) Chan et al. (2015)	38 F 29 F	Clozapine Lithium Venlafaxine Clozapine	250 700	11 d 7 d	Febrile onset	Creatinine 13.6 mg dL⁻¹. Biopsy: AIN Creatinine 4.0 mg dL⁻¹. Biopsy: tubulointerstitial nephritis with eosinophil-rich interstitial infiltrates and occasional granulomas	Vomiting, oliguria. Urea 92 mg dL⁻¹ Fever, eosinophilia	All drugs ceased Clozapine stopped	Creatinine normal 15 d after stopping clozapine Creatinine normal 4 w after stopping clozapine

AIN, acute interstitial nephritis; *CRP*, C-reactive protein; *M*, male; *F*, female; *IN*, interstitial nephritis; *IV*, intravenous; *LVEF*, left ventricular ejection fraction; *U/S*, ultrasound; *d*, days; *w*, weeks; *mo*, months; *yr*, years.

Siddiqui et al. (2008) noted that the case they described also developed cardiomyopathy, with reduced left ventricular ejection fraction (40%). Hence, they proposed an IgE mediated hypersensitivity reaction as suggested by Kilian et al. (1999) for clozapine-induced myocarditis (see Chapter 2, Myocarditis and Cardiomyopathy). In this regard, it is relevant to note that cardiac involvement is described in nine of the reports to the TGA (2015) of interstitial nephritis, acute kidney injury, or kidney failure, and five of these list myocarditis (Table 13.1).

13.1.4 Clinical and Laboratory Features

The common clinical features of the published cases are pyrexia and tachycardia, and some had gastrointestinal symptoms, diarrhea, and/or vomiting (Au et al., 2004; Southall and Fernando, 2000; Table 13.2). Although rash is regarded as a classical feature (Beck and Salant, 2012), it is described in none of these cases. Creatinine was invariably elevated and proteinuria may develop. Eosinophilia occurred in some, but not all, and CRP was substantially elevated. Urinalysis may reveal the presence of red blood cells and eosinophils (Chan et al., 2015). In the presence of documented evidence of renal dysfunction and raised inflammatory markers, renal biopsy is not required to confirm the diagnosis for clinical purposes (Beck and Salant, 2012; Perazella and Markowitz, 2010). This will be reassuring to psychiatrists treating psychotic patients.

13.1.5 Differential Diagnosis

Suspected clozapine-induced interstitial nephritis responding to withdrawal of clozapine will be an indication of cause. For cases not improving following clozapine discontinuation, renal biopsy will indicate whether the patient has interstitial nephritis, but may not clarify whether the condition is substance-related (Beck and Salant, 2012).

13.1.6 Management

If renal injury is not severe, the patient may improve and recover without treatment (Elias et al., 1999), but most published cases have been treated with a corticosteroid (Estébanez et al., 2002; Fraser and Jibani, 2000; Parekh et al., 2014). The value of this intervention has not been demonstrated in clinical trials (Perazella and Markowitz, 2010), but it appears to be beneficial in hastening recovery in severe cases (Parekh et al., 2014). Interstitial nephritis may progress to end-stage renal disease if the causative agent is not withdrawn (Martuseviciene et al., 2006). In somewhat less severe cases with prolonged exposure and severe tubular atrophy and interstitial fibrosis, renal damage may not be completely reversible (Beck and Salant, 2012). The effect of corticosteroid treatment on prognosis is unclear.

13.1.7 Prevention

The authors of the case reports have variously recommended monitoring strategies for kidney dysfunction in patients commencing clozapine (Mohan et al., 2013; Au et al., 2004; Fraser and Jibani, 2000; Kanofsky et al., 2011). The strategies include checking renal parameters if eosinophil count is elevated or fever develops. Unfortunately, both of these events frequently occur benignly in patients commencing clozapine. Given the evidence that interstitial nephritis with clozapine is very rare, recommending active surveillance specifically for this entity would seem unreasonable. However, many of the features, particularly fever and raised CRP, are the same as those accompanying myocarditis and the two adverse events may occur together. The best advice is to follow the monitoring guidelines for myocarditis (see Chapter 2, Myocarditis and Cardiomyopathy, Section 2.10 and Fig. 2.4). If the patient is unwell with fever and CRP greater than 100 mg L^{-1}, but no cardiac involvement has been found after checking troponin and conducting echocardiography, investigation of serum creatinine may hold the key. Alternatively, if after diagnosis of myocarditis and withdrawal of clozapine, the patient continues to be severely unwell despite improvement in markers of cardiac function, interstitial nephritis should be considered as an additional diagnosis.

13.2 INTERSTITIAL LUNG DISEASE

13.2.1 Definition

Drug-induced interstitial lung disease may be immune-mediated or toxic in nature. The term interstitial lung disease applies to a group of diseases affecting the tissue and spaces around the pulmonary air sacs and distinguishes these diseases from obstructive airways disease. Drug-induced interstitial lung disease is diagnosed when cough, fever, dyspnea, and/or pleuritic chest pain develop; diffuse alveolar damage, interstitial pneumonia, eosinophilic pneumonia, hypersensitivity pneumonitis, and/or granulomatous lung disease are revealed by radiology; other causes including congestive cardiac failure, infection, or malignancy are absent; and drug withdrawal is followed by symptom subsidence (Matsuno, 2012; Box 13.2).

BOX 13.2 Interstitial Lung Disease

- There is little evidence of a causal relationship between antipsychotics and interstitial lung disease with one exception.
- It appears that interstitial pneumonitis may occur rarely in the context of the hypersensitivity events occurring with initiation of clozapine.
- The apparent rarity may be a true reflection of occurrence or it may be a consequence of failure to investigate for pulmonary disease.

13.2.2 Epidemiology

Against a background of use by tens of thousands of people, a total of 33 cases of clozapine-related interstitial lung disease (Table 13.3) have been published in the medical literature and reported to the Australian Therapeutic Goods Administration (TGA) (2015) and to the United Kingdom Medicines and Healthcare products Regulatory Agency (MHRA) (2015). Similarly, for other antipsychotics, very few cases have been reported, despite use by large numbers of patients. Some cases of interstitial lung disease from other causes might be expected among the users.

One published case with clozapine was suspected to be allergic alveolitis and myocarditis, where the time to onset, 15 days, was consistent with that expected for myocarditis (Benning, 1998). The symptoms were pyrexia, lethargy, cough, and dyspnea. X-ray revealed widespread reticular and linear markings in both lungs, consistent with an inflammatory process. Computerized tomography (CT) indicated interstitial shadowing. Echocardiography was unremarkable. Elevated erythrocyte sedimentation rate (ESR) (90 mm h^{-1}) and eosinophilia were present. The patient responded to discontinuation of clozapine and conservative management.

In the other published case associated with clozapine, a 41-year-old woman who had been taking clozapine for 2 months developed mild dyspnea (Arias et al., 2011). On bronchoalveolar lavage, lymphocytes were 54% and eosinophils 2%. CT revealed diffuse bilateral ground-glass opacity. Lung biopsy indicated mild chronic inflammation without granulomas. Liver function test results were elevated and ESR increased (130 mm h^{-1}), but peripheral eosinophilia was absent. Viral, bacterial, and mycobacterial cultures were negative. Two months after tapering and discontinuing clozapine, chest CT indicated resolution of pathology.

Five of the Australian cases (allergic alveolitis $n = 2$, pneumonitis $n = 2$, lung infiltration) occurred within 2−3 weeks after commencing clozapine (Hill, R. Personal communication. July 14, 2015). The inflammatory event appeared to be a manifestation of the hypersensitivity reaction which can follow initiation of clozapine. All five either recovered on withdrawal of clozapine or were recovering at the time of reporting. The three other reports with clozapine have scant information, including with respect to time to onset. The details of the two Australian cases of interstitial lung disease with olanzapine do not give confidence of a causal association, because of prolonged duration of exposure and drug abuse, respectively. The report of pneumonitis with amisulpride came with little information.

In the published case attributed to haloperidol, the patient was given a range of medication because her psychiatric condition was unstable (Sato and Takeichi, 1990). Transbronchial biopsy revealed lymphocyte proliferation with fibroblastic and fibroelastic thickening of the alveolar walls. The condition was attributed to haloperidol because the patient improved as this drug was down titrated. The case of interstitial lung disease with chlorpromazine

TABLE 13.3 Summary of Reports of Interstitial Lung Disease With Antipsychotics Published in the Literature, and Reported to the Australian Therapeutic Goods Administration (TGA) (2015) and the United Kingdom Medicines and Healthcare products Regulatory Agency (MHRA) (2015). The number of cases is specified in the left hand column under each source.

Literature		TGA		MHRA	
Clozapine		Clozapine (total reports 7875)		Clozapine (total reports 12568)	
1	Allergic alveolitis	2	Allergic alveolitis	1	Alveolitis
1	Lymphocytic alveolitis	1	Lung infiltration	8	Pulmonary fibrosis
		2	Pulmonary fibrosis	9	Interstitial lung disease
		1	Interstitial lung disease	5	Pneumonitis; 1 fatal
		2	Pneumonitis	Olanzapine (total reports 3303)	
		Olanzapine (total reports 1717)		1	Pneumonitis
		2	Pulmonary fibrosis; 1 fatal	Chlorpromazine (total reports 1126)	
Chlorpromazine		Amisulpride (total reports 306)		1	Allergic alveolitis
1	Interstitial lung disease	1	Pneumonitis	Quetiapine (total reports 2169)	
Haloperidol				1	Pneumonitis
1	Interstitial pneumonitis			Risperidone (total reports 4166)	
				3	Pulmonary fibrosis
				1	Interstitial lung disease

involved significant fibrosis with cubic metaplasia of the alveoli epithelium, although clinical examination revealed no abnormality besides bilateral crepitations (Clerici et al., 1986).

13.2.3   Conclusion

In summary, then, it appears that interstitial lung disease may occur in the context of the response to initiation of clozapine, frequently involving fever, tachycardia, and eosinophilia, and occasionally myocarditis (see Chapter 2, Myocarditis and Cardiomyopathy) (Ronaldson et al., 2011). The very low number of reported cases may indicate rare occurrence, or may be a consequence of a failure to investigate for pulmonary disease in view of more obvious or more widely recognized reasons for the signs and symptoms; cough, dyspnea, chest pain, and fever occur with myocarditis (Ronaldson et al., 2011). Interstitial lung disease appears to be vanishingly rare with other antipsychotics, if indeed there is a causal relationship.

REFERENCES

Interstitial Nephritis

Au, A.F., Luthra, V., Stern, R., 2004. Clozapine-induced acute interstitial nephritis. Am. J. Psychiatry 161, 1501.

Beck, L.H., Salant, D.J., 2012. Chapter 285. Tubulointerstitial diseases of the kidney. In: Longo, D.L., Fauci, A.S., Kasper, D.L., et al., Harrison's Principles of Internal Medicine, 18th ed. McGraw-Hill Medical, New York.

Chan, S.Y., Cheung, C.Y., Chan, P.T., Chau, K.F., 2015. Clozapine-induced acute interstitial nephritis. Hong Kong Med. J. 21 (4), 372−374.

Elias, T.J., Bannister, K.M., Clarkson, A.R., et al., 1999. Clozapine-induced acute interstitial nephritis. Lancet 354, 1180−1181.

Estébanez, C., Fernandez Reyes, M.J., Sanchez Hernandez, R., et al., 2002. Acute interstitial nephritis caused by clozapine [Spanish]. Nefrologia 22, 277−281.

Fraser, D., Jibani, M., 2000. An unexpected and serious complication of treatment with the atypical antipsychotic drug clozapine. Clin. Nephrol. 54, 78−80.

Fukuda, Y., Watanabe, H., Ohtomo, Y., et al., 1996. Immunologically mediated chronic tubulo-interstitial nephritis caused by valproate therapy. Nephron 72, 328−329.

He, L., Peng, Y., Fu, X., et al., 2013. Dibenzodiazepine derivative quetiapine- and olanzapine-induced chronic interstitial nephritis. Renal Failure 35, 657−659.

Hunter, R., Gaughan, T., Queirazza, F., et al., 2009. Clozapine-induced interstitial nephritis − a rare but important complication: a case report. J. Med. Case Rep. 3, 8574.

Kanofsky, J.D., Woesner, M.E., Harris, A.Z., et al., 2011. A case of acute renal failure in a patient recently treated with clozapine and a review of previously reported cases. Pim. Care Companion CNS Disord. 13 (3). Available from: http://dx.doi.org/10.4088/PCC.10br01091.

Kilian, J.G., Kerr, K., Lawrence, C., et al., 1999. Myocarditis and cardiomyopathy associated with clozapine. Lancet 354, 1841−1845.

Liang, C.S., Bai, Y.M., Liou, Y.J., et al., 2012. Acute renal failure after paliperidone overdose: a case report. J. Clin. Psychopharmacol. 32, 128.

Martuseviciene, G., Kamper, A.L., Horn, T., 2006. A severe case of interstitial nephritis caused by sodium valproate [Danish]. Ugeskrift for Laeger 168, 3729–3730.

Mohan, T., Chua, J., Kartika, J., et al., 2013. Clozapine-induced nephritis and monitoring implications. Aust. N.Z. J. Psychiatry 47, 586–587.

Parekh, R., Fattah, Z., Sahota, D., et al., 2014. Clozapine induced tubulointerstitial nephritis in a patient with paranoid schizophrenia. BMJ Case Rep. (online). Available from: http://dx.doi.org/10.1136/bcr-2013-203502

Perazella, M.A., Markowitz, G.S., 2010. Drug-induced acute interstitial nephritis. Nat. Rev. Nephrol. 6, 461–470.

Ronaldson, K.J., Taylor, A.J., Fitzgerald, P.B., et al., 2011. A new monitoring protocol for clozapine induced myocarditis based on an analysis of 75 cases and 94 controls. Aust. N.Z. J. Psychiatry 45, 458–465.

Ronaldson, K.J., Fitzgerald, P.B., Taylor, A.J., et al., 2012. Rapid clozapine dose titration and concomitant sodium valproate increase the risk of myocarditis with clozapine: a case-control study. Schizophr. Res. 141, 173–178.

Siddiqui, B.K., Asim, S., Shamim, A., et al., 2008. Simultaneous allergic interstitial nephritis and cardiomyopathy in a patient on clozapine. Clin. Kidney J. 1, 55–56.

Southall, K.E., Fernando, S.N., 2000. A case of interstitial nephritis on clozapine. Aust. N.Z. J. Psychiatry 34, 697–698.

Therapeutic Goods Administration, Australian Government. Database of Adverse Event Notifications (DAEN). Retrieved (June 5, 2015). from: https://www.tga.gov.au/databaseadverse-event-notifications-daen.

Watanabe, T., Yoshikawa, H., Yamazaki, S., et al., 2005. Secondary renal Fanconi syndrome caused by valproate therapy. Pediatr. Nephrol. 20, 814–817.

Interstitial Lung Disease

Arias, S.A., Cohen, P., Kwon, J.S., 2011. Clozapine-induced lymphocytic alveolitis. Am. J. Psychiatry 168, 210–211.

Benning, T.B., 1998. Clozapine-induced extrinsic allergic alveolitis. Br. J. Psychiatry 173, 440–441.

Clerici, C., Lacronique, J., Kemeny, J., 1986. Bioclinical conference in pneumology. Hopital Laennec. Case n. 4--February 1985. Interstitial pneumopathy associated with pulmonary infiltration by foamy macrophages [French]. Revue de Pneumologie Clinique 42, 300–305.

Matsuno, O., 2012. Drug-induced interstitial lung disease: mechanisms and best diagnostic approaches. Respir. Res. 13, 39.

Medicines and Healthcare products Regulatory Agency (MHRA), United Kingdom Government. Drug Analysis Prints. Retrieved (July 13, 2015) from http://www.mhra.gov.uk/Safetyinformation/Howwemonitorthesafetyofproducts/Medicines/TheYellowCardScheme/YellowCarddata/Druganalysisprints/index.htm.

Ronaldson, K.J., Taylor, A.J., Fitzgerald, P.B., et al., 2011. A new monitoring protocol for clozapine induced myocarditis based on an analysis of 75 cases and 94 controls. Aust. N.Z. J. Psychiatry 45, 458–465.

Sato, T., Takeichi, M., 1990. Drug-induced pneumonitis associated with haloperidol. A case report. Gen. Hosp. Psychiatry 12, 341–343.

Therapeutic Goods Administration, 2015. Australian Government. Database of Adverse Event Notifications (DAEN). Retrieved (July 13, 2015) from https://www.tga.gov.au/database-adverse-event-notifications-daen.

Part VII

Clinical and Forensic Challenges in the Use of Antipsychotic Drugs

The Benefits of Antipsychotic Drugs: Symptom Control and Improved Quality of Life

Jian-Ping Zhang

Hofstra Northwell School of Medicine, Hempstead, NY, United States

14.1 THERAPEUTIC OBJECTIVES IN SCHIZOPHRENIA

Schizophrenia is a chronic and debilitating mental disorder, characterized by both positive and negative symptoms such as hallucinations, delusions, thought disorders, disorganized behavior, avolition, and social withdraw, as well as cognitive and functional impairment (van Os and Kapur, 2009). The life-time prevalence of schizophrenia ranges from 0.30% to 0.66% worldwide (McGrath et al., 2008), up to 2.3% including other psychotic disorders (Perala et al., 2007). Schizophrenia carries significant medical comorbidity and increased mortality, with an average life-span shortened by as much as 10−25 years (Goff et al., 2005; Colton and Manderscheid, 2006). The etiology of schizophrenia is considered multifactorial, with both genetic and environmental factors playing important roles. Illness onset typically occurs in late adolescence to young adulthood and its course is commonly chronic and severely disabling. The broad objectives of treatment are to reduce symptoms, restore social functioning, and prevent symptom relapse, so these patients usually require life-time treatment which causes significant public health and economic burden (Rice, 1999).

When Emil Kraepelin (1919) first described the concept of schizophrenia a century ago, he noted "the treatment of dementia praecox offers few points of intervention." Prior to the 1950s, this statement largely remained true. Either experimental drug treatment or psychoanalytic therapy was not effective, and most schizophrenia patients stayed in state institutions for many years. Electroconvulsive therapy was effective in reducing symptoms, but it was not widely used due to side effects at that time. In the early 1950s, an

Life-Threatening Effects of Antipsychotic Drugs. DOI: http://dx.doi.org/10.1016/B978-0-12-803376-0.00014-9
© 2016 Elsevier Inc. All rights reserved.

antihistamine, chlorpromazine, was serendipitously found to have a strong calming effects on psychotic patients although it was initially used to prevent postsurgical shock. This opened up a new era of modern psychopharmacology, and it quickly became a mainstream therapy for schizophrenia. Within a short time span, millions of patients with schizophrenia around world had been treated with this medication. Many other similar antipsychotic drugs were developed and used in clinical practice, contributing partly to the deinstitutionalization movement in the 1960s and 1970s. The discovery that dopamine D2 receptor antagonism played a critical role in these drugs' antipsychotic efficacy (Kapur and Mamo, 2003) led to the formulation of dopamine theory of schizophrenia, which in turn sparked development of more antipsychotic drugs that are primarily D2 antagonists (first-generation antipsychotics, FGA). After clozapine was introduced in Europe and North America as an atypical antipsychotic drug with minimal side effects of extrapyramidal symptoms (EPSs) and tardive dyskinesia (TD), efforts to produce similar drugs created the second-generation antipsychotics (SGAs) characterized by serotonin receptor modulation in addition to D2 blockade. However, recent works suggested that different SGAs have varying degrees of antipsychotic efficacy and different side effect profiles, challenging the classification of SGAs versus FGAs grouping (Leucht et al., 2013). Nevertheless, SGAs have been widely used in treating not only schizophrenia, but also bipolar affective disorder, major depressive disorder (MDD), and many other mental disorders in off-label use (Maher et al., 2011; Olfson et al., 2012). In 2010, about 1−2% of the adult population in the United States was prescribed antipsychotics, and the percentage of antipsychotic use in the older population was even higher due to dementia-related diagnoses (Olfson et al., 2015). Recent evidence shows that antipsychotic drugs are generally safe to use during pregnancy (Vigod et al., 2015).

This chapter will briefly discuss the pharmacology of current antipsychotic agents and summarize available evidence on the efficacy of antipsychotic drugs in treating schizophrenia and related psychotic disorders, as well as other mental disorders. Although these drugs can cause significant adverse events, those will be discussed in other chapters.

14.2 PHARMACOLOGY OF ANTIPSYCHOTIC DRUGS

Antipsychotic drugs as a class bind to receptors and modulate functions of multiple neurotransmitter systems in the brain, including but not limited to dopamine, serotonin, glutamate, adrenaline, acetylcholine, and histamine (Correll, 2010). These actions likely contribute to both clinical efficacy and adverse reactions. Table 14.1 lists the receptor binding profiles for commonly used antipsychotic drugs.

The main mechanism of action of antipsychotics is dopamine D2 receptor antagonism (Kapur and Mamo, 2003). The dopamine hypothesis of

TABLE 14.1 Relative Affinity to Neurotransmitter Receptors for Commonly Used Antipsychotics at Therapeutic Doses

	D1	D2	D3	D4	5-HT$_{1A}$	5-HT$_{2A}$	5-HT$_{2C}$	5-HT$_6$	5-HT$_7$	α$_1$	α$_2$	H$_1$	M$_1$
FGAs													
Chlorpromazine	++	+	++	++	−	+	++	+	+	+++	+++	++++	+++
Haloperidol	+	++++	+++	+++	−	+	−	−	−	+++	+	−	−
Perphenazine	−	+++	++	−	+	++	+	−	−	+++	−	+++	−
Sulpride	−	++++	++	−	−	−	−	−	−	−	−	−	−
Zotepine	+	++	++	+	++	+++	++	++	++	++	++	++	+
SGAs													
Clozapine	+	+	+	++	−	+++	++	++	++	+++	+	+++	++++
Olanzapine	++	++	+	++	−	+++	++	++	−	++	+	+++	+++
Risperidone	+	+++	++	−	−	++++	++	−	+++	+++	++	−	−
Quetiapine	−	+	−	−	+	++	−	+	−	+++	−	++	++
Ziprasidone	+	+++	++	++	+++	++++	++++	+	++	++	+	++	−
Aripiprazole	−	++++	++	+	++	+++	+	+	++	+	+	+	−
Lurasidone	+	++++	+	+	+++	+++	+	+	++++	+	++	−	−
Amisulpride	−	++++	++	−	−	−	+	+	−	−	−	−	−

−, Minimal to none; +, low; ++, moderate; +++, high; ++++, very high.

Source: Adapted from Correll, C.U., 2010. From receptor pharmacology to improved outcomes: individualising the selection, dosing, and switching of antipsychotics. Eur. Psychiatry 25 (Suppl. 2), S12–S21 (Correll, 2010); Miyamoto, S., Duncan, G.E., et al., 2005. Treatments for schizophrenia: a critical review of pharmacology and mechanisms of action of antipsychotic drugs. Mol. Psychiatry 10 (1), 79–104 (Miyamoto et al., 2005); and Kusumi, I., Boku, S., et al., 2015. Psychopharmacology of atypical antipsychotic drugs: from the receptor binding profile to neuroprotection and neurogenesis. Psychiatry Clin. Neurosci. 69 (5), 243–258 (Kusumi et al., 2015).

schizophrenia states that there is dysregulation of neurotransmission in brain dopaminergic circuits with excessive dopaminergic signaling in the mesolimbic pathway (causing positive symptoms) and reduced signaling in the mesocortical pathway (resulting in negative symptoms) (Miyamoto et al., 2012). Blockade of D2 receptors in the mesolimbic pathway will reduce dopamine activity and therefore decrease positive symptoms. Brain imaging studies have shown that an in vivo striatal D2 receptor occupancy of 65−70% is required to achieve antipsychotic effects, at least for some FGAs, and that D2 occupancy of greater than 80% significantly increases the risk of EPSs, a common side effect of antipsychotic drugs (Remington and Kapur, 1999). These have led researchers to hypothesize that D2 antagonism may be "necessary and sufficient" for antipsychotic efficacy (Kapur and Mamo, 2003), because all known antipsychotic drugs bind to the D2 receptor and drugs that have targeted non-D2 receptors without at least some element of D2 blockade have not been proven effective in treating schizophrenia.

The discovery that clozapine is superior than other drugs in treating refractory schizophrenia (Kane et al., 1988) and that it has only weak D2 affinity led to the development of SGAs. One of the hypotheses about SGAs was that they act more on serotonergic receptors and that a high ratio of affinities for $5\text{-}HT_{2A}$ to D2 receptors is a critical feature of the "atypicality" of SGAs (Meltzer et al., 1989). Others argued that SGAs tend to bind to D2 receptors then disassociate quickly and that these "fast-off" characteristics define low EPS liability among SGAs (Kapur and Seeman, 2001). Each model seems to explain only part of the antipsychotic drug actions, and it is likely that both dopaminergic and serotonergic binding play important roles in antipsychotic efficacy. In contrast, binding profiles to other neurotransmitter receptors are able to predict drug-induced side effects. For example, strong affinities to histamine H_1, adrenergic α_1, and muscarinic M_1 receptors are associated with sedation, orthostatic hypotension, and anticholinergic effects. In clinical practice, it is important to recognize the different pharmacodynamic and pharmacokinetic properties of each antipsychotic drug and understand how these factors impact clinical efficacy and adverse reactions.

14.3   SYMPTOM REDUCTION IN SCHIZOPHRENIA

Schizophrenia is characterized by its prominent positive symptoms including auditory and visual hallucinations, paranoia and delusions, as well as disorganized behavior and thinking, which are primarily responsible for a patient's functional impairment, agitation, aggression, loss of productivity, institutionalization, and increased risks of self-harm as well as harm to others. Antipsychotic drugs, both FGAs and SGAs, have been shown to be efficacious in reducing these symptoms, thus helping patients to recover from the illness and integrate back to the community. Evidence of antipsychotic efficacy mostly comes from (1) early placebo-controlled studies conducted by the National Institute of Mental Health (NIMH), (2) Phase 3 clinical trials of new drugs sponsored by pharmaceutical companies for FDA registration purposes, and (3) head-to-head comparative efficacy trials of two or more antipsychotic agents. Very few recent placebo-controlled studies (except new drug registration trials) were conducted due to ethical concerns that an acutely psychotic patient should not be given placebo while multiple efficacious drugs are available to treat the patient.

An early NIMH study provided initial evidence to support the strong effects of antipsychotic drugs (Cole et al., 1964). In this largely first episode schizophrenia cohort ($n = 334$), 61% of patients on chlorpromazine responded to treatment, whereas only 22% of patients on placebo had significant reduction in symptoms. This resulted in a response rate difference of 39% or a Number Needed to Treat (NNT) of $2-3$, which is a large effect size by any measure. Davis and colleagues (1989) summarized approximately 100 double-blind studies conducted before 1989 comparing an FGA and placebo in the acute treatment of schizophrenia, and found that FGAs were more effective than placebo in most studies. Overall, 75% of patients treated with phenothiazines were much improved after 6 weeks compared with less than 25% of placebo-treated patients. Based on this and other reviews, the Schizophrenia Patient Outcome Research Team (PORT), convened by the Agency for Health Care Policy and Research and NIMH in 1992 to improve the quality of care for psychiatric patients, concluded that antipsychotic drugs were helpful in controlling positive symptoms of schizophrenia and had significantly reduced its morbidity and mortality (Dixon et al., 1995). Many of these studies reviewed used chlorpromazine and other low potency antipsychotics as the active drug. Other reviews have examined the efficacy of high potency drugs such as haloperidol and found them equally efficacious. A Cochrane review on haloperidol (Joy et al., 2006) showed a pronounced superiority over placebo, with an NNT of 3 in both short-term and medium-term studies, with a response rate of 43.8% in haloperidol versus 14.4% in placebo groups.

When clozapine, olanzapine, risperidone, and other SGAs came on the market in the 1990s, they were initially considered as more efficacious than FGAs with fewer side effects. However, later studies largely discredited the claim of SGA's superiority, except clozapine, in treating refractory schizophrenia. Compared to studies conducted in the 1960s to 1980s, recent studies showed an emerging trend that placebo response rate became increasingly higher (Rutherford et al., 2014), which may contribute to the relatively modest effect sizes associated with SGAs. Nevertheless, the evidence is clear that SGAs are efficacious in reducing psychotic symptoms. A comprehensive meta-analysis on 38 randomized placebo-control trials with 7323 patients demonstrated that the overall effect size was 0.51 (Cohen's d) for psychotic symptom reduction, with 41% response rate in SGAs group and 24% response rate in placebo group (Leucht et al., 2009). Although this resulted in a modest NNT of 6, SGAs have been the dominant force in treating schizophrenia, bipolar disorder, and other psychotic spectrum disorders in the past two decades, due to their relatively mild side effect profile in EPS and TD and aggressive marketing efforts by the pharmaceutical companies.

Although evidence supports the efficacy of antipsychotic drugs in reducing positive symptoms of schizophrenia, not all drugs were created equal. A recent review examined the 15 most prescribed antipsychotic drugs in comparative efficacy and tolerability in 212 trials (including placebo-controlled and head-to-head trials) with 43,049 patients (Leucht et al., 2013). The authors found that these drugs were all significantly more efficacious than placebo, but some drugs were more efficacious than others. Clozapine was the most effective drug with an effect size of 0.88 compared to placebo, and was more effective than all other drugs. This is not surprising because clozapine has been recommended as the first choice for treatment refractory schizophrenia for almost 30 years (Kane et al., 1988). After clozapine, amisulpride, olanzapine, and risperidone were significantly more effective than the other drugs except paliperidone and zotepine. The differences in efficacy were small, but side effects differed substantially among drugs. Another meta-analysis on first episode schizophrenia treatment trials showed that although SGAs had similar efficacy to FGAs in symptoms reduction and response rate, SGAs were slightly superior to FGAs in reducing negative symptoms and depression, as well as improving cognitive impairment, and patients on SGAs were less likely to stop their medications (Zhang et al., 2013). Consistent with other reviews, it seemed that olanzapine and amisulpride may be more efficacious than FGAs in treating first episode schizophrenia given available evidence.

In summary, most antipsychotic drugs are efficacious in treating psychotic symptoms. However, heterogeneity among drugs is too large to warrant the straightforward classification of FGAs versus SGAs. Antipsychotic treatment still needs to be tailored to an individual patient's need, considering both efficacy and side effects.

14.4   RELAPSE PREVENTION AND ANTIPSYCHOTIC MAINTENANCE TREATMENT

Schizophrenia is a chronic illness and requires life-long drug therapy. Without treatment, up to 80% of patients will have at least one episode of psychotic relapse (e.g., increase in psychotic symptoms and rehospitalization) within 5 years (Shepherd et al., 1989; Robinson et al., 1999). Early randomized placebo-control studies showed that after being stabilized on antipsychotics, patients switching to placebo experienced significantly higher rates of rehospitalization than patients continuing to receive medications (Engelhardt et al., 1967).

Leucht and colleagues (2012) systematically reviewed the literature from 1959 to 2011 on the role of antipsychotic drugs in relapse prevention in schizophrenia, and included 65 randomized controlled studies with 6493 patients. For all major outcomes including relapse, rehospitalization, dropping out of treatment, and aggressive behavior, patients with continued drug treatment did significantly better than patients who went on placebo treatment. 22% of patients on medications relapsed, compared to 57% of patients on placebo. Ten percent of patients on medications were readmitted to the hospital, whereas 26% of patients on placebo were rehospitalized. The review also examined individual antipsychotic drugs used in the trials, including chlorpromazine, haloperidol, quetiapine, paliperidone, and ziprasidone, and the evidence was quite clear that antipsychotics were effective in preventing relapse, regardless of which drug is used. It was concluded that antipsychotic maintenance treatment substantially reduces relapse risks in all schizophrenic patients for up to 2 years of follow-up.

Studies have investigated which type of antipsychotic drugs may be more effective in preventing relapse in schizophrenia, SGAs versus FGAs, as well as depot formulation versus oral medications. A recent meta-analysis reviewed 23 studies with 4504 patients comparing SGAs and FGAs in relapse prevention in schizophrenia (Kishimoto et al., 2013a,b). Although individual SGAs did not statistically outperform FGA comparators, SGAs as a whole were associated with lower relapse rate (29%) than were FGAs (37.5%). Because treatment nonadherence is a significant predictor of relapse (Robinson et al., 1999), there has been a considerable amount of interest in using long-acting injectable (LAI) depot formulations of antipsychotic medications. However, recent large randomized clinical trials comparing LAIs and oral medications could not find significant advantage of LAIs over oral drugs in preventing psychotic relapse (Rosenheck et al., 2011; Buckley et al., 2015). The negative results may be due to several factors such as lack of selection for prior nonadherence, intense assessment schedule, and free oral medication. Therefore, whether these findings can be applied to real-world practice has been called into question. To overcome the limitations of these studies, a meta-analysis of mirror-image studies, which compare a period of oral antipsychotic treatment with a subsequent period of LAI treatment for the same patients, was conducted to further explore the impact of LAIs on relapse prevention. The systematic review included 25 studies with 5940 patients, and found that LAIs showed strong superiority over oral antipsychotics in preventing rehospitalization and decreasing the number of hospitalization (Kishimoto et al., 2013a,b). Patients on oral medications were twice more likely to be hospitalized than patients on LAIs.

In summary, the available evidence is quite clear that antipsychotic drugs are beneficial in preventing psychotic relapse in patients with schizophrenia, and that LAIs may be advantageous over oral medications in achieving this goal.

14.5   IMPROVING QUALITY OF LIFE IN PATIENTS WITH SCHIZOPHRENIA

For patients with schizophrenia, psychosis usually starts in late adolescence and early adulthood, which is a critical period for personal, occupational, and social development. Because of psychotic symptoms, both positive and negative symptoms, patients cannot function normally at home and in the society, leading to life-long functional impairment and poor quality of life. Although antipsychotic drugs are efficacious in reducing positive symptoms, they have limited effects on negative symptoms and cognitive impairment, both of which play important roles in an individual's functional status. In addition, side effects of antipsychotic drugs, such as annoying EPSs, irreversible TD, and significant weight gain, have negatively impacted on a patient's quality of life and sense of well-being, often leading to medication nonadherence, which, in turn, causes psychotic relapse and further decline in functional status. As such, it is critical in clinical practice to balance the benefits and risks of medications to maximize the chance of treatment success, which ultimately results in functional recovery and improved quality of life.

Compared to the literature on the effects of antipsychotic drugs on symptom reduction and relapse prevention, there have been relatively fewer studies on patients self-reported functional outcomes, such as quality of life. Most of the early placebo-controlled studies did not include any quality of life measures, and other studies used quality of life as a secondary or tertiary outcome. Two randomized placebo-controlled studies (total $n = 406$) found that olanzapine significantly improved patients' quality of life more than placebo (Beasley et al., 1996; Lecrubier et al., 2006). In a pooled analysis of three phase 3 registration trials (total $n = 1306$), paliperidone was associated with large improvement in social and personal performance compared to placebo with an effect size of $0.52-0.85$, and the gain was sustained throughout 52 weeks of follow-up (Patrick et al. 2010). However, other studies did not find significant advantage of antipsychotic drugs over placebo on improving quality of life (Moller et al., 2004; Nasrallah et al., 2008).

Because of relatively benign neuromuscular side effects of SGAs and their slight advantages in treating negative symptoms and cognitive impairment (Zhang et al., 2013), it was thought that SGAs may be able to contribute more to quality of life in patients with schizophrenia. An early study with 230 patients reinforced this claim, in which SGAs including olanzapine, risperidone, quetiapine, and clozapine seemed to outperform FGAs in patient-reported quality of life (Voruganti et al., 2000). However, a more recent randomized controlled clinical trial with 227 schizophrenia patients was designed to specifically test whether SGAs were superior to FGAs in improving quality of life, and did not find any statistical significance between the two groups of drugs (Jones et al., 2006). If anything, patients on FGAs were slightly better on quality of life than those on SGAs, but the difference did not reach statistical significance.

Therefore, the evidence on antipsychotic drugs and patient-reported quality of life is inconsistent. This may be due to conceptualization issues and measurement difficulties of the quality of life construct, multiple scales used in different studies, and a lack of studies that are designed to assess quality of life as primary outcomes (Awad and Voruganti, 2004, 2013). With increased interests in patient-centered outcomes in medical research in recent years and a new mandate from the US Food and Drug Administration (FDA) on new drug development, it is expected that there will be more studies on using antipsychotic drugs to improve quality of life in patients with schizophrenia in the near future.

14.6 ANTIPSYCHOTIC DRUGS IN TREATING OTHER PSYCHIATRIC DISORDERS

Since the debut of chlorpromazine more than 60 years ago, antipsychotic drugs have evolved to be not only the mainstay therapy for schizophrenia, they have also become an important part of treatment strategies for many other psychiatric disorders. Most SGAs have obtained FDA approval as monotherapy in treating acute mania in bipolar affective disorder, and several were also indicated as augmentation therapy for MDD. Furthermore, antipsychotic drugs have been widely used off-label in many psychiatric conditions including anxiety, insomnia, obsessive-compulsive disorder, agitation, conduct disorder, personality disorders, eating disorder, and posttraumatic stress disorder. This section summarizes the available evidence for the benefits of antipsychotic drugs in treating other psychiatric disorders.

The manic phase of bipolar affective disorder is characterized by elevated mood, grandiosity, decreased need of sleep, increased goal-directed behavior, pressured speech, and reckless risky behavior, often requiring hospital admission for stabilization. For a long time, lithium and antiepileptic drugs were primarily used during treatment for acute mania. FGAs were attempted to treat bipolar disorder with mixed results, due to concerns of inducing depressive episodes and side effects of EPS (Esparon et al., 1986; Cavazzoni et al., 2006). However, SGAs have emerged as a major force of bipolar disorder treatment in the past two decades. Several treatment guidelines from various organizations recommend SGAs as one of the first line treatments for acute mania, either alone or combining with a mood stabilizer, and to a lesser degree, maintenance treatment for bipolar disorder (Connolly and Thase, 2011). Scherk and colleagues (2007) reviewed the evidence for SGAs' efficacy of treating acute mania. Twelve studies with over 2773 patients compared SGA monotherapy including aripiprazole, olanzapine, quetiapine, risperidone, and ziprasidone, to placebo, and found that all of these drugs significantly decreased manic symptoms than did placebo. Risperidone had the largest effect size with a Cohen's d of 0.66. Five studies with 633 patients comparing an SGA (olanzapine, quetiapine, and risperidone) to a mood stabilizer (either lithium or valproate sodium) showed that SGAs might have slight advantage over mood stabilizers in acute mania treatment. The combination therapy of an SGA adding to a mood stabilizer was also significantly better than a placebo in reducing manic symptoms in six studies with 1317 patients. A more recently updated meta-analysis examined the comparative efficacy of 13 commonly used agents in 68 randomized controlled trials with 16,073 patients (Cipriani et al., 2011). They found that antipsychotic drugs seem to be better than anticonvulsants and lithium in treating acute mania, and concluded that olanzapine, risperidone, and haloperidol should be considered as among the best options for mania treatment.

Although treatment of bipolar depression is controversial and can be clinically challenging, several SGAs have gained FDA approval for bipolar depression, including quetiapine, olanzapine (in combination with fluoxetine), and lurasidone. In a meta-analytic review of the evidence on SGAs in bipolar depression treatment, 29 studies with 8331 patients were included (Taylor et al., 2014). It was found that olanzapine monotherapy or the combination of olanzapine and fluoxetine had the best efficacy in improving depressive symptoms, although ziprasidone and quetiapine were associated with fewer switch to mania. Lurasidone had the second highest response rate next to the olanzapine/fluoxetine combo therapy. In a separate review of various classes of medications in treating bipolar depression, lurasidone, olanzapine/fluoxetine combination therapy, and quetiapine were found to be more effective than placebo, with NNT all less than 10, whereas aripiprazole and ziprasidone were not as effective (Vazquez et al., 2015). Although antidepressants and anticonvulsants are still mainstay treatment for bipolar depression, the evidence is clear that certain antipsychotic drugs are viable options in treating the depressive phase of bipolar disorder. Among different antipsychotic agents, differences in efficacy are relatively small, but differences in and drug-induced adverse events are large. Balancing risks and benefits, it seems that lurasidone may have the best risk/benefit ratio with both good efficacy and tolerability (Gao et al., 2015; Vazquez et al., 2015).

Antipsychotic drugs are also an important part of treatment strategies for MDD, both MDD with psychotic features and treatment refractory MDD. Three drugs, aripiprazole, olanzapine, and quetiapine (XR formulation), have gained FDA approval for adjunctive treatment of MDD in conjunction with antidepressants (Table 14.2). The use of SGAs to augment antidepressant treatment increased dramatically in the past two decades. One study found that from 1999 to 2000 SGA prescription in MDD treatment was up from 4.6% to 12.5% (Gerhard et al., 2014). Nelson and Papakostas (2009) reviewed 16 randomized, placebo-controlled studies of SGAs as augmentation treatment to antidepressants in 3480 patients. Four SGAs were used: olanzapine, risperidone, quetiapine, and aripiprazole. Although risperidone does not have FDA indication for MDD adjunctive therapy, it was still significantly better than placebo in both treatment response rate and remission

TABLE 14.2 FDA-Approved Indications for Selected FGAs and SGAs

	Schizophrenia	Schizoaffective Disorder	BAD (Manic/Mixed)	BAD (Depression)	BAD (Maintenance)	MDD (Adjunctive)
Chlorpromazine	X		X			
Fluphenazine	X					
Haloperidol	X					
Perphenazine	X					
Aripiprazole	X		X		X	X
Asenapine	X		X			
Clozapine	X					
Iloperidone	X					
Lurasidone	X			X		
Olanzapine	X		X	X[a]	X	X
Paliperidone	X	X				
Quetiapine	X		X	X	X	X
Risperidone	X		X		X	
Ziprasidone	X		X		X	

BAD, bipolar affective disorder; MDD, major depressive disorder.
[a]In combination with fluoxetine.

rate. Combining all 16 studies, all SGAs significantly outperformed placebo in augmenting antidepressant treatment. The overall pooled response rate in SGA groups was 44.2%, compared to 29.9% for placebo. The pooled remission rates were 30.7% for SGAs and 17.2% for placebo. Clearly, some antipsychotics can be beneficial as an adjunctive treatment for patients with MDD who have failed to respond to antidepressant monotherapy.

In addition to bipolar disorder and MDD, antipsychotic drugs are also widely used off-label to treat a variety of psychiatric conditions. Often, these uses are not supported by empirical evidence (i.e., randomized controlled clinical trials), although these drugs are frequently utilized to treat certain symptoms such as agitation, aggression, and hyperactivity that may present in many different diagnostic categories. Maher and colleagues (2011) reviewed literature on the efficacy of SGAs for off-label use in dementia, anxiety, Obsessive Compulsive Disorder (OCD), eating disorder, Post-traumatic Stress Disorder (PTSD), insomnia, personality disorders, depression, and substance abuse. They found that SGAs including aripiprazole, olanzapine, and risperidone had statistically significant, albeit modest, effects in treating elderly patients with dementia who presented with psychosis, mood alterations, and aggression in 14 placebo-controlled studies, although their use was associated with increased mortality rate and other drug-related adverse events. In addition, their meta-analysis found that quetiapine demonstrated significant benefits in treating generalized anxiety disorder, and risperidone showed advantages over placebo in treating OCD. The evidence for using SGAs to treat other psychiatric conditions was inconclusive.

Taken together, evidence supports that antipsychotic drugs can be an important part of treatment strategies for many psychiatric conditions. However, these drugs are associated with significant side effects. Risk and benefit analysis must be carefully considered when planning to use antipsychotics in treating other conditions. More research is needed to examine the efficacy and risks of these drugs in treating non-FDA indicated psychiatric conditions.

REFERENCES

Awad, A.G., Voruganti, L.N., 2004. Impact of atypical antipsychotics on quality of life in patients with schizophrenia. CNS Drugs 18 (13), 877–893.

Awad, A.G., Voruganti, L.N., 2013. The impact of newer atypical antipsychotics on patient-reported outcomes in schizophrenia. CNS Drugs 27 (8), 625–636.

Beasley Jr., C.M., Sanger, T., et al., 1996. Olanzapine versus placebo: results of a double-blind, fixed-dose olanzapine trial. Psychopharmacology (Berl.) 124 (1–2), 159–167.

Buckley, P.F., Schooler, N.R., et al., 2015. Comparison of SGA oral medications and a long-acting injectable SGA: the PROACTIVE study. Schizophr. Bull. 41 (2), 449–459.

Cavazzoni, P.A., Berg, P.H., et al., 2006. Comparison of treatment-emergent extrapyramidal symptoms in patients with bipolar mania or schizophrenia during olanzapine clinical trials. J. Clin. Psychiatry 67 (1), 107–113.

Cipriani, A., Barbui, C., et al., 2011. Comparative efficacy and acceptability of antimanic drugs in acute mania: a multiple-treatments meta-analysis. Lancet 378 (9799), 1306–1315.

Cole, J.O., Goldberg, S.C., et al., 1964. Phenothiazine treatment in acute schizophrenia. Arch. Gen. Psychiatry 10, 246–261.

Colton, C.W., Manderscheid, R.W., 2006. Congruencies in increased mortality rates, years of potential life lost, and causes of death among public mental health clients in eight states. Prev. Chronic. Dis. 3 (2), A42.

Connolly, K.R., Thase, M.E., 2011. The clinical management of bipolar disorder: a review of evidence-based guidelines. Prim. Care Companion CNS Disord. 13 (4).

Correll, C.U., 2010. From receptor pharmacology to improved outcomes: individualising the selection, dosing, and switching of antipsychotics. Eur. Psychiatry 25 (Suppl. 2), S12–S21.

Davis, J.M., Barter, J.T., et al., 1989. Antipsychotic drugs. In: Kaplan, H.I., Sadock, B.J. (Eds.), Comprehensive Textbook of Psychiatry, 5. Williams & Wilkins, Baltimore, MD, pp. 1591–1626.

Dixon, L.B., Lehman, A.F., et al., 1995. Conventional antipsychotic medications for schizophrenia. Schizophr. Bull. 21 (4), 567–577.

Engelhardt, D.M., Rosen, B., et al., 1967. Phenothiazines in prevention of psychiatric hospitalization. IV. Delay or prevention of hospitalization—a reevaluation. Arch. Gen. Psychiatry 16 (1), 98–101.

Esparon, J., Kolloori, J., et al., 1986. Comparison of the prophylactic action of flupenthixol with placebo in lithium treated manic-depressive patients. Br. J. Psychiatry 148, 723–725.

Gao, K., Yuan, C., et al., 2015. Important clinical features of atypical antipsychotics in acute bipolar depression that inform routine clinical care: a review of pivotal studies with number needed to treat. Neurosci. Bull. 31 (5), 572–588.

Gerhard, T., Akincigil, A., et al., 2014. National trends in second-generation antipsychotic augmentation for nonpsychotic depression. J. Clin. Psychiatry 75 (5), 490–497.

Goff, D.C., Cather, C., et al., 2005. Medical morbidity and mortality in schizophrenia: guidelines for psychiatrists. J. Clin. Psychiatry 66 (2), 183–194, quiz 147, 273–274.

Jones, P.B., Barnes, T.R., et al., 2006. Randomized controlled trial of the effect on Quality of Life of second- vs first-generation antipsychotic drugs in schizophrenia: Cost Utility of the Latest Antipsychotic Drugs in Schizophrenia Study (CUtLASS 1). Arch. Gen. Psychiatry 63 (10), 1079–1087.

Joy, C.B., Adams, C.E., et al., 2006. Haloperidol versus placebo for schizophrenia. Cochrane Database Syst. Rev. 4, CD003082.

Kane, J., Honigfeld, G., et al., 1988. Clozapine for the treatment-resistant schizophrenic. A double-blind comparison with chlorpromazine. Arch. Gen. Psychiatry 45 (9), 789–796.

Kapur, S., Mamo, D., 2003. Half a century of antipsychotics and still a central role for dopamine D2 receptors. Prog. Neuropsychopharmacol. Biol. Psychiatry 27 (7), 1081–1090.

Kapur, S., Seeman, P., 2001. Does fast dissociation from the dopamine d(2) receptor explain the action of atypical antipsychotics? A new hypothesis. Am. J. Psychiatry 158 (3), 360–369.

Kishimoto, T., Nitta, M., et al., 2013a. Long-acting injectable versus oral antipsychotics in schizophrenia: a systematic review and meta-analysis of mirror-image studies. J. Clin. Psychiatry 74 (10), 957–965.

Kishimoto, T., Agarwal, V., et al., 2013b. Relapse prevention in schizophrenia: a systematic review and meta-analysis of second-generation antipsychotics versus first-generation antipsychotics. Mol. Psychiatry 18 (1), 53–66.

Kraepelin, E., 1919. Dementia Praecox and Paraphrenia. Krieger, New York, NY.

Kusumi, I., Boku, S., et al., 2015. Psychopharmacology of atypical antipsychotic drugs: from the receptor binding profile to neuroprotection and neurogenesis. Psychiatry Clin. Neurosci. 69 (5), 243–258.

Lecrubier, Y., Quintin, P., et al., 2006. The treatment of negative symptoms and deficit states of chronic schizophrenia: olanzapine compared to amisulpride and placebo in a 6-month double-blind controlled clinical trial. Acta Psychiatr. Scand. 114 (5), 319–327.

Leucht, S., Arbter, D., et al., 2009. How effective are second-generation antipsychotic drugs? A meta-analysis of placebo-controlled trials. Mol. Psychiatry 14 (4), 429–447.

Leucht, S., Tardy, M., et al., 2012. Antipsychotic drugs versus placebo for relapse prevention in schizophrenia: a systematic review and meta-analysis. Lancet 379 (9831), 2063–2071.

Leucht, S., Cipriani, A., et al., 2013. Comparative efficacy and tolerability of 15 antipsychotic drugs in schizophrenia: a multiple-treatments meta-analysis. Lancet 382 (9896), 951–962.

Maher, A.R., Maglione, M., et al., 2011. Efficacy and comparative effectiveness of atypical antipsychotic medications for off-label uses in adults: a systematic review and meta-analysis. JAMA 306 (12), 1359–1369.

McGrath, J., Saha, S., et al., 2008. Schizophrenia: a concise overview of incidence, prevalence, and mortality. Epidemiol. Rev. 30, 67–76.

Meltzer, H.Y., Matsubara, S., et al., 1989. The ratios of serotonin2 and dopamine2 affinities differentiate atypical and typical antipsychotic drugs. Psychopharmacol. Bull. 25 (3), 390–392.

Miyamoto, S., Duncan, G.E., et al., 2005. Treatments for schizophrenia: a critical review of pharmacology and mechanisms of action of antipsychotic drugs. Mol. Psychiatry 10 (1), 79–104.

Miyamoto, S., Miyake, N., et al., 2012. Pharmacological treatment of schizophrenia: a critical review of the pharmacology and clinical effects of current and future therapeutic agents. Mol. Psychiatry 17 (12), 1206–1227.

Moller, H.J., Riedel, M., et al., 2004. Zotepine versus placebo in the treatment of schizophrenic patients with stable primary negative symptoms: a randomized double-blind multicenter trial. Pharmacopsychiatry 37 (6), 270–278.

Nasrallah, H., Morosini, P., et al., 2008. Reliability, validity and ability to detect change of the Personal and Social Performance scale in patients with stable schizophrenia. Psychiatry Res. 161 (2), 213–224.

Nelson, J.C., Papakostas, G.I., 2009. Atypical antipsychotic augmentation in major depressive disorder: a meta-analysis of placebo-controlled randomized trials. Am. J. Psychiatry 166 (9), 980–991.

Olfson, M., Blanco, C., et al., 2012. National trends in the office-based treatment of children, adolescents, and adults with antipsychotics. Arch. Gen. Psychiatry 69 (12), 1247–1256.

Olfson, M., King, M., et al., 2015. Antipsychotic treatment of adults in the United States. J. Clin. Psychiatry 76 (10), 1346–1353.

Patrick, D.L., Burns, T., et al., 2010. Measuring social functioning with the personal and social performance scale in patients with acute symptoms of schizophrenia: interpretation of results of a pooled analysis of three Phase III trials of paliperidone extended-release tablets. Clin. Ther. 32 (2), 275–292.

Perala, J., Suvisaari, J., et al., 2007. Lifetime prevalence of psychotic and bipolar I disorders in a general population. Arch. Gen. Psychiatry 64 (1), 19–28.

Remington, G., Kapur, S., 1999. D2 and 5-HT2 receptor effects of antipsychotics: bridging basic and clinical findings using PET. J. Clin. Psychiatry 60 (Suppl. 10), 15–19.

Rice, D.P., 1999. The economic impact of schizophrenia. J. Clin. Psychiatry 60 (Suppl. 1), 4–6, discussion 28–30.

Robinson, D., Woerner, M.G., et al., 1999. Predictors of relapse following response from a first episode of schizophrenia or schizoaffective disorder. Arch. Gen. Psychiatry 56 (3), 241–247.

Rosenheck, R.A., Krystal, J.H., et al., 2011. Long-acting risperidone and oral antipsychotics in unstable schizophrenia. N. Engl. J. Med. 364 (9), 842–851.

Rutherford, B.R., Pott, E., et al., 2014. Placebo response in antipsychotic clinical trials: a meta-analysis. JAMA Psychiatry 71 (12), 1409–1421.

Scherk, H., Pajonk, F.G., et al., 2007. Second-generation antipsychotic agents in the treatment of acute mania: a systematic review and meta-analysis of randomized controlled trials. Arch. Gen. Psychiatry 64 (4), 442–455.

Shepherd, M., Watt, D., et al., 1989. The natural history of schizophrenia: a five-year follow-up study of outcome and prediction in a representative sample of schizophrenics. Psychol. Med. Monogr. Suppl. 15, 1–46.

Taylor, D.M., Cornelius, V., et al., 2014. Comparative efficacy and acceptability of drug treatments for bipolar depression: a multiple-treatments meta-analysis. Acta Psychiatr. Scand. 130 (6), 452–469.

van Os, J., Kapur, S., 2009. Schizophrenia. Lancet 374 (9690), 635–645.

Vazquez, G.H., Holtzman, J.N., et al., 2015. Efficacy and tolerability of treatments for bipolar depression. J. Affect. Disord. 183, 258–262.

Vigod, S.N., Gomes, T., et al., 2015. Antipsychotic drug use in pregnancy: high dimensional, propensity matched, population based cohort study. BMJ 350, h2298.

Voruganti, L., Cortese, L., et al., 2000. Comparative evaluation of conventional and novel antipsychotic drugs with reference to their subjective tolerability, side-effect profile and impact on quality of life. Schizophr. Res. 43 (2–3), 135–145.

Zhang, J.P., Gallego, J.A., et al., 2013. Efficacy and safety of individual second-generation vs. first-generation antipsychotics in first-episode psychosis: a systematic review and meta-analysis. Int. J. Neuropsychopharmacol. 16 (6), 1205–1218.

Chapter 15

Antipsychotic-Related Mortality: Risk and Strategy for Improved Clinical Management

Dan Cohen

Mental Health Services North-Holland North, Heerhugowaard, The Netherlands; University of Groningen, Groningen, The Netherlands

15.1 REDUCED LIFE-EXPECTANCY WITH SEVERE MENTAL ILLNESS (SMI)

The reduced life expectancy in schizophrenia and, in general in severe mental disorders, constitutes exactly the opposite of what doctors aim at, namely recuperation of the patient by curing the illness, restoring the status quo before the outbreak of the illness, prolongation of life expectancy, and ideally normalization of the life expectancy to that of the general population.

The reduced life expectancy does not result from underdevelopment of the country involved: it is found in countries with highly sophisticated and developed health care systems such as Denmark (Wahlbeck et al., 2011; Laursen et al., 2013), Finland (Tiihonen et al., 2009), Israel (Kodesh et al., 2012), the United States (Colton and Manderscheid, 2006), and Sweden (Ösby et al., 2000). The size of the reduced life expectancy, expressed in years of potential life lost (YPLL), is not trivial: the mean reduction is between 15 and 20 years, with outliers above and below the range. The lower reductions of life expectancy, found for instance in Israel at 12 years (Kodesh et al., 2012) or in Denmark at 11−20 years (Wahlbeck et al., 2011) qualify as relatively favorable compared to other countries, despite being not good enough. These are in contrast to outliers at the other extreme, such as Finland with 22.5−25 YPLL or Arizona which tops the list with 32 YPLL (Colton and Manderscheid, 2006).

Increased suicide rates contribute less to this outcome than might be expected. A recent Swedish study of mortality in bipolar illness found an

8-fold increase in men and a 10-fold increase in women (Crump et al., 2013b). Since the prevalence of suicide in the nonpsychiatric population is low, the absolute contribution of suicide to mortality in bipolar disorder is small, and the proportion dying of suicide is: 5.4% (34/626) for females and 9.6% (43/ 450) for males. On the other hand, compared to the suicide mortality rate, the increase in cardiovascular mortality in severe mental illness (SMI) is relatively modest. In one cohort study conducted in the United Kingdom, the hazard ratio (HR) for coronary heart disease mortality in SMI was 3.22 (95% confidence interval (CI) 1.99−5.21) for those aged 18−49 years, 1.86 (95% CI 1.63−2.12) for those aged 50−75 years, and 1.05 (95% CI 0.92−1.19), with adjustment for age, sex, and calendar period, but not for smoking status and social deprivation (Osborn et al., 2007). The risk of death from stroke was similarly increased with SMI. Since cardiovascular disease is the cause of around 35% of deaths in developed countries, this indicates an excessive absolute burden of death from cardiovascular disease.

Since the seminal publication of Brown et al. (1999), lifestyle issues have dominated the discussion, and for good reason. Increased smoking rates, varying between 50% (Mitchell et al., 2013) and 72% (Brown et al., 2010), and increased prevalence of the metabolic syndrome—dependent on the definition—varying between 28.6% and 35.3%, have been well documented (Mitchell et al., 2013).

15.1.1   Cardiovascular Disease Mortality

The absolute mortality from cardiovascular disease and the increase in mortality relative to the general population are compelling reasons to explore causes. To illustrate this point: in a multinational meta-analysis, Saha et al. (2007) found a twofold standardized mortality ratio (SMR) from cardiovascular disease among people with schizophrenia. A Swedish study (Ösby, 2008) detailed the SMRs for cardiovascular deaths in schizophrenia; all SMRs were around two (Table 15.1).

These figures become more disturbing when absolute numbers are considered: for the Ösby (2008) study they represent a total *excess* deaths of 12,083, of which 3410 were from cardiovascular causes. Further, Ösby noted

TABLE 15.1 Standardized Mortality Ratios in Schizophrenia (Ösby, 2008)

	Cardiovascular Disease	Coronary Heart Disease	Myocardial Infarction	All Causes of Death
Men	2.08	1.91	1.75	2.33
Women	2.15	2.06	1.86	2.35

that the SMR for all causes of death for patients with schizophrenia had increased significantly over the study period, 1970–2003 ($p < 0.0001$), as the benefits from medical advances in the prevention and treatment of cardiovascular disease had not been experienced by this population.

15.1.2 Sudden Cardiac Death

Increased risk of SCD in schizophrenia has been found in patients treated with FGAs and with SGAs (see Chapter 1, Sudden Cardiac Death and Ventricular Arrhythmias). The rates of SCD were associated with antipsychotic drug use in a dose-dependent way, with incidence rate ratios indicating a possibly greater risk for SGAs than for FGAs: compared to nonusers the incidence rate ratio of SCD was 1.31 (low dose), 2.01 (moderate dose), and 2.41 (high dose) in users of FGAs and 1.59 (low dose), 2.13 (moderate dose), and 2.86 (high dose) in users of SGAs (Ray et al., 2009). The increased risk is ascribed to blockade of potassium channels and prolongation of cardiac repolarization. Nevertheless, not only high, but also low, doses of antipsychotics are associated with a significantly increased risk of SCD, and this risk is found in persons who use antipsychotics for indications other than schizophrenia. (Straus et al., 2004).

15.1.3 QTc-Prolongation

For over two decades, repolarization disorder, especially prolongation of the QT-interval, has been at the forefront of cardiac safety of antipsychotic drugs. The issue of prolongation of the QT-interval is not only of theoretical importance: witness the worldwide withdrawal of the first-generation antipsychotic (FGA), thioridazine, in 2005 (Lothian, 2014) and of the second-generation antipsychotic (SGA), sertindole, in 1998 (NHS). While prolongation of the QT-interval in itself is not dangerous, the possibly resulting *torsade de pointes* (TdP) are. A recent comprehensive review of the relation between QTc-prolongation and TdP with SGA (Husnain and Vieweg, 2014) draws conclusions based on both studies and individual cases. The studies allow for two conclusions. First, it is not possible to categorize any of the nine antipsychotics studied for their risk of causing TdP. Second, all nine antipsychotics have the potential to cause QTc-prolongation. In toxicology studies TdP was more likely to occur in overdosage with amisulpride, than with clozapine, risperidone, quetiapine, and ziprasidone. From case reports, TdP is a rare adverse effect that has been reported to occur with therapeutic dosages, with modest dosage increase and with a QTc interval below 500 ms. The conclusion is that, in users of antipsychotics, individual vulnerability and the presence or absence of other risk factors determine the development of QTc-prolongation and TdP. A second conclusion is that the relation between the QT-prolongation, TdP, and sudden cardiac death (SCD) is unclear as has been previously suggested (Koponen et al., 2008). Not only has the exact role of QTc-prolongation in the development of TdP not been established, but neither has its role in ventricular arrhythmias, and SCD, nor are the roles of dose and the presence or absence of a psychiatric disease known.

15.1.3.1   Screening for QTc-Prolongation

It would be beneficial if screening by ECG for risk of QTc-prolongation were viable. A recent retrospective study in 97 hospitalized nonpsychiatric patients (mean age 67 years) who were treated with low-dose haloperidol (mean 2.6 mg; standard deviation 2.2 mg), yielded two surprising results (Blom et al., 2011). First, 94% of the patients with potentially dangerous QTc-prolongation during haloperidol had normal pretreatment QTc-duration. Second, most patients with borderline or abnormal pretreatment QTc-duration developed a shortening of the QTc-duration during haloperidol treatment. Both results were unexpected and, although they are the results of only one study in less than 100 patients without psychiatric illness, they nevertheless throw doubt on the predictive value of ECG-screening. Furthermore, a recent study found that results varied from none to clinically significant prolongation of the QTc-interval depending on the correction method used and whether correction was made for heart rate (Noordam et al., 2015). These studies indicate that a thorough re-evaluation of the significance of the QTc interval, how it is measured and its contribution to cardiovascular mortality with or without psychotropic use is required.

15.1.4   Brugada Syndrome

The Brugada syndrome (BS) is an inherited syndrome associated with an increased risk of SCD attributable to ECG abnormalities (Brugada and Brugada, 1992). BS is uncommon in the general population: its worldwide prevalence is estimated at 0.02−0.05% or 1 in 2000−5000 persons (Postema, 2012). Its key pathophysiologic mechanism is disrupted cardiac depolarization. A mutation in SCN5A, the gene encoding the α-subunit of the sodium channel that drives depolarization, was found in approximately 20% of BS patients (Chen, 1998; Kapplinger et al., 2010). Analysis of ECG data in 275 outpatients with schizophrenia or schizoaffective disorder found a prevalence of 11.6% of BS compared with 1.1% among individuals without schizophrenia (Blom et al., 2014). While patients with schizophrenia who have BS may be susceptible to the arrhythmia-causing effects of antipsychotic medication (blockade of depolarization) (Postema et al., 2009), two things need to be noticed. First, 50% of the patients with a Brugada-ECG did not use sodium channel blocking medication. Second, it is unlikely that the use of sodium channel blocking medication alone results in a Brugada-ECG when an innate factor is absent (Yap et al., 2009). Therefore, this study points to a vulnerability that is present in patients with schizophrenia (Blom et al., 2014).

15.2 SUICIDE REDUCED WITH CLOZAPINE

At the other end of the spectrum of antipsychotic-related deaths are the life-saving effects of antipsychotic drugs. This point is, in particular, relevant for the reduction of the suicide rate by clozapine, a topic that, according to some (Sinyor and Remington, 2012), has "unjustifiably been ignored." The pertinent questions in this context are: what is the scale of the problem, what is the contribution by clozapine, and what are the obstacles for the use of clozapine?

The cumulative risk of suicide after 10 years is 2.05−4.1% and 3.23−6.55% after 20 years (Table 15.2). What exactly do these risks and percentages mean, to the psychiatrist, to the patients, and the family and friends involved? When we consider the suicide rate for 1 year of 0.31%, reported by Dutta et al. (2010), we find that the SMR (total number of cases observed divided by the total expected numbers) is 11.1. In plain language: in the first year after the first psychotic episode the suicide rate is 11.1 times higher than in the nonpsychotic general population. The 10-year cumulative rate of suicide was found to vary, 2.05−4.1% (SMR for lowest cumulative risk, 3.92). Translated to number of patients affected, this rate indicates that after 10 years every 25th−50th patient with the diagnosis of schizophrenia has committed suicide.

The next question is what does clozapine contribute to the suicide rate in schizophrenia? In their milestone study in 67,072 current and former clozapine users, Walker et al. (1997) found a statistically significant and clinically relevant lowered suicide mortality rate (risk ratio (RR) = 0.17; 95% CI: 0.10−0.30) in current compared to past clozapine users. In a population-based Swedish study of 26,000 patients with schizophrenia, and including 2138 patients using clozapine, the fully adjusted (including adjustment for psychiatric and somatic diagnoses and previous suicide attempts) odds ratio (OR) for suicide attempts relative to that for haloperidol was statistically significantly reduced only with clozapine (OR 0.52; 95% CI: 0.32−0.84)

TABLE 15.2 Cumulative Suicide Risk in Schizophrenia or Related Disorders

	N	Length of Follow-Up (years)	Cumulative Risk of Suicide After		
			1 Year	10 Years	20 Years
Palmer et al. (2005)	22,598	20 (max)	n.r.	n.r.	5.6%
Dutta et al. (2010)	2723	11.5 (mean)	0.31%	2.05%	3.23%
Nordentoft et al. (2011)	22,011	36 (max)	n.r.	n.r.	6.55%
Limousin et al. (2007)	3434	10 (max)	n.r.	4.1%	n.r.

n.r., not reported.

(Ringbäck Weitoft et al., 2014). The fully adjusted ORs for death by suicide showed significant protection with zuclopenthixol (OR 0.38; 95% CI: 0.15−0.98) and aripiprazole (OR 0.21; 95% CI: 0.05−0.94), but not for clozapine (OR 0.51; 95% CI: 0.23−1.13). The wide CI for clozapine indicates that only a small number of patients taking clozapine died by suicide. Etiological fraction calculation determined that 95 suicide attempts would have been prevented during the study period (2006−09) with use of clozapine rather than traditional drugs.

A Finnish study found that clozapine was associated with the lowest risk of death from any cause and from suicide of any antipsychotic (adjusted HR relative to perphenazine 0.74; 95% CI: 0.60−0.91 and 0.34; 95% CI: 0.20−0.57, respectively) and despite metabolic syndrome affecting many patients taking clozapine, the risk of death from ischemic heart disease was not raised (0.78; 95% CI: 0.54−1.12) (Tiihonen et al., 2009).

This brings us to the comparison of all-cause mortality in clozapine treatment versus nonclozapine treatment. In a Swedish cohort study of all-cause mortality in 8277 patients with schizophrenia followed for 7 years, relative to the perphenazine reference group, the HRs for patients on clozapine monotherapy ($N = 1420$) were elevated, but narrowly failed to reach statistically significance: 1.29 (95% CI: 0.99−1.68) (Crump et al., 2013a). Other studies have considered all-cause mortality as well. In a large ($N = 14,754$; 748 on clozapine) London study of people with serious mental illness, mortality over 5 years in the clozapine group was significantly lower, for both natural causes (HR 0.5; 95% CI: 0.2−0.9) and unnatural causes (HR 0.2; 95% CI: 0.05−0.9) (Hayes et al., 2014). A US study, that compared mortality within 1 year of initiating clozapine treatment ($N = 3123$) or standard oral antipsychotic medication in a same sized propensity score-matched cohort, found no significant increase (HR 1.38; 95% CI: 0.55−3.45) (Stroup et al., 2016).

With a 10-year cumulative rate of death from suicide of 2.05−4.1%, suicide constitutes a major mortality threat in schizophrenia. Treatment with clozapine is associated with lowered suicides rates in most, but not in all, studies. Clozapine treatment was not associated with increased all-cause mortality, and Tiihonen et al. (2009) found no increase in mortality specifically in relation to cardiovascular disease. Thus there are no grounds for the fear that clozapine may prevent death from suicide while increasing death from other causes. Therefore, as far as the contribution of antipsychotic drugs to the risk of suicide is concerned, clozapine has the most favorable data and on this ground patients should be given a fair chance of a trial with clozapine.

15.3   AN OBSTACLE TO CLOZAPINE PRESCRIBING: AGRANULOCYTOSIS

In a study of psychiatrists' attitude, the risk of agranulocytosis was found to be a major reason that puts psychiatrists off from clozapine (Nielsen et al., 2010), so a look at the factual basis, that is, the actual risks involved, does not seem superfluous. First the incidence rates: all studies on the incidence of agranulocytosis have figures below the 1% level, somewhere in the range 0.21−0.8% of the study population. As far as mortality is concerned, the strict monitoring practiced in the Western world seems to bear fruit: the mortality of cases of is 2.2−4.2%—the 10 times higher mortality rate in China is probably due to lacuna monitoring practices or ineffective treatment (see Table 15.3)—which means that 95.8% or more of the cases survive. Looked at from the perspective of the whole treated population, mortality due to agranulocytosis is 0.1−0.3%. Whichever interpretation of the data one may give, the bottom line is that mortality from agranulocytosis in clozapine-treated populations worldwide is remarkably consistent, and very low, namely 0.3‰ or below, which corresponds with between 1 and 3 in every 10,000 clozapine-treated patients.

Weighing the risk of agranulocytosis against the benefit of reduced suicide rates, one is confronted with a sharp and worrisome contrast: with a cumulative 10-year suicide risk varying between 2% and 4%, suicide will affect a mean 3 persons out of every 100. Mortality due to agranulocytosis, which is mainly restricted to the first year of treatment, amounts to 1−3 deaths per 10,000 patients. So the choice is to avoid the 1−3 deaths per 10,000 patients at a cost of 200−400 deaths due to suicide. Further, we have already established that mortality from other causes is not significantly increased.

The conclusion seems unavoidable that not only is the doctors' fear of prescribing clozapine irrational (Cohen, 2014; Meltzer, 2005), but it is also

TABLE 15.3 Agranulocytosis: Cumulative Incidence (per 1000 Patients) and Mortality (per 100 Patients)

	Population (N)	Agranulocytosis		Mortality Rate		
		Cases (n)	Incidence (‰)	Number	Study Population (‰)	Affected Cases (%)
Alvir et al. (1993)	11,555	73	8.0	2	0.2	2.7
Atkin et al. (1996)	6316	43	8.0	2	0.3	4.2
Munro et al. (1999)	12,760	93	7.3	2	0.2	2.2
Honigfeld et al. (1998)	99,502	382	3.8	12	0.1	3.1
Tang et al. (2008)	43,302	92	2.1	21[a]	0.04	33.9

[a]Outcome was unreported in 30 patients; mortality rate was calculated based on the reported 92 cases.

negligent and in a way cruel. Withholding a potentially beneficial treatment from the most severely affected mentally ill patients means refusing to relieve patients' suffering when this could be achieved. Plus this policy costs the loss of hundreds of lives that could have been saved.

15.4 DIABETIC KETOACIDOSIS: POOR OUTCOMES WITH SEVERE MENTAL ILLNESS (SMI)

Diabetic ketoacidosis (DKA) is characterized by the triad of hyperglycemia, anion gap, metabolic acidosis, and ketosis. Metabolic acidosis is often the major finding. The serum glucose concentration is usually higher than 500 mg dL^{-1} (28 mmol L^{-1}) but lower than 800 mg dL^{-1} (44 mmol L^{-1}). However, serum glucose concentrations may exceed 900 mg dL^{-1} (50 mmol L^{-1}) in patients with DKA who are comatose (Kitabchi et al., 2006). Untreated or late detection can result in the death of the patient.

DKA, in itself a rare phenomenon, has for the past two decades been on a slow but steady increase: its incidence in the United States rose from 3.2/10,000 in 1988 to 4.6/10,000 in 2009 (Table 15.4) (Centers for Disease Control and Prevention, 2012a). However, the incidence in other populations may be lower, for example, a Danish study of 1999 data, found an incidence of 1.29 per 10,000, with a small sex difference (male 1.44, female 1.14) (Henriksen et al., 2007).

Published cases of DKA associated with FGA are rare. A fatal case of neuroleptic malignant syndrome and DKA with chlorpromazine and a single dose of intramuscular zuclopenthixol 3 days before death has been described (de Boer and Gate, 1992). A second case, reported more than 10 years later, was a patient with acute pancreatitis with valproate, who developed DKA after addition of chlorpromazine and haloperidol. In this case, DKA was not fatal: both pancreatitis and DKA subsided completely after 6 weeks (Laghate and Gupta, 2004).

TABLE 15.4 Incidence/10,000 Person-Years of Diabetic Ketoacidosis

General Population		Schizophrenia	
Denmark[a] (Henriksen et al., 2007)	USA (Nationwide)[b] (Centers for Disease Control and Prevention, 2012a)	USA (Leslie and Rosenheck, 2004)	USA (Henderson et al., 2007)
1.29	4.6	15.5	15

[a]1999.
[b]2009.

From 1996 onward cases of treatment-emergent DKA in patients with schizophrenia treated with the atypical antipsychotics, clozapine, olanzapine, risperidone, and quetiapine, have been reported (Cohen, 2004). In clozapine treatment, analysis of 26 cases showed that DKA developed quickly: 61% within the first 3 months of treatment. African descent was found to be a risk factor (Nihalani et al., 2007). A comparable short time to onset and racial risk were also found in nonclozapine associated DKA (Cohen, 2004).

The main questions in this context are: Is treatment-emergent DKA restricted to SGA or does it also occur with FGA? Is there a difference in DKA rate between individual antipsychotics and do the incidence and mortality rates of DKA in antipsychotic treated patients with schizophrenia differ from the rates found in the general population?

In the period 1993−2000 a total number of 20 cases of DKA were reported to the US Food and Drug Administration (Baker et al., 2009). Analysis of the FDA case reports for antipsychotic drugs 1993−2006 showed that DKA was reported for all seven analyzed antipsychotics (aripiprazole, clozapine, haloperidol, olanzapine, quetiapine, risperidone, and ziprasidone) with an increased tendency for DKA in five out of the seven antipsychotics: clozapine, haloperidol, olanzapine, quetiapine, and risperidone (Baker et al., 2009). So clearly DKA occurs with both FGA and SGA but rates with SGA use are disproportionately higher and therefore warrant particular attention in clinical practice. Two US population-wide studies have calculated the incidence of DKA in schizophrenia. A 12-month study (Sep. 2000−Sep. 2001) in a Veteran Administration (VA) population of 56,849 patients with schizophrenia, found that 88 patients were hospitalized for DKA, which corresponds to a hospitalization rate for DKA of 15.5/10,000 person-years (Leslie and Rosenheck, 2004). A second US study compared the hospitalization rate for DKA of the general population with that of patients with schizophrenia or schizoaffective disorders during a 7-year period, 1995−2001. In 0.138% of the patients (1132 out of a total of 819,308 persons) of the general population, DKA was the discharge diagnosis. With schizophrenia or schizoaffective disorder, the DKA-discharge rate increased more than threefold: 0.47% (23/4850), which corresponds with a DKA incidence rate per 10,000 person-years of 15 (Henderson et al., 2007).

In a comprehensive review of case reports of DKA in atypical antipsychotic treatment, 69 cases were identified with a mean age of 37.5, and mortality was 7.5% (Guenette et al., 2013). In four consecutive reviews, Koller analyzed the incidence of hyperglycemia and mortality from DKA for each individual atypical antipsychotic using data from the medical drug surveillance system of the Food and Drug Administration. The case fatality from DKA was 31% (25/80) with clozapine (Koller et al., 2001), 11% (9/80) with olanzapine (Koller and Doraiswamy, 2002), 33% (7/21) with quetiapine (Koller et al., 2004), and 15% (4/26) with risperidone (Koller et al., 2003) (Table 15.5).

TABLE 15.5 Case Fatality With Diabetic Ketoacidosis

	Mean Age (years)	Whole Population	30–50 Years	>70 Years	
Denmark	n.a.	4%	2%	15%	Henriksen et al., 2007
USA (nationwide)	n.a.	7.5%	NA	NA	CDC., 2012b
Case reports	38	n.a.	7%	n.a.	Guenette et al., 2013
Clozapine	39	n.a.	31%	n.a.	Koller et al., 2001
Olanzapine	40	n.a.	11%	n.a.	Koller and Doraiswamy, 2002
Quetiapine	35	n.a.	33%	n.a.	Koller et al., 2004
Risperidone	40	n.a.	15%	n.a.	Koller et al., 2003

CDC, Centers for Disease Control and Prevention; n.a., not applicable; NA, not available.

In contrast, the case fatality from DKA in the general Danish population was 4%, showing a strong effect of age: in patients >70 years, case fatality was 15%, seven times higher than the 2% in patients 30–50 years (Henriksen et al., 2007). Consideration of the mortality rates in DKA shows three findings. First, the mortality rates in schizophrenia are increased compared with the same-aged patients in the general population. Second, even the lowest mortality rate in schizophrenia (7.5%) (Guenette et al., 2013) is higher than the mortality of 4% for the whole study group in the general population. Third, the four studies by Koller et al. that resemble a population-wide study, such as the Danish Henriksen et al. (2007) study, all have case fatalities of 11% or above, that is, rates that are similar to or greater than the case fatality of persons more than 70 years of age in the general population. In other words, DKA has mortality rates in schizophrenia patients aged below 40 years comparable with that of patients aged more than 70 years in the general population.

Several factors may contribute to these differences. First, there may be differences in awareness in care providers. In patients with diagnosed diabetes it is only logical for the care provider to be aware of possible complications of the diabetes. On the other hand, as DKA occurrence is concentrated in the initial phase of antipsychotic treatment, both patients and care providers are caught unaware, which might delay the diagnostic process. A further complicating factor might be somatic undertreatment in schizophrenia that has been documented for other somatic illnesses (Lambert et al., 2003).

15.5 STRATEGY FOR IMPROVED OUTCOMES

15.5.1 Poor Care of Somatic Illness in Severe Mental Illness (SMI)

Care for patients with the diagnosis of schizophrenia has drastically been transformed in the past decades. Here, but a few developments from among many are named. Early detection and the prevention of transition from ultra-high risk to psychosis has seen a rapid advancement in the past two decades, with contributions from both drug treatment (Wunderink et al., 2013) and cognitive therapy (Morrison et al., 2014). Psychiatric care has shifted from inpatient care, centered around psychiatric wards, to community based outpatient care with the focus on rehabilitation. However impressive the improvements and the progress, the level of medical nonpsychiatric care seems largely unaffected by these developments. In so far as the gap in life expectancy between schizophrenia patients and the general population has changed, it has worsened (Saha et al., 2007). The results of a Finnish cohort study in 12,939 patients with schizophrenia exemplifies this state of affairs. The authors found an increased coronary heart disease morbidity and mortality and at the same time a lowered prescription rate of cardioprotective drug treatment, such as antihypertensive and lipid-lowering drugs (Lahti et al., 2012). Similar findings have been reported in relation to coronary revascularization procedures (Laursen et al., 2013; Lawrence et al., 2003).

What is needed, is a multipronged approach. First and foremost a change of attitude in the medical profession, especially in psychiatrists, is needed. Patients with schizophrenia need to be considered to suffer from a complex disease that can have deleterious effects on many, if not all, aspects of functioning in life. Looked at from a somatic point of view, schizophrenia is a potentially life-threatening disease, both in itself and as a result of treatment-related side-effects. Somatic diagnosis and treatment in patients with schizophrenia is complicated by several factors. One such factor is the disability in organization and planning, that is associated with schizophrenia. A second is different levels of self-neglect that may negatively affect the presentation of relevant complaints in the doctor's office.

The second point, relates to the locus of responsibility for adequate diagnosis and treatment of somatic pathologies. Of course, the family doctor has the knowledge and responsibility for somatic care, but there is a major but. Not only might patients with schizophrenia not turn up for years at the family doctor's office (Cradock-O'Leary et al., 2002), but also the basic approach of the family doctor is that they diagnose and treat patients who seek help. But psychiatric patients might not seek help.

An example may illustrate the intricacies involved: an intelligent 50-year-old patient showed up at my office for his penfluridol (an oral antipsychotic drug taken once a week). As he had also been diagnosed with type 2 diabetes mellitus, I checked—out of personal curiosity (Cohen, 2006)—his latest laboratory results. It turned out that he had not visited the laboratory for a whole year, neither had he visited the family doctor's diabetes nurse. When asked for an explanation, he confirmed the state of affairs and explained that his legs hurt too much to walk the 15 minutes distance from his home to the laboratory and that, in consequence, visits to the diabetes nurse did not make sense as no new laboratory results would be available. Without these it would be impossible to evaluate the past 3 months adequately and to adapt responsively the dosing regimens of the antidiabetic drugs. When phoned, the family doctor's office confirmed that he had been invited for the quarterly visit to the diabetes nurse but that he had not shown up, not at the regular appointments nor at the extra appointments. All appointment notifications had been sent to his home.

What can we learn from this example? As background knowledge: diabetes care by a diabetes nurse, specifically appointed for that purpose, in the family doctor's office, is one of the most intensive ways of monitoring a somatic disease in outpatients in the Netherlands. Still this care proved to be insufficient in this patient: as far as diabetes care was concerned he should be considered a drop-out. Despite his intelligence, he had not called upon the diabetes nurse to tell her that his claudication prevented him from visiting the laboratory, nor had he called in help from his brother or sister to transport him to the laboratory. First and foremost this example illustrates the adequacy for the psychiatric patient of the medical model based on the patient taking the initiative to seek help. This behavior is one of the obstacles that is often present in patients with schizophrenia.

Diabetes care in the Netherlands is provided by diabetes nurses who have been trained to autonomously monitor diabetes patients in the GP practice. This model works brilliantly for patients with diabetes from the general population. Nevertheless, this model fell short in this example because it presupposes a patient who is fully responsible for their help-seeking behavior. If a patient does not show up, the patient, not the care provider, is to blame. What is missing is an assertive approach that would easily have detected and remedied the apparent lack of cooperation in this case.

15.5.2 Assertive Care for Mental Illness

In psychiatric care of patients with SMI, Flexible Assertive Community Treatment (FACT), a so-called Dutch variant of assertive community treatment, has been developed (van Veldhuizen, 2007) and successfully implemented. Recently the first results have been reported: against the current of national increase in acute forced admission, an actual decrease was reported in areas where FACT-care had been introduced (Broer et al., 2015). The 9% increase in psychiatric remission rate is a second, clinically relevant, though statistically insignificant, finding (Nugter et al., 2015).

FACT covers many divergent areas, from psychiatric crisis interventions, prescription of psychotropic drugs, detection and treatment of double diagnosis (SMI plus substance dependence or abuse), rehabilitation and participation by peer specialists. Notwithstanding the great advantages and improvements of this model, its focus is mostly—and understandably—on all aspects of psychiatric care in the broadest sense. The implication of the focus being on psychiatry is that the somatic aspects (diagnosis, treatment, and care) and the responsibility thereof are left out of consideration and remain based on the traditional medical model: a patient who needs medical help needs to show help-seeking behavior. As we have seen, this model does not work for the patient with SMI.

In our example, the FACT-model with its deep-rooted assertive attitude would easily have remedied the impasse. In the assertive model, care providers do not restrict their proactive actions to sending notifications of new appointments to patients. When a patient does not show up and/or is not being heard from, the "F" of flexibility translates into an upscaling of care; in combination with the "A" of assertiveness, this will result in a phone call being made and/or a home visit being paid in order to explore the patients' reasons and explanations for not showing up. That would or could not be the end of the affair: the required 3-monthly laboratory tests needed to be performed and measures would be taken to ensure regular blood sampling. In our example, the FACT staff member would discuss with the patient and his family whether he could be taken to the laboratory, by either his family or his psychiatric case manager, or whether the laboratory assistant would pay home visits for the required blood sampling. This case further illustrates that a patient's drive for seeking medical help and solving problems are not directly related to the patient's intelligence.

15.5.3 Difficulties for Medical Practitioners

In short, while for SMI-patients extensive models have been developed to manage the complex psychiatric, cognitive, and psychological issues plus problems of rehabilitation, early detection, and dual diagnosis, the accessory model for medical issues has largely remained unchanged. If this continues, the inevitable result will be a continuation of the appalling gap in life expectancy between people with and without SMI or, the current trend may continue and the gap increase further (Saha et al., 2007). Decreased mortality due to physical causes has been found among patients with schizophrenia with community treatment orders, compared with a similar group of patients without community treatment orders. The community treatment orders imposed compulsory treatment and the reduced mortality was thought to be due to increased outpatient and community contacts with psychiatric services (Kisely et al., 2013). It goes without saying that if the general practitioner's somatic care falls short in patients with SMI, the treatment of medical specialists, with their inpatient orientation, will almost certainly fall short in this patient population. Specialists' consultations reports regularly state "we didn't make a follow-up appointment."

A point of interest is that the incidence rates of the adverse effects discussed earlier—independent of whether they are disease-related, drug-related or both—occur at a rate of a few per 1000, or 10,000, rather than per hundred, as can be seen in Tables 15.3 and 15.4. The same applies to adverse effects that have not been discussed, such as fatal pulmonary embolus (see Chapter 3, Pulmonary Embolism). The incidence rates of venous thrombo-embolism (fatal and nonfatal) for clozapine, the drug with the highest rates, have been reported to vary between 1 per 2000−6000 (Hägg et al., 2000) and 2.9−3.6 per 10,000 patients, corresponding to 1 per 3000−3500 patients (Jönsson et al., 2012).

The question to be discussed here is: what are the implications of these adverse effects for clinical practice? These are at least twofold: first, it has to be realized that treating—that is, to say drug-prescribing—psychiatrists need to be aware of and have detailed knowledge of a wide array of life-threatening adverse effects, which cover many different major branches of internal medicine, such as cardiology (sudden (cardiac) death), vascular diseases (pulmonary embolism), hematology (agranulocytosis), endocrinology (diabetes mellitus), and digestive diseases (ileus). Second, and partly in contrast, the incidence rates being what they are, the chances that treating psychiatrists will encounter one of these adverse effects in their own practice, even during a life-long career, are very small. This brings us to the following step, that is, if this situation applies for the psychiatrists, whose profession it is to treat patients with SMI and to prescribe them antipsychotic drugs, what can we expect from a family doctor since SMI occurs in 5% or less of the general patient population? In short, where specialists' expertise is required, only general practitioners' knowledge at best is provided. So here is one aspect of the dilemma. Further, monitoring for somatic disease is beyond the requirements and skills of a psychiatrist, justifying referral to the family doctor, where however the approach needed for this vulnerable population is missing. In addition, there are no clinically useful predictors for the development of serious adverse effects. The only and best thing to remedy for this lack is to monitor in an indiscriminate, population-based way.

Psychiatrists' attitude to somatic aspects of medicine is also an issue. The case of clozapine (Nielsen et al., 2010) testifies to psychiatrists' ignorance of the risk and symptoms of the serious, potentially lethal somatic complications of their treatment. Moreover, these psychiatrists were reluctant to prescribe clozapine, because of concern about its adverse effects, even in cases where the patient had failed to respond to two previous trials of anti-psychotics, and were more likely to resort to "nonevidence based treatments." If psychiatrists' actions are so controlled by fear of somatic adverse effects as to deny the best treatment available to those whose illness is the most severe and debilitating—those who according to national and international guidelines should be prescribed this treatment—then psychiatrists cannot be expected to take any responsibility for somatic disease in patients with less serious psychiatric illness.

15.5.4 Assertive Care for Somatic Illness

What is needed is an extension of the position statement and intention statement on cardiovascular disease (De Hert et al., 2009), both in scope as well as in commitment. The aim and scope is simple, namely a reduction of mortality in schizophrenia to the level of the general population. Phrased otherwise, its aim is normalization of the life expectancy of the SMI population. The means by which this aim can be attained is a more difficult subject, but it will first and foremost require a health service which takes full responsibility for adequate somatic care of psychiatric patients. Obstacles from different sources will need to be addressed, be it the patients' inappropriately infrequent general practitioners' visits (van Hasselt et al., 2013) or health care professionals' attitude. All these result in the same outcome, namely that "assessment and treatment of common physical health problems in people with schizophrenia falls well below acceptable standards" (Crawford et al., 2014). Cooperation and communication between primary and secondary care services needs to improve if premature mortality is to be reduced, and technological obstacles that stand in the way of coordinated somatic care, such as a lack of current data on the patient's health status and treatment, need to be removed. A shared IT system is essential (Johansson, 2015).

Several options have been implemented and tested (Kisely and Lawrence, 2010). Although not unequivocally evidence-based, several strings of evidence argue in favor of incorporating assertive somatic treatment within the assertive community treatment (ACT approaches). As stated already, the first obstacle to remove is the reactive approach of GPs, responding to and treating only patients who present to them with physical complaints.

An example may clarify what is at issue. A 59-year-old Caucasian male patient with a schizoaffective disorder, obesity, hypothyroid function, and normocytic anemia, moved from the capital Amsterdam to a more rural community. He found a new GP who prescribed both psychiatric medications, specifically in this case lithium and clozapine, and treatment for somatic conditions. The once per year monitoring of leukocytes and clozapine and lithium plasma levels yielded normal results. Three years later, this patient was referred to FACT-care, where he was found to be mentally stable but with deterioration in his somatic condition. His BMI had changed only slightly (from 32.7 to 33.2), but his treatment for diabetes, high dose metformin, had been discontinued. His diabetes markers were seriously raised: fasting plasma glucose level 16.5−18.7 mmol L^{-1} (N: 3.3−6.1 mmol L^{-1}); HbA1c 91−93 mmol L^{-1} (N: 20−42 mmol L^{-1}). His cholesterol results were normal, except for a hypertriglyceridemia of 5.9 mmol L^{-1} (N: 0.6−2.2 mmol L^{-1}). His hemoglobin measured 7.6−8.0 mmol L^{-1} (N: 8.5−11 mmol L^{-1}), which was consistent with the descriptive diagnosis of normocytic anemia. In short, within the framework of the reactive approach of the GP, this patient received not only minimal psychiatric care and monitoring but also severely deficient, or completely lacking, care of his physical disease. The lack of felt need by the patient to seek help (Cradock-O'Leary et al., 2002), the superficially good presentation, and his stoic attitude contributed and all led to the same result. This example graphically illustrates how medical underconsumption functions in daily practice in the most severely affected psychiatric patient population and how it can lead in the long run to the shortening of life-expectancy (Colton and Manderscheid, 2006).

The second reason is practical: GP's work within a certain but rather strict time frame, that leaves little room for SMI patients who have several impediments in their help-seeking behavior, such as disorganization, which might result in their showing up much too late or not at all, aberrant day-night rhythm, which prevents them from attending during the regular GP office hours. A third reason is that the psychiatric pathology often results in a fragmentary and/or lacuna presentation of the complaints, which sometimes omits the main symptoms. A fourth reason is both practical and economic: GPs are not motivated to be trained to care adequately for the physical needs of psychiatric patients. Thus, time and money are better invested in training a restricted number of motivated psychiatric nurses to become well-educated in certain aspects of somatic diagnosis and treatment than a 100-fold of not intrinsically motivated GPs.

Last but not least, most psychiatrists do not have, nor do they have ready access to, specialized expertise on the widely divergent, possibly life-threatening effects of antipsychotics; hence the need for this volume. If psychiatrists are not well-informed in this regard, GPs are far less so, and with good reason: only a small proportion of their patients have SMI and/or are treated with antipsychotic medication.

The implication of this vision is indeed that major components of primary health care for the SMI populations will have to be transferred from the GP to the ACT-teams, more specifically to psychiatric nurse practitioners working in the (F-)ACT-teams. It goes without saying that those nurses will need to be well-trained and well-versed in the diagnosis and treatment of common health care problems in the SMI population (Cohen, 2015). I believe that only a concerted effort by a multidisciplinary team with both up-to-date knowledge on adverse effects of antipsychotic medication and an assertive attitude to both psychiatric health (with all its bifurcations) and, with equal emphasis, to somatic health. I consider that the first and foremost task of providers of health care to psychiatric patients is to normalize their life expectancy. The best way to do this is to keep them healthy within the framework of assertive somatic care, as part of the service provided by teams delivering assertive psychiatric care.

15.5.5 Conclusion: Increase Clozapine Prescribing

As has been argued earlier, clozapine prescription probably lowers suicide rates without at the same time negatively affecting the overall or cardiovascular mortality rate. As prescription of clozapine is and has for many years been low in many countries, a concerted effort is needed to increase clozapine prescription. Currently two different approaches, one passive and the other active, have been described and documented. In a naturalistic New Zealand study over a 4.5-year period, the overall rate of clozapine prescription saw a 50% rise, from 21% to 33% (Wheeler et al., 2013). The second model is the approach adopted by the Dutch Clozapine Collaboration Group (Cohen, 2014), a national clozapine expertise center. It offers an information service, free of charge, to mental health professionals on all questions that are somehow related to clozapine and is also engaged in educating mental health professionals by lecturing programs at work and scientific meetings, by providing educational materials, such as patient information, algorithms for frequently encountered or potentially dangerous situations and by providing a national guideline on clozapine treatment. The 10 years of its existence saw a 56% increase in clozapine prescription compared to a 19% increase in the prescription of other antipsychotics during the same period (Bogers et al., 2016).

REFERENCES

Alvir, J.M., Lieberman, J.A., Safferman, A.Z., Schwimmer, J.L., Schaaf, J.A., 1993. Clozapine-induced agranulocytosis. Incidence and risk factors in the United States. N. Engl. J. Med. 329, 162–167.

Atkin, K., Kendall, F., Gould, D., Freeman, H., Liberman, J., O'Sullivan, D., 1996. Neutropenia and agranulocytosis in patients receiving clozapine in the UK and Ireland. Br. J. Psychiatry 169, 483–488.

Baker, R.A., Pikalov, A., Tran, Q.-V., Kremenets, T., Arani, R.B., Doraiswamy, P.M., 2009. Atypical antipsychotic drugs and diabetes mellitus in the US Food and Drug Administration adverse event database: a systematic Bayesian signal detection analysis. Psychopharmacol. Bull. 42, 11–31.

Blom, M.T., Bardai, A., van Munster, B.C., Nieuwland, M.I., de Jong, H., van Hoeijen, D.A., et al., 2011. Differential changes in QTc duration during in-hospital haloperidol use. PLoS One 6, e23728.

Blom, M.T., Cohen, D., Seldenrijk, A., Penninx, B.W., Nijpels, G., Stehouwer, C.D., et al., 2014. Brugada syndrome ECG is highly prevalent in schizophrenia. Circ. Arrhythm. Electrophysiol. 7, 384–391.

Bogers, J.P.A.M., Cohen, D., Dijk, D., van Bakker, B., Schulte, P.F.J., 2016. Clozapine underutilization in the treatment of schizophrenia: how can clozapine prescription rates be improved? J. Clin. Psychopharmacol. 36 (2), 109−111.

Brugada, P., Brugada, J., 1992. Right bundle branch block, persistent ST segment elevation and sudden cardiac death: a distinct clinical and electrocardiographic syndrome. A multicenter report. J. Am. Coll. Cardiol. 20, 1391−1396.

Broer, J., Koetsier, H., Mulder, C.L., 2015. The number of compulsory admissions continues to rise: implications for the new Dutch law on obligatory mental health care. Tijdschr. Psychiatr. 57, 240−247.

Brown, S., Birtwistle, J., Roe, L., Thompson, C., 1999. The unhealthy lifestyle of people with schizophrenia. Psychol. Med. 29, 697−701.

Brown, S., Kim, M., Mitchell, C., Inskip, H., 2010. Twenty-five year mortality of a community cohort with schizophrenia. Br. J. Psychiatry 196, 116−121.

Centers for Disease Control and Prevention, 2012a. Age-Adjusted Hospital Discharge Rates for Diabetic Ketoacidosis (DKA) as First-Listed Diagnosis per 10,000 Population, United States, 1988−2009. <http://www.cdc.gov/diabetes/statistics/dkafirst/fig7.htm>.

Centers for Disease Control and Prevention, 2012b. Death Rates for Hyperglycemic Crises as Underlying Cause per 1,000,000 General Population, by Age, United States, 1980−2009. < http://www.cdc.gov/diabetes/statistics/mortalitydka/tRateDKADiabPopByCensus.htm >.

Chen, Q., Kirsch, G.E., Zhang, D., Brugada, R., Brugada, J., Brugada, P., et al., 1998. Genetic basis and molecular mechanism for idiopathic ventricular fibrillation. Nature 392, 293−296.

Cohen, D., 2004. Atypical antipsychotics and new onset diabetes mellitus. An overview of the literature. Pharmacopsychiatry 37, 1−11.

Cohen, D., 2006. Diabetes Mellitus in Schizophrenia and Schizoaffective Disorder: An Iatrogenic or Endogenic Problem? (thesis). Utrecht.

Cohen, D., 2014. Prescribers fear as a major side effect of clozapine. Acta Psychiatr. Scand. 130, 154−155.

Cohen, D., 2015. Severe mental illness shortens life expectancy. [Een ernstige psychiatrische aandoening verkort de levensverwachting]. Huisarts Wet. 58, 16−18.

Colton, C.W., Manderscheid, R.W., 2006. Congruencies in increased mortality rates, years of potential life lost, and causes of death among public mental health clients in eight states. Prev. Chronic Dis. 3, A42.

Cradock-O'Leary, J., Young, A.S., Yano, E.M., Wang, M., Lee, M.L., 2002. Use of general medical services by VA patients with psychiatric disorders. Psychiatr. Serv. 53, 874−878.

Crawford, M.J., Jayakumar, S., Lemmey, S.J., Zalewska, K., Patel, M.X., Cooper, S.J., et al., 2014. Assessment and treatment of physical health problems among people with schizophrenia: national cross-sectional study. Br. J. Psychiatry 205, 473−477.

Crump, C., Winkleby, M.A., Sundquist, K., Sundquist, J., 2013a. Comorbidities and mortality in persons with schizophrenia: a Swedish national cohort study. Am. J. Psychiatry 170, 324−333.

Crump, C., Sundquist, K., Winkleby, M.A., Sundquist, J., 2013b. Comorbidities and mortality in bipolar disorder: a Swedish national cohort study. JAMA Psychiatry 70, 931−939.

De Boer, C., Gate, H.P., 1992. Neuroleptic malignant syndrome and diabetic keto-acidosis. Br. J. Psychiatry 161, 856−858.

De Hert, M., Dekker, J.M., Wood, D., Kahl, K.G., Holt, R.I., Möller, H.J., 2009. Cardiovascular disease and diabetes in people with severe mental illness position statement from the European Psychiatric Association (EPA), supported by the European Association for the Study of Diabetes (EASD) and the European Society of Cardiology (ESC). Eur. Psychiatry 24, 412−424.

Dutta, R., Murray, R.M., Hotopf, M., Allardyce, J., Jones, P.B., Boydell, J., 2010. Reassessing the long-term risk of suicide after the first episode of psychosis. Arch. Gen. Psychiatry 67, 1230–1237.

Guenette, M.D., Hahn, M., Cohn, T.A., Teo, C., Remington, G.J., 2013. Atypical antipsychotics and diabetic ketoacidosis: a review. Psychopharmacology 226, 1–12.

Hägg, S., Spigset, O., Söderström, T.G., 2000. Association of venous thromboembolism and clozapine. Lancet 355 (9210), 1155–1156.

Hasnain, M., Vieweg, W.V., 2014. QTc interval prolongation and torsade de pointes associated with second-generation antipsychotics and antidepressants: a comprehensive review. CNS Drugs 28, 887–920.

Hayes, R.D., Downs, J., Chang, C.K., Jackson, R.G., Shetty, H., Broadbent, M., et al., 2014. The effect of clozapine on premature mortality: an assessment of clinical monitoring and other potential confounders. Schizophr. Bull. 41, 644–655.

Henderson, D.C., Cagliero, E., Copeland, P.M., Louie, P.M., Borba, C.P., Fan, X., et al., 2007. Elevated hemoglobin A1c as a possible indicator of diabetes mellitus and diabetic ketoacidosis in schizophrenia patients receiving atypical antipsychotics. J. Clin. Psychiatry 2007 (68), 533–541.

Henriksen, O.M., Røder, M.E., Prahl, J.B., Svendsen, O.L., 2007. Diabetic ketoacidosis in Denmark incidence and mortality estimated from public health registries. Diabetes Res. Clin. Pract. 76, 51–56.

Honigfeld, G., Arellano, F., Sethi, J., Bianchini, A., Schein, J., 1998. Reducing clozapine-related morbidity and mortality: 5 years of experience with the Clozaril National Registry. J. Clin. Psychiatry 59 (Suppl. 3), 3–7.

Johansson, F., 2015. Improving assessment and treatment of physical health problems in people with severe mental illness: the case for a shared IT system. Br. J. Psychiatry 206, 435–436.

Jönsson, A.K., Spigset, O., Hägg, S., 2012. Venous thromboembolism in recipients of antipsychotics. CNS Drugs 26, 649–662.

Kapplinger, J.D., Tester, D.J., Alders, M., Benito, B., Berthet, M., Brugada, J., et al., 2010. An international compendium of mutations in the SCN5A-encoded cardiac sodium channel in patients referred for Brugada syndrome genetic testing. Heart Rhythm. 7, 33–46.

Kisely, S., Lawrence, D., 2010. Inequalities in healthcare provision for people with severe mental illness. J. Psychopharmacol. 24 (Suppl. 4), 61–68.

Kisely, S., Preston, N., Xiao, J., Lawrence, D., Louise, S., Crowe, E., 2013. Reducing all-cause mortality among patients with psychiatric disorders: a population-based study. Can. Med. Assoc. J. 185, E50–E55.

Kitabchi, A.E., Umpierrez, G.E., Murphy, M.B., Kreisberg, R.A., 2006. Hyperglycemic crises in adult patients with diabetes: a consensus statement from the American Diabetes Association. Diabetes Care 29, 2739–2748.

Kodesh, A., Goldshtein, I., Gelkopf, M., Goren, I., Chodick, G., Shalev, V., 2012. Epidemiology and comorbidity of severe mental illnesses in the community: findings from a computerized mental health registry in a large Israeli health organization. Soc. Psychiatry Psychiatr. Epidemiol. 47, 1775–1782.

Koller, E., Schneider, B., Bennett, K., Dubitsky, G., 2001. Clozapine-associated diabetes. Am. J. Med. 111, 716–723.

Koller, E.A., Doraiswamy, P.M., 2002. Olanzapine-associated diabetes mellitus. Pharmacotherapy 22, 841–852.

Koller, E.A., Cross, J.T., Doraiswamy, P.M., Schneider, B.S., 2003. Risperidone-associated diabetes mellitus: a pharmacovigilance study. Pharmacotherapy 23, 735–744.

Koller, E.A., Weber, J., Doraiswamy, P.M., Schneider, B.S., 2004. A survey of reports of quetiapine-associated hyperglycemia and diabetes mellitus. J. Clin. Psychiatry 65, 857−863.

Koponen, H., Alaräisänen, A., Saari, K., Pelkonen, O., Huikuri, H., Raatikainen, M.J., et al., 2008. Schizophrenia and sudden cardiac death: a review. Nord. J. Psychiatry 62, 342−345.

Laghate, V.D., Gupta, S.B., 2004. Acute pancreatitis and diabetic ketoacidosis in non-diabetic person while on treatment with sodium valproate, chlorpromazine and haloperidol. J. Assoc. Physicians India 52, 257−258.

Lahti, M., Tiihonen, J., Wildgust, H., Beary, M., Hodgson, R., Kajantie, E., et al., 2012. Cardiovascular morbidity, mortality and pharmacotherapy in patients with schizophrenia. Psychol. Med. 42, 2275−2285.

Lambert, T.J.R., Velakoulis, D., Pantellis, C., 2003. Medical comorbidity in schizophrenia. Med. J. Aust. 178, S67−S70.

Laursen, T.M., Wahlbeck, K., Hällgren, J., Westman, J., Ösby, U., Alinaghizadeh, H., et al., 2013. Life expectancy and death by diseases of the circulatory system in patients with bipolar disorder or schizophrenia in the Nordic countries. PLoS One 8 (6), e67133.

Lawrence, D.M., Holman, C.D., Jablensky, A.V., Hobbs, M.S., 2003. Death rate from ischaemic heart disease in Western Australian psychiatric patients, 1980−1998. Br. J. Psychiatry 182, 31−36.

Leslie, D.L., Rosenheck, R.A., 2004. Incidence of newly diagnosed diabetes attributable to atypical antipsychotic medications. Am. J. Psychiatry 161, 1709−1711.

Limousin, F., Loze, J.Y., Philippe, A., 2007. Ten-year prospective follow-up study of mortality by suicide in schizophrenic patients. Schizophr. Res. 94, 23−28.

Lothian National Health Service. Shared Care Agreement 2014. <http://www.ljf.scot.nhs.uk/SharedCareofMedicines/Shared%20Care%20Agreements/SCA/SCA%20Thioridazine%20v1%200%20Final.pdf>.

Meltzer, H.Y., 2005. Suicide in schizophrenia, clozapine and adoption of evidence-based medicine. J. Clin. Psychiatry 66, 530−533.

Mitchell, A.J., Vancampfort, D., Sweers, K., Winkel, R., van, Yu, W., De Hert, M., 2013. Prevalence of metabolic syndrome and metabolic abnormalities in schizophrenia and related disorders—a systematic review and meta-analysis. Schizophr. Bull. 39, 306−318.

Morrison, A.P., Turkington, D., Pyle, M., Spencer, H., Brabban, A., Dunn, G., et al., 2014. Cognitive therapy for people with schizophrenia spectrum disorders not taking antipsychotic drugs: a single-blind randomised controlled trial. Lancet 383 (9926), 1395−1403.

Munro, J., O'Sullivan, D., Andrews, C., Arana, A., Mortimer, A., Kerwin, R., 1999. Active monitoring of 12,760 clozapine recipients in the UK and Ireland. Beyond pharmacovigilance. Br. J. Psychiatry 175, 576−580.

NHS [National electronic Library for Medicines]. EU CHMP recommends lifting ban on atypical antipsychotic Serdolect (sertindole).

Nielsen, J., Dahm, M., Lublin, H., Taylor, D., 2010. Psychiatrists' attitude towards and knowledge of clozapine treatment. J. Psychopharmacol. 24, 965−971.

Nihalani, N.D., Tu, X., Lamberti, J.S., Olson, D., Olivares, T., Costea, G.O., et al., 2007. Diabetic ketoacidosis among patients receiving clozapine: a case series and review of sociodemographic risk factors. Ann. Clin. Psychiatry 19, 105−112.

Noordam, R., van den Berg, M.E., Niemeijer, M.N., Aarts, N., Leening, M.J., Deckers, J.W., et al., 2015. Assessing prolongation of the heart rate corrected QT interval in users of tricyclic antidepressants: advice to use Fridericia rather than Bazett's correction. J. Clin. Psychopharmacol. 35, 260−265.

Nordentoft, M., Mortensen, P.B., Pedersen, C.B., 2011. Absolute risk of suicide after first hospital contact in mental disorder. Arch. Gen. Psychiatry 68, 1058–1064.

Nugter, M.A., Engelsbel, F., Bähler, M., Keet, R., van Veldhuizen, R., 2015. Outcomes of Flexible Assertive Community Treatment (FACT) implementation: a prospective real life study. Community Ment. Health J. Available from: http://dx.doi.org/10.1007/s10597-015-9831-2.

Osborn, D.P., Levy, G., Nazareth, I., Petersen, I., Islam, A., King, M.B., 2007. Relative risk of cardiovascular and cancer mortality in people with severe mental illness from the United Kingdom's General Practice Research Database. Arch. Gen. Psychiatry 64, 242–249.

Ösby, U., 2008. Cardiovascular outcome and schizophrenia in Sweden. Schizophr. Res. 102 (Suppl. 2), 18.

Ösby, U., Correia, N., Brandt, L., Ekbom, A., Sparén, P., 2000. Time trends in schizophrenia mortality in Stockholm county, Sweden: cohort study. Br. Med. J. 321, 483–484.

Palmer, B.A., Pankratz, V.S., Bostwick, J.M., 2005. The lifetime risk of suicide in schizophrenia: a reexamination. Arch. Gen. Psychiatry 62, 247–253.

Postema, P.G., 2012. About Brugada syndrome and its prevalence. Europace 2012 (14), 925–928.

Postema, P.G., Wolpert, C., Amin, A.S., Probst, V., Borggrefe, M., Roden, D.M., et al. (2009) Drugs and Brugada syndrome patients: review of the literature, recommendations, and an up-to-date website (www.brugadadrugs.org). Heart Rhythm. 6(9):1335–1341.

Ray, W.A., Chung, C.P., Murray, K.T., Hall, K., Stein, M.C., 2009. Atypical antipsychotic drugs and the risk of sudden cardiac death. N. Engl. J. Med. 360, 225–235.

Ringbäck Weitoft, G., Berglund, M., Lindström, E.A., Nilsson, M., Salmi, P., Rosén, M., 2014. Mortality, attempted suicide, re-hospitalisation and prescription refill for clozapine and other antipsychotics in Sweden—a register-based study. Pharmacoepidemiol. Drug Saf. 23, 290–298.

Saha, S., Chant, D., McGrath, J., 2007. A systematic review of mortality in schizophrenia: is the differential mortality gap worsening over time? Arch. Gen. Psychiatry 64, 1123–1131.

Sinyor, M., Remington, G., 2012. Is psychiatry ignoring suicide? The case for clozapine. J. Clin. Psychopharmacol. 32, 307–308.

Straus, S.M.J.M., Bleumink, G.S., Dieleman, J.P., van der Lei, J., t Jong, G.W., Kingma, J., et al., 2004. Antipsychotics and the risk of sudden cardiac death. Arch. Intern. Med. 164, 1293–1297.

Stroup, T.S., Gerhard, T., Crystal, S., Huang, C., Olfson, M., 2016. Comparative effectiveness of clozapine and standard antipsychotic treatment in adults with schizophrenia. Am. J. Psychiatry 173 (2), 166–173.

Tang, Y.L., Mao, P.X., Jiang, F., Chen, Q., Wang, C.Y., Cai, Z.J., et al., 2008. Clozapine in China. Pharmacopsychiatry 41, 1–9.

Tiihonen, J., Lönnqvist, J., Wahlbeck, K., Klaukka, T., Niskanen, L., Tanskanen, A., et al., 2009. 11-year follow-up of mortality in patients with schizophrenia: a population-based cohort study (FIN11 study). Lancet 374, 620–627.

van Hasselt, F.M., Schorr, S.G., Mookhoek, E.J., Brouwers, J.R., Loonen, A.J., Taxis, K., 2013. Gaps in health care for the somatic health of outpatients with severe mental illness. Int. J. Ment. Health Nurs. 22, 249–255.

Van Veldhuizen, J.R., 2007. FACT: a Dutch version of ACT. Community Ment. Health 43, 421–433.

Wahlbeck, K., Wetsman, J., Nordentoft, M., Gissler, M., Laursen, T.M., 2011. Outcomes of Nordic mental health systems: life expectancy of patients with mental health disorders. Br. J. Psychiatry 199, 453–458.

Walker, A.M., Lanza, L.L., Arellano, F., Rothman, K.J., 1997. Mortality in current and former users of clozapine. Epidemiology 8, 671–677.

Wheeler, A., Humberstone, V., Robinson, G., 2013. Outcomes for schizophrenia patients with clozapine treatment: how good does it get? J. Psychopharmacol. 23, 957–965.

Wunderink, L., Nieboer, R.M., Wiersma, D., Sytema, S., Nienhuis, F.J., 2013. Recovery in remitted first-episode psychosis at 7 years of follow-up of an early dose reduction/discontinuation or maintenance treatment strategy: long-term follow-up of a 2-year randomized clinical trial. JAMA Psychiatry 70, 913–920.

Yap, Y.G., Behr, E.R., Camm, A.J., 2009. Drug-induced Brugada syndrome. Europace 11, 989–994.

FURTHER READING

Bushe, C.J., Taylor, M., Haukka, J., 2010. Mortality in schizophrenia: a measurable clinical endpoint. J. Psychopharmacol. 24, 17–25.

De Hert, M., Correll, C.U., Cohen, D., 2011. Do antipsychotic medications reduce or increase mortality in schizophrenia? A critical appraisal of the FIN-11 study. Schizophr. Res. 117, 68–74.

Gallego, J.A., Nielsen, J., De Hert, M., Kane, J.M., Correll, C.U., 2012. Safety and tolerability of antipsychotic polypharmacy. Expert Opin. Drug Saf. 11, 527–542.

Gören, J.L., Meterko, M., Williams, S., Young, G.J., Baker, E., Chou, C.-H., et al., 2013. Antipsychotic prescribing pathways, polypharmacy, and clozapine use in treatment of schizophrenia. Psychiatr. Serv. 64, 527–533.

Grohmann, R., Hippius, H., Helmchen, H., Rüther, E., Schmidt, L.G., 2004. The AMUP study for drug surveillance in psychiatry—a summary of inpatient data. Pharmacopsychiatry 37 (Suppl. 1), S16–S26.

Hennen, J., Baldessarini, R.J., 2005. Suicidal risk during treatment with clozapine: a meta-analysis. Schizophr. Res. 73, 139–145.

Honkola, J., Hookana, E., Malinen, S., Kaikkonen, K.S., Junttila, M.J., Isohanni, M., et al., 2012. Psychotropic medications and the risk of sudden cardiac death during an acute coronary event. Eur. Heart. J. 33, 745–751.

Kelly, D.L., McMahon, R.P., Liu, F., Love, R.C., Wehring, H.J., Shim, J.C., et al., 2010. Cardiovascular disease mortality in patients with chronic schizophrenia treated with clozapine: a retrospective cohort study. J. Clin. Psychiatry 71, 304–311.

Kiviniemi, M., Suvisaari, J., Koivumaa-Honkanen, H., Häkkinen, U., Isohanni, M., Hakko, H., 2013. Antipsychotics and mortality in first-onset schizophrenia: prospective Finnish register study with 5-year follow-up. Schizophr. Res. 150, 274–280.

Laursen, T.L., Munk-Olsen, T., Agerbo, E., Gasse, C., Mortenson, P.B., 2009. Somatic hospital contacts, invasive cardiac procedures, and mortality from heart disease in patients with severe mental disorder. Arch. Gen. Psychiatry 66, 1713–1720.

Chapter 16

Forensic Investigation of Antipsychotic-Related Deaths

Robert J. Flanagan[1] and Peter Manu[2,3]

[1]*King's College Hospital, London, United Kingdom,* [2]*Hofstra Northwell School of Medicine, Hempstead, NY, United States,* [3]*South Oaks Hospital, Amityville, NY, United States*

16.1 INTRODUCTION

The causality framework for deaths occurring in persons taking antipsychotic drugs has four main components: accidental deaths; natural deaths, not-related to the antipsychotic treatment; adverse effects of antipsychotic drugs taken in therapeutic doses; voluntary or involuntary antipsychotic drug poisoning. However, the cause and mechanism of death in patients treated with antipsychotic drugs have not been thoroughly investigated. Without exception, all of the large-scale epidemiological studies on fatality rates presented earlier in this book have relied on clinical assessments, rather than on complete forensic evaluation that included a careful autopsy and accurate toxicological measurements. If death is clearly by self-inflicted trauma, for example, then the choice or adequacy of treatment (drug, dosage, adherence) may be called into question. In all cases the pharmacology and toxicology, not only of the antipsychotic(s) prescribed, but in many cases also of other drugs/poisons that may have contributed to the death and/or been prescribed for the deceased are important factors in the investigation, which often extends to study of clinical and nursing records, macroscopic postmortem findings, and postmortem biochemistry and histology. Accurate diagnosis of the cause of death in such circumstances is important not only for the families of the deceased, but also to enable accurate epidemiological data to be gathered with the aim, if possible, of preventing future deaths.

Life-Threatening Effects of Antipsychotic Drugs. DOI: http://dx.doi.org/10.1016/B978-0-12-803376-0.00016-2
© 2016 Elsevier Inc. All rights reserved.

16.2 CLINICAL AND PATHOLOGICAL CORRELATIONS

From an empirical vantage point, the main causes of deaths produced by adverse effects of antipsychotic drugs prescribed, administered, and taken in therapeutic dosages are relatively straightforward (Table 16.1). The antipsychotic-induced delay in myocardial repolarization is a necessary condition for the emergence of *torsades de pointes*, which can lead to ventricular fibrillation and sudden cardiac death. Patients who die during the course of clozapine-induced myocarditis have severe left ventricular dysfunction progression to cardiogenic shock. Low output heart failure may also be present in patients with massive pulmonary thromboembolism, but in this case the mechanism of death includes severe hypoxia. Patients with agranulocytosis and severe neutropenia, as well as those with bowel ischemia, are at risk of dying in septic shock. Postictal arousal failure followed by respiratory arrest is the mechanism of death in patients who had a drug-induced tonic−clonic seizure (Bozorgi and Lhatoo, 2013). The metabolic complications of antipsychotic treatment accelerate atherosclerosis and increase substantially the risk of fatal myocardial ischemia or cerebral thrombosis. Asphyxia is the mode of death in patients with airway obstruction produced by laryngeal spasm or oropharyngeal dysphagia. Finally, in patients with severe drug-induced liver or renal failure, death may be preceded by coma related to metabolic encephalopathy or by catastrophic bleeding.

TABLE 16.1 Main Causes of Deaths Produced by Adverse Effects of Antipsychotic Drugs

Drug-Related Effect	Main Cause(s) of Death
Delayed myocardial repolarization	Ventricular fibrillation
Myocarditis, cardiomyopathy	Pump failure, cardiogenic shock
Pulmonary embolism, alveolitis	Gas-exchange failure
Agranulocytosis, pancreatitis, bowel perforation	Septic shock
Seizure	Postictal arousal failure
Hyperglycemia	Diabetic ketoacidosis, hyperosmolar state
Metabolic syndrome	Coronary occlusion, stroke
Laryngospastic dystonia, oropharyngeal dysphagia	Airway obstruction
Liver failure	Metabolic encephalopathy, hemorrhagic shock

In structured root-cause analyses performed by a multidisciplinary team on 100 consecutive cases of sudden death that occurred among psychiatric patients 19–74 years of age cared for in a single behavioral health institution in New York City (119,500 patients-years), a cause of death was identified in 48% of the cases (Manu et al., 2011). Limited autopsies were performed in 18 patients. These patients died suddenly of a large variety of conditions, including acute coronary syndrome, upper airway obstruction, pulmonary embolism, pneumonia, bronchial asthma, thrombotic stroke, brain hemorrhage, heart failure, aortic dissection, myocarditis, *commotio cordis*, diabetic ketoacidosis (DKA), septic shock, seizure, and gastrointestinal hemorrhage. In the remaining 52 patients the cause of sudden death remained unexplained. The cases with explained and unexplained sudden death were similar with respect to age, gender, psychiatric diagnoses, and exposure to conventional and atypical antipsychotics, but significantly more subjects from the unexplained sudden death group had a history of dyslipidemia and diabetes (19.2% vs 2.1%), and dyslipidemia and hypertension (23.1% vs 8.3%), which are major risk factors for coronary artery disease. While significantly better than death certificates for establishing the cause of death, root-cause analyses are have shortcomings compared with autopsy data. For instance, a diagnosis of pulmonary thromboembolism is sometimes missed in patients who die after developing wheezing and shortness of breath and are thought to have suffered a fatal asthma attack (Byard, 2011).

As expected, autopsy series have a lower proportion of unexplained deaths. In a recent report of results of autopsies performed in 51 of 57 patients with schizophrenia treated with antipsychotic drugs who died suddenly during admission to a psychiatric hospital (Ifteni et al., 2014), autopsy-based causes of sudden death were most commonly cardiovascular disorders (62.8%), with a myocardial infarction identified in a majority of patients (52.9%). Other causes present in more than 1 patient each included pneumonia (11.8%), airway obstruction (7.8%), and myocarditis (5.9%). The death remained unexplained in 6 (11.8%) patients, but anatomical abnormalities were identified in 5 of them, and included extensive coronary arteriosclerosis, fibro-fatty myocardial changes and chronic pericarditis. A problem is the fact that some of the pathological findings may not have been lethal, but simply represent incidental findings. The issue is of particular importance for a forensic diagnosis of myocarditis, when careful grading must be applied to myocyte necrosis, neutrophilic infiltration, perivascular cuffs, and interstitial edema (Casali et al., 2012).

16.3 TOXICOLOGICAL ASSESSMENTS

If there is a clear cause of death such as trauma in someone prescribed antipsychotics then the coroner's verdict may be straightforward. However, toxicological investigation of samples of blood, for example, collected at the postmortem examination is usually performed to ascertain not only if the presence of drugs such as ethanol may have influenced a decision to self-harm, for example, but also to help assess adherence and possibly adequacy of treatment. At the other extreme, if someone being treated with antipsychotics dies unexpectedly and the postmortem examination is inconclusive as to the cause of death, toxicological examination of specimens of body fluids taken at the autopsy may yield valuable information that is not available from other sources. Such investigations assume added importance if, for example, death occurred in hospital and/or the deceased was detained by the state at the time of death.

16.3.1 Postmortem Toxicology

It used to be assumed that concentrations of drugs and other poisons measured in blood obtained at autopsy reflected the situation at the time of death, hence interpretation of results could be made simply by comparison with "normal" or "therapeutic" plasma drug/drug metabolite concentration data. However, we now know that interpretation of postmortem toxicology results must take into consideration the clinical pharmacology of the agents in question, the circumstances under which death occurred including the mode (route) of exposure, and other factors such as how the body was stored prior to sampling and the age of the deceased (Drummer, 2007; Gruszecki et al., 2007). Further important considerations include the changes that might occur in the composition of blood or other body fluids after death, the nature of the specimens sent for analysis, the stability of the analytes, and the suitability of the analytical methods employed (Pélissier-Alicot et al., 2003; Skopp, 2004; Ferner, 2008).

Recommended practice for blood collection postmortem is to sample a peripheral, usually femoral, vein by needle aspiration after ligating the vein proximally before opening the body (Dinis-Oliveira et al., 2010). However, it is not generally appreciated that this procedure is rarely followed, and indeed may not be possible if there has been trauma, for example. Even if the recommended procedure is adhered to, other changes may serve to alter the composition of the "blood" sampled from that circulating at the time of death. Such changes may be brought about by prolonged attempts at resuscitation, or by diffusion from tissues into blood as autolysis proceeds, possibly also by diffusion from the gastrointestinal tract, from inhaled vomit, or simply by sample contamination with, for example, gut contents or urine (Table 16.2). This phenomenon is referred to generally as postmortem redistribution, and with lipid-soluble drugs such as antipsychotics, that is, drugs with a relatively high volume of distribution (V) administered chronically, an increase in the blood concentration of the drug and any plasma metabolites after death may occur, although subsequent decreases have also been reported with certain drugs (Saar et al., 2012). In the case of clozapine,

TABLE 16.2 Factors Influencing the Likelihood of Postmortem Change in Blood Drug/Poison Concentrations

Factor	Comment
Site of collection	Central sites (heart, vena cava, or "subclavian" blood) more likely to show changes than peripheral sites (e.g., femoral vein after appropriate isolation). Blood from left ventricle of heart more likely to show change than blood from right ventricle
Time between death and specimen collection	A longer elapsed time gives more potential for changes as tissue pH decreases and autolysis proceeds
Medical intervention	Attempted resuscitation may result in aspiration of stomach contents, release of drug from tissues, such as lung due to trauma, and/or movement of blood from central to peripheral sites after death. Drugs may also be administered
Position of body when found	May result in blood draining from central sites to peripheral sites
Transport of the body	May promote movement of blood from central site to peripheral sites
Body storage temperature	The higher the temperature, the greater the potential for change
Method of sampling	Needle aspiration less likely to result in sample contamination with tissue fluid, for example. "Cavity blood" (blood remaining when the central organs have been removed) likely to be useful only for qualitative work due to contamination by other fluids
Specimen preservation	Sodium fluoride needed to help stabilize certain analytes (e.g., ethanol, cocaine, 6-acetylmorphine) does not reverse any precollection changes
Headspace in specimen tube	Volatile analytes will equilibrate between sample and headspace; opening the tube when cold (4°C) will minimize losses
Volume of blood collected	A larger specimen volume less likely to be influenced by localized changes in blood composition
Nature of poison	Lipophilic compounds more likely to show increase than lipophobic compounds; volatile or otherwise unstable compounds likely to show decrease; ethanol concentration may increase, or decrease depending on circumstance
Presence of poison in the airways, GI tract, or bladder	Postmortem diffusion may alter concentrations in blood and in adjacent tissues (sample liver from deep inside right lobe as furthest from stomach)

increases averaging 400–500% have been observed (Flanagan et al., 2005). In the case of injectable antipsychotics it is self-evident that the injection site may be near to the site of blood collection at postmortem. A further consideration with chlorpromazine and also with olanzapine is that these drugs not only are likely to undergo postmortem redistribution, but also are notoriously unstable in postmortem blood, rendering any attempt at the interpretation of quantitative data equivocal at best. Moreover, in the case of chlorpromazine there are a number of likely pharmacologically-active, but likewise unstable metabolites to complicate the picture.

Blood concentrations of water-soluble analytes with a relatively small V such as lithium may change minimally after death, although continued absorption from the gastrointestinal tract may take place postmortem even with such compounds and this may be reflected in blood sampled from central sites, such as the vena cava. Similarly, although free (unconjugated, i.e., unmetabolized) morphine concentrations in ventricular postmortem blood are consistently higher than those at peripheral sites, especially at concentrations >0.3 mg L^{-1}, there appears to be on average little change in morphine concentrations with time after death in blood specimens obtained from either central, or peripheral sites.

Many deaths that become the subject of postmortem investigation occur outside hospital and it may be some days before the body is found and samples collected for analysis. Postmortem blood is thus highly variable in composition. There is always a degree of hemolysis and sedimentation of cells. Clot formation, contamination with tissue fluid, or putrefaction may have occurred. Dehydration may have resulted from exposure to heat during a fire or dilution may have occurred in bodies recovered from water, a phenomenon perhaps more apparent in bodies recovered from fresh water than from sea water. Nevertheless, whole blood is commonly used in postmortem toxicology because (1) it is relatively easy to collect, (2) it is relatively homogeneous making it easier to dispense in the laboratory, and (3) there are often data on the plasma or serum (or sometimes even whole blood) concentrations of many analytes measured during normal therapy in adults to provide at least some basis for the interpretation of results. The data compilation by Baselt (2014) is the standard reference work in this area. However, even the obvious comparison with plasma analyte concentrations measured in life must be performed with considerable caution, in part because the whole blood:plasma (b:p) ratio may not be unity. Very strongly plasma protein bound compounds are often largely restricted to the plasma and have b:p ratios of 0.5–0.6, while substances such as ethanol that are highly water-soluble and do not bind to protein generally have b:p ratios of 0.8–0.9. Of course, these values vary somewhat depending on packed cell volume (hematocrit). Other compounds such as chloroquine are associated mainly with platelets and granulocytes, while carbon monoxide, and lead and other heavy metals are associated primarily with erythrocytes. In the case of quinine, the proportions of drug present in plasma and in red cells can change markedly during the course of an infection.

Clearly where there is no obvious indication of poisoning and there are the possibilities (1) that a patient or victim may have developed tolerance to some of the actions of the drug and/or (2) that postmortem changes in blood analyte concentrations may have occurred, the availability of additional information such as the results of tissue analyses may provide some information on the nature and magnitude of exposure, although comparative data are sparse. Measurement of poison concentrations in a representative specimen of gastric contents can give an estimate of unabsorbed dose if the total volume of contents is known. However, simply detecting a basic drug in gastric contents does not prove recent ingestion, since many drugs are excreted in saliva, and ion-trapping of basic drugs that diffuse from blood into the stomach can occur. If the patient was admitted to hospital there may be antemortem specimens available for analysis, but the availability of such samples should not preclude appropriate sampling at autopsy.

16.3.2   Accuracy of a Diagnosis of Poisoning

The circumstances in which exposure to a toxic agent may have occurred are crucial in assessing the possible involvement of the agent in a death. Coingestion of alcohol exacerbates the respiratory depressant effects of many drugs. Secondly, patients become tolerant to some of the toxic effects of medication on chronic exposure, hence a moderate, perhaps unintentional, overdose or incautious resumption of chronic therapy with a toxic drug may have much more serious consequences if the patient has been nonadherent in the preceding days or weeks. Tolerance cannot be measured in retrospect, although hair or nail analysis can sometimes be employed to attempt to assess prior exposure to toxic metals, illicit drug use, or adherence to prescribed medication in the weeks or months before death. Hair is well preserved even after burial, but an analysis gives no information as regards fatal poisoning, and qualitative information on exposure may be all that can be gleaned (Box 16.1). Importantly, it is now known that so-called "decontamination" (washing) procedures that were claimed to remove contaminants from the surface of hair prior to cutting into segments and digestion to give a time course of exposure simply transport the contaminants (drugs or drug breakdown products) into the medulla of the hair rendering any attempt to generate a time-course speculative at best (Cuypers et al., 2016).

The effects of tolerance are most clearly seen with clozapine, where the potentially fatal dose in a healthy adult is as little as 25 mg by mouth (Pokorny et al., 1994), yet after cautious dose escalation some patients may require more than the British National Formulary recommended maximum of 900 mg per day to achieve symptom control (MacCall et al., 2009). In a patient not prescribed clozapine who died after insisting on taking another patient's

---

BOX 16.1 Potential Origin of Drugs/Metabolites/Decomposition Products on/in Hair

- Deliberate administration (self or other)
- Inhalation (secondary smoke, exhaled air)
- Deposition from contaminated atmosphere (dust, etc.)
- Accidental exposure from contaminated surfaces via food/fingers, etc.
- Sweat after single large exposure
- Endogenous production, e.g., in the case of γ-hydroxybutyrate

---

medication, concentrations of clozapine and its N-desmethyl metabolite norclozapine in a femoral blood sample obtained postmortem were 0.48 and 0.20 mg L^{-1}, respectively (Stanworth et al., 2012). By way of comparison, audit of 104,127 plasma samples (26,796 patients) assayed for therapeutic drug monitoring purposes in the period 1993–2007 showed plasma clozapine 0.6 mg L^{-1} or more in 20% samples (8.4% 1 mg L^{-1} or more) (Couchman et al., 2010). The highest plasma clozapine and norclozapine concentrations that have been encountered in life during operation of our clozapine therapeutic drug monitoring service have been 6.05 and 1.72 mg L^{-1}, respectively. The patient was a 42-year-old male smoker prescribed 750 mg per day clozapine (predose sample, assay request form stated: "Dose correct? Poor/noncompliance?"). Obviously these elevated concentrations overlap dramatically with the postmortem blood concentrations observed in clozapine self-poisoning hence it is clear that other evidence, if available, has to be taken into account in individual cases.

To give a further practical example, postmortem blood olanzapine concentrations of 1 mg L^{-1} or above have been reported after olanzapine self-poisoning (Elian, 1998; Stephens et al., 1998). In addition, Merrick et al. (2001) reported the death of a male aged 25 who had been prescribed olanzapine. The postmortem (heart) blood olanzapine concentration was reported as 0.40 mg L^{-1} and death was attributed to accidental olanzapine poisoning in the absence of any other identifiable cause of death. Plasma olanzapine may well have been lower, or higher, at death in all these cases—with olanzapine, only plasma collected and stored appropriately is likely to give reliable quantitative results (Fisher et al., 2013). In clinical cases plasma olanzapine (12 hour postdose sample) is normally <0.1 mg L^{-1} (100 μg L^{-1}), but higher concentrations are often encountered especially at doses >20 mg per day. For example, a plasma olanzapine concentration of 0.48 mg L^{-1} was encountered in a female patient aged 44 years prescribed 30 mg per day olanzapine in whom nonadherence was suspected (Patel et al., 2011). Moreover, serum olanzapine concentrations of up to 1 mg L^{-1} have been reported in patients ingesting 150–1000 mg olanzapine with only mild manifestations of toxicity such as lethargy, ataxia, disorientation, miosis, and slurred speech (Cohen et al., 1999; O'Malley et al.,

1999; Shrestha et al., 2001; Singh et al., 2012). Indeed, there are few corroborating human data to indicate that olanzapine is particularly toxic in the amounts usually taken in self-poisoning episodes (Capel et al., 2000; Chue and Singer, 2003; Palenzona et al., 2004; Lennestål et al., 2007; Tse et al., 2008) and there are relatively few reports of olanzapine-related fatal poisoning (Elian, 1998; Stephens et al., 1998; Gerber and Cawthon, 2000; Schreinzer et al., 2001; Merrick et al., 2001; Davis et al., 2005; Singh et al., 2012).

The introduction of olanzapine long-acting injection (LAI) in 2004 was accompanied by reports of postinjection delirium/sedation syndrome (PDSS), which appears likely to be due to intravascular rather than intramuscular delivery of the injection (Lindenmayer, 2010). The clinical features described include sedation, dizziness, confusion, slurred speech, altered gait, weakness, muscle spasms, and/or unconsciousness in association with very high (1 mg L^{-1} or so) plasma olanzapine concentrations. Such events have not been reported with other injectable antipsychotics. In one survey (669 patients) there were 24 occurrences of PDSS (Anand et al., 2015). All patients recovered within 72 hours after receiving the injection, and there were no fatalities. Of the patients who experienced these events, 19 (83%) continued to receive further injections of olanzapine LAI. The incidence of PDSS per injection was 0.07%. No deaths have been reported.

Nowadays, quetiapine is licensed not only for the treatment of schizophrenia, but also for use in depression and in bipolar disorder. It is also increasingly misused (Malekshahi et al., 2015; Pilgrim and Drummer, 2013). Although this drug may not always prolong the QT interval after overdosage (Vivek, 2004; Hunfeld et al., 2006; Berling and Isbister, 2015), coma, respiratory depression, and seizures may occur (Balit et al., 2003; Reichert et al., 2014), and there have been a number of reports of fatalities principally involving this drug (Mainland et al., 2001; Fernandes and Marcil, 2002; Trenton et al., 2003; Hopenwasser et al., 2004; Langman et al., 2004). A factor in the clinical toxicology of quetiapine may be that after ingestion this drug is extensively metabolized in the first pass through the liver, a process that may be saturated after overdosage. A further consideration, however, is that at ordinary doses quetiapine sulfoxide is the principal plasma metabolite of quetiapine (Fisher et al., 2012), and this may decompose to give quetiapine on storage in postmortem blood.

As to amisulpride, after overdosage this drug has reportedly a similar risk of QT prolongation to that of thioridazine (Berling and Isbister, 2015). There are, however, very few unequivocal reports of fatal amisulpride poisoning (Isbister et al., 2006).

16.3.3 Postmortem Biochemistry

Vitreous humor is preferred to blood for most postmortem biochemistry (Table 16.2) since it is thought far less susceptible to autolytic change, is less likely to be subject to postmortem contamination by diffusion of drugs or other poisons that may be present at high concentration in the thorax or abdomen at death, and lies within the relatively protected environment of the eye socket (Thierauf et al., 2009). Aspiration must be gentle to avoid as far as possible contamination with retinal fragments. After death, however, potassium quickly leaks from the retina and hence vitreous potassium is not a reliable indicator of antemortem plasma potassium and is of minimal value in the diagnosis of exogenous potassium administration. The possibility of concurrent vitreous disease confounding the results must also be remembered (Parsons et al., 2003).

Vitreous sodium and chloride concentrations may fall after death at rates of up to 1 mmol L^{-1} per hour, whereas potassium increases at a rate of $0.14-0.19 \text{ mmol L}^{-1}$ per hour. Be this as it may, if the potassium concentration is $<15 \text{ mmol L}^{-1}$, then the sodium and chloride concentrations are thought likely to reflect the situation at death. Urea and creatinine, on the other hand, are relatively stable in postmortem specimens. If vitreous sodium, chloride, and urea are >155, >115, and $>10 \text{ mmol L}^{-1}$, respectively, this may indicate antemortem dehydration. If the urea concentration is $>20 \text{ mmol L}^{-1}$ and creatinine $>200 \text{ µmol L}^{-1}$ with sodium and chloride being within the normally accepted range, this indicates uremia was present before death. An especially difficult area is attempting to distinguish between hypernatremic dehydration and sodium chloride poisoning in infants and children and due caution must be exercised in interpreting results (Coulthard and Haycock, 2003).

16.4 SYSTEM-SPECIFIC FORENSIC CONSIDERATIONS

16.4.1 Antipsychotics and Sudden Unexpected Death

Particular problems may arise when the need to assess exposure to drugs or other poisons is only raised after the autopsy has been completed, since either specimens may not have been collected, or not all appropriate specimens may have been obtained. Further factors that may complicate the investigation of antipsychotic-related deaths are (1) that there is thought to be a risk of fatal toxicity with many centrally acting drugs at normally used doses (Witchel et al., 2003) and (2) many people with mental health problems, most notably schizophrenia, also smoke tobacco and some use alcohol, illicit drugs, herbal (natural) remedies, anabolic steroids, synthetic cannabinoids, and so-called "legal highs" (new or novel pharmaceutical substances, NPS). While toxicological screening methods usually pick up use of traditionally-misused drugs, they are largely useless with respect to herbal toxins unless a traditional drug, such as sildenafil, or a toxic metal salt is the active component of the product. Likewise anabolic steroids, many NPS, and synthetic cannabinoids are outwith the scope of most toxicology screens and have to be looked for "on request" via a specialist laboratory. Even then, successful detection is not guaranteed and simply finding a synthetic cannabinoid, for example, in a biological sample does not necessarily mean that the compound found was involved in causing the death.

It is known that smokers are at increased risk of sudden death when compared with nonsmokers. Furthermore, schizophrenia and affective disorders are themselves associated with increased mortality as compared to the general population (Ruschena et al., 1998), although there is uncertainty as to whether there is a greater risk of sudden, unexpected death in schizophrenic patients and whether these deaths are related to antipsychotic medication (Barnes and Kerwin, 2003; Royal College of Psychiatrists, 1997).

One consideration in the use of antipsychotics is that all such drugs have potentially toxic effects on the heart. However, it is unclear whether the apparent increase in deaths attributable to a fatal arrhythmia in patients with schizophrenia is due to drug treatment, or to the underlying disease, an event such as a fatal arrhythmia leaving no evidence postmortem (Flanagan, 2008). With antipsychotics, although it seems likely that other antipsychotic drugs exert similar effects (Ray and Meador, 2002), concerns as to cardiotoxicity in normal use of thioridazine (Thompson, 1994; Reilly et al., 2000, 2002; Witchel et al., 2003) led to the restriction of the use of this drug in the UK in December 2000 (MHRA, 2000) and to the voluntary withdrawal of droperidol in March 2001. As far as can be ascertained, these changes have had no effect on the incidence of sudden unexpected death in schizophrenia (Handley et al., 2016).

Given that the terminal event of life is cessation of the heartbeat, diagnosis of an antipsychotic-induced fatal arrhythmia as the cause of a death is perforce one of exclusion of all possible underlying causes of death. The presence of cardiomyopathy, for example, is a clear risk factor for a fatal arrhythmia, a risk that could be exacerbated by the presence of a proarrhythmic drug such as an antipsychotic or an antidepressant. Indeed, the risk could be multiplied if more than one proarrhythmic drug has been used. On the other hand, prescription of a drug does not necessarily mean that the patient has been taking it as prescribed in the days or weeks before death. The clinical features of cardiomyopathy are nonspecific and include fever, fatigue, lethargy, and drowsiness. In some cases drug treatment is implicated if the condition resolves after withdrawing the drug (Wooltorton, 2002). However, other possible causes of cardiomyopathy include chronic alcohol consumption and hypertension, itself possibly caused by drug-induced weight gain, and it is sometimes impossible to nominate a single underlying cause of death in such cases.

US FDA have warned healthcare providers and patients about the risk of quetiapine-induced QT interval prolongation and torsade de pointes when using this drug within its product licence (Hasnain et al., 2014). However, how this warning translates into clinical practice is unknown as comparable data from patients not prescribed quetiapine are lacking. In the case of haloperidol there was no difference in cardiac-related mortality in a group of patients prescribed this drug as compared to a control group (Ifteni et al., 2015).

16.4.2   Diabetes-Related Deaths

Chronic treatment with clozapine and olanzapine especially is associated with an increased risk of metabolic disorder including diabetes. Untreated DKA and hyperosmolar hyperglycemic syndrome (HHS) have mortality rates of 2–5% and 15–20%, respectively (Pasquel and Umpierrez, 2014; Corwell et al., 2014). After death, acetone is normally detected on gas chromatographic analysis of blood/urine ethanol, and measurement of blood β-hydroxybutyrate (Table 16.3) is used to confirm DKA as a likely cause of death. HHS patients do not produce acetone or other biochemical markers that can be tested for postmortem, and the only clue as to the presence of hyperglycemia in life may be a raised vitreous glucose concentration (Table 16.3).

16.4.3   Seizure-Related Deaths

Many centrally acting drugs including antipsychotics tend to lower the seizure threshold. As in the case of a fatal arrhythmia, a seizure-related death may leave no clear evidence postmortem. Investigation of possible seizure-related deaths usually include (1) clinical history and circumstances of the death, and any relevant autopsy findings, (2) use of nonprescribed drugs, (3) assessment of current drug therapy, including dosage and duration of therapy, and any recent changes in dosage, (4) assessment of adherence not only with possibly proconvulsant drugs, but also with any antiepileptic therapy, and (5) perhaps most importantly exclusion of other possible causes of death.

16.4.4   Other Potential Causes of Unexpected Death

In addition to arrhythmia and epileptic seizure, there are a range of conditions that death may be attributed to in the absence of a clear metabolic, mechanical, infection-related, or pharmacological cause of death. Lobar pneumonia can cause sudden collapse in the absence of clinical indicators of infection (Ifteni et al., 2014). Sleep apnea (Khoo et al., 2009) and positional asphyxia may need to be considered as an underlying cause of death based on either history, or postmortem findings. Neuroleptic malignant syndrome and heat stroke are also diagnoses of exclusion that lack pathognomonic features (Kerwin et al., 2004; Sheil et al., 2007).

TABLE 16.3 Postmortem Biochemistry: Interpretation of Results

Analyte	Matrix	Reference Range	Interpretation of Raised Concentration
Chloride	Vitreous humor	95–105 mmol L^{-1}	Salt poisoning; dehydration (interpret in conjunction with creatinine and urea)
Creatinine	Vitreous humor	<100 μmol L^{-1}	Poor renal function; high protein intake; large muscle mass; heat shock
Glucose	Vitreous humor	After death vitreous humor glucose falls rapidly therefore any detectable glucose requires investigation	(Drug induced) hyperglycemia, diabetic ketoacidosis, stress response (interpret in conjunction with lactate)
Hemoglobin A1c (HbA1c)	Blood	27–67 mmol mol^{-1} Hb	Poor long term (2–8 weeks) blood glucose control
β-Hydroxybutyrate	Blood, vitreous humor	0.1–1.0 mmol L^{-1}	Fasting, prolonged alcohol abuse, diabetic ketoacidosis, stress response (e.g., hypothermia)
Lactate	Vitreous humor	<10 mmol L^{-1}	Interpret in conjunction with glucose
Potassium	Vitreous humor	After death vitreous humor potassium increases rapidly. Concentrations >15 mmol L^{-1} suggest postmortem decomposition	Postmortem decomposition, little interpretative value
Sodium	Vitreous humor	135–145 mmol L^{-1}	Salt poisoning; dehydration (interpret in conjunction with creatinine and urea)
Tryptase	Blood	<100 μmol L^{-1}	Anaphylactic shock
Urea	Vitreous humor	<10 mmol L^{-1}	Renal function; upper GI hemorrhage

Source: Belsey and Flanagan, 2016.

16.5 CONCLUSIONS

Finding an antipsychotic in samples of blood or other tissues obtained post-mortem from a patient prescribed such a drug is of course not unexpected. A decision may be required on whether there is any evidence that dosage was excessive, which could indicate dose-related toxicity (acute, chronic, or acute-on-chronic) or self-poisoning as the cause of, or a contributory factor toward, the death. It must not be assumed that all those charged with investigating antipsychotic- or other drug-related deaths are familiar with all the information discussed in this chapter. Clinicians and others who may be asked to help in such enquiries are strongly advised to seek specialist advice especially as regards the clinical interpretation of postmortem biochemistry and toxicology results.

REFERENCES

Anand, E., Berggren, L., Deix, C., Tóth, Á., McDonnell, D.P., 2015. A 6-year open-label study of the efficacy and safety of olanzapine long-acting injection in patients with schizophrenia: a post hoc analysis based on the European label recommendation. Neuropsychiatr. Dis. Treat. 11, 1349–1357.

Balit, C.R., Isbister, G.K., Hackett, L.P., Whyte, I.M., 2003. Quetiapine poisoning: a case series. Ann. Emerg. Med. 2003 (42), 751–758.

Barnes, T.R.E., Kerwin, R., 2003. Mortality and sudden death in schizophrenia. In: Camm, J. (Ed.), Cardiovascular Risk Associated With Schizophrenia and Its Treatment. Galliard Healthcare Communications, London, pp. 7–23.

Baselt, R.C., 2014. Disposition of Toxic Drugs and Chemicals in Man, 10th edition, Biomedical Publications, Seal Beach, CA.

Belsey, S., Flanagan, R.J., 2016. Postmortem biochemistry: Current applications. J. Forensic Leg. Med. 41, 49–57.

Berling, I., Isbister, G.K., 2015. Prolonged QT risk assessment in antipsychotic overdose using the QT nomogram. Ann. Emerg. Med. 66, 154–164.

Bozorgi, A., Lhatoo, S.D., 2013. Seizures, cerebral shutdown, and SUDEP. Epilepsy Curr. 13, 236–240.

Byard, R.W., 2011. All that wheezes is not asthma—alternative findings at autopsy. J. Forensic Sci. 56, 252–255.

Capel, M.M., Colbridge, M.G., Henry, J.A., 2000. Overdose profiles of new antipsychotic agents. Int. J. Neuropsychopharmacol. 3, 51–54.

Casali, M.B., Lazzaro, A., Gentile, G., Blandino, A., Ronchi, E., Zoja, R., 2012. Forensic grading of myocarditis: an experimental contribution to the distinction between lethal myocarditis and incidental myocarditis. Forensic Sci. Int. 223, 78–86.

Chue, P., Singer, P., 2003. A review of olanzapine-associated toxicity and fatality in overdose. J. Psychiatr. Neurosci. 28, 253–261.

Cohen, L.G., Fatalo, A., Thompson, B.T., Di Centes Bergeron, G., Flood, J.G., Poupolo, P.R., 1999. Olanzapine overdose with serum concentrations. Ann. Emerg. Med. 34, 275–278.

Corwell, B., Knight, B., Olivieri, L., Willis, G.C., 2014. Current diagnosis and treatment of hyperglycemic emergencies. Emerg. Med. Clin. North Am. 32, 437–452.

Couchman, L., Morgan, P.E., Spencer, E.P., Flanagan, R.J., 2010. Plasma clozapine, norcloza-pine, and the clozapine:norclozapine ratio in relation to prescribed dose and other factors: data from a therapeutic drug monitoring service, 1993–2007. Ther. Drug Monit. 32, 438–447.

Coulthard, M.G., Haycock, G.B., 2003. Distinguishing between salt poisoning and hypernatrae-mic dehydration in children. Br. Med. J. 326, 157–160.

Cuypers, E., Flinders, B., Boone, C.M., Bosman, I.J., Lusthof, K.J., van Asten, A.C., et al., 2016. Consequences of Decontamination Procedures in Forensic Hair Analysis Using Metal-Assisted Secondary Ion Mass Spectrometry Analysis. Anal. Chem. Available from: http://dx. doi.org/10.1021/acs.analchem.5b03979.

Davis, L.E., Becher, M.W., Tlomak, W., Benson, B.E., Lee, R.R., Fisher, E.C., 2005. Persistent choreoathetosis in a fatal olanzapine overdose: drug kinetics, neuroimaging, and neuropa-thology. Am. J. Psychiatry 162, 28–33.

Dinis-Oliveira, R.J., Carvalho, F., Duarte, J.A., Remião, F., Marques, A., Santos, A., et al., 2010. Collection of biological samples in forensic toxicology. Toxicol. Mech. Methods 20, 363–414.

Drummer, O.H., 2007. Post-mortem toxicology. Forensic Sci. Int. 165, 199–203.

Elian, A.A., 1998. Fatal overdose of olanzapine. Forensic Sci. Int. 91, 231–235.

Fernandes, P.P., Marcil, W.A., 2002. Death associated with quetiapine overdose. Am. J. Psychiatry 159, 2114.

Ferner, R.E., 2008. Post-mortem clinical pharmacology. Br. J. Clin. Pharmacol. 66, 430–443.

Fisher, D., Handley, S., Flanagan, R.J., Taylor, D., 2012. Plasma concentrations of quetiapine, N-desalkylquetiapine, O-desalkylquetiapine, 7-hydroxyquetiapine and quetiapine sulfoxide in relation to quetiapine dose, formulation and other factors. Ther. Drug Monit. 34, 415–421.

Fisher, D.S., Partridge, S.J., Handley, S.A., Flanagan, R.J., 2013. Stability of some atypical anti-psychotics in human plasma, human serum, calf serum, oral fluid and haemolysed whole blood. Forensic Sci. Int. 229, 151–156.

Flanagan, R.J., 2008. Fatal toxicity of drugs used in psychiatry. Hum. Psychopharmacol. 23 (S1), S43–S51.

Flanagan, R.J., Spencer, E.P., Morgan, P.E., Barnes, T.R.E., Dunk, L., 2005. Suspected cloza-pine poisoning in the UK/Eire, 1992–2003. Forensic Sci. Int. 155, 91–99.

Gerber, J.E., Cawthon, B., 2000. Overdose and death with olanzapine: two case reports. Am. J. Forensic Med. Pathol. 21, 249–251.

Gruszecki, A.C., Booth, J., Davis, G.G., 2007. The predictive value of history and scene investi-gation for toxicology results in a medical examiner population. Am. J. Forensic Med. Pathol. 28, 103–106.

Handley, S., Patel, M.X., Flanagan, R.J., 2016. Antipsychotic-related fatal poisoning, England and Wales, 1993–2013: impact of the withdrawal of thioridazine. Clin Toxicol (Phila).1–10, Mar 29.

Hasnain, M., Vieweg, W.V., Howland, R.H., Kogut, C., Breden Crouse, E.L., Koneru, J.N., et al., 2014. Quetiapine, QTc interval prolongation, and torsade de pointes: a review of case reports. Ther. Adv. Psychopharmacol. 4, 130–138.

Hopenwasser, J., Mozayani, A., Danielson, T.J., Harbin, J., Narula, H.S., Posey, D.H., et al., 2004. Postmortem distribution of the novel antipsychotic drug quetiapine. J. Anal. Toxicol. 28, 264–267.

Hunfeld, N.G., Westerman, E.M., Boswijk, D.J., de Haas, J.A., van Putten, M.J., Touw, D.J., 2006. Quetiapine in overdosage: a clinical and pharmacokinetic analysis of 14 cases. Ther. Drug Monit. 28, 185–189.

Ifteni, P., Correll, C.U., Burtea, V., Kane, J.M., Manu, P., 2014. Sudden unexpected death in schizophrenia: autopsy findings in psychiatric inpatients. Schizophr. Res. 155, 72–76.

Ifteni, P., Grudnikoff, E., Koppel, J., Kremen, N., Correll, C.U., Kane, J.M., et al., 2015. Haloperidol and sudden cardiac death in dementia: autopsy findings in psychiatric inpatients. Int. J. Geriatr. Psychiatry 30 (12), 1224–1229.

Isbister, G.K., Murray, L., John, S., Hackett, L.P., Haider, T., et al., 2006. Amisulpride deliberate self-poisoning causing severe cardiac toxicity including QT prolongation and torsades de pointes. Med. J. Aust. 184, 354–356.

Kerwin, R.W., Osborne, S., Sainz-Fuertes, R., 2004. Heat stroke in schizophrenia during clozapine treatment: rapid recognition and management. J. Psychopharmacol. 18, 121–123.

Khoo, S.M., Mukherjee, J.J., Phua, J., Shi, D.X., 2009. Obstructive sleep apnea presenting as recurrent cardiopulmonary arrest. Sleep Breath. 13, 89–92.

Langman, L.J., Kaliciak, H.A., Carlyle, S., 2004. Fatal overdoses associated with quetiapine. J. Anal. Toxicol. 28, 520–525.

Lennestål, R., Asplund, C., Nilsson, M., Lakso, H.A., Mjörndal, T., Hägg, S., 2007. Serum levels of olanzapine in a non-fatal overdose. J. Anal. Toxicol. 31, 119–121.

Lindenmayer, J.P., 2010. Long-acting injectable antipsychotics: focus on olanzapine pamoate. Neuropsychiatr. Dis. Treat. 6, 261–267.

MacCall, C., Billcliff, N., Igbrude, W., Natynczuk, S., Spencer, E.P., Flanagan, R.J., 2009. Clozapine: more than 900 mg/day may be needed. J. Psychopharmacol. 23, 206–210.

Mainland, M.K., Wagner, M.A., Gock, S.B., Wong, S.H., 2001. Quetiapine-related fatalities. J. Analyt. Toxicol. 25, 381–382.

Malekshahi, T., Tioleco, N., Ahmed, N., Campbell, A.N., Haller, D., 2015. Misuse of atypical antipsychotics in conjunction with alcohol and other drugs of abuse. J. Subst. Abuse Treat. 48, 8–12.

Manu, P., Kane, J.M., Correll, C.U., 2011. Sudden deaths in psychiatric patients. J. Clin. Psychiatry 72, 936–941.

Merrick, T.C., Felo, J.A., Jenkins, A.J., 2001. Tissue distribution of olanzapine in a postmortem case. Am. J. Forensic Med. Pathol. 22, 270–274.

MHRA, 2000. Medicines and Healthcare Products Regulatory Agency (medicines) Restricts the Use of Thioridazine. Press release 2000/0734.

O'Malley, G.F., Seifert, S., Heard, K., Daly, F., Dart, R.C., 1999. Olanzapine overdose mimicking opioid intoxication. Ann. Emerg. Med. 34, 279–281.

Palenzona, S., Meier, P.J., Kupferschmidt, H., Rauber-Luethy, C., 2004. The clinical picture of olanzapine poisoning with special reference to fluctuating mental status. J. Toxicol. Clin. Toxicol. 42, 27–32.

Parsons, M.A., Start, R.D., Forrest, A.R., 2003. Concurrent vitreous disease may produce abnormal vitreous humour biochemistry and toxicology. J. Clin. Pathol. 56, 720.

Pasquel, F.J., Umpierrez, G.E., 2014. Hyperosmolar hyperglycemic state: a historic review of the clinical presentation, diagnosis, and treatment. Diabetes Care 37, 3124–3131.

Patel, M.X., Bowskill, S., Couchman, L., Lay, V., Taylor, D., Spencer, E.P., et al., 2011. Plasma olanzapine in relation to prescribed dose and other factors: data from a therapeutic drug monitoring service, 1999–2009. J. Clin. Psychopharmacol. 31, 411–417.

Pélissier-Alicot, A.L., Gaulier, J.M., Champsaur, P., Marquet, P., 2003. Mechanisms underlying postmortem redistribution of drugs: a review. J. Anal. Toxicol. 27, 533–544.

Pilgrim, J.L., Drummer, O.H., 2013. The toxicology and comorbidities of fatal cases involving quetiapine. Forensic Sci. Med. Pathol. 9, 170–176.

Pokorny, R., Finkel, M.J., Robinson, W.T., 1994. Normal volunteers should not be used for bioavailability or bioequivalence studies of clozapine. Pharm. Res. 11, 1221.

Ray, W.A., Meador, K.G., 2002. Antipsychotics and sudden death: is thioridazine the only bad actor? Br. J. Psychiatry 180, 483−484.

Reichert, C., Reichert, P., Monnet-Tschudi, F., Kupferschmidt, H., Ceschi, A., Rauber-Lüthy, C., 2014. Seizures after single-agent overdose with pharmaceutical drugs: analysis of cases reported to a poison center. Clin. Toxicol. (Phila.) 52, 629−634.

Reilly, J.G., Ayis, S.A., Ferrier, I.N., Jones, S.J., Thomas, S.H., 2000. QTc-interval abnormalities and psychotropic drug therapy in psychiatric patients. Lancet 355, 1048−1052.

Reilly, J.G., Ayis, S.A., Ferrier, I.N., Jones, S.J., Thomas, S.H., 2002. Thioridazine and sudden unexplained death in psychiatric in-patients. Br. J. Psychiatry 180, 515−522.

Royal College of Psychiatrists, 1997. The Association Between Antipsychotic Drugs and Sudden Death. Council Report CR57. Royal College of Psychiatrists, London.

Ruschena, D., Mullen, P.E., Burgess, P., Cordner, S.M., Barry-Walsh, J., Drummer, O.H., et al., 1998. Sudden death in psychiatric patients. Br. J. Psychiatry 172, 331−336.

Saar, E., Beyer, J., Gerostamoulos, D., Drummer, O.H., 2012. The time-dependant post-mortem redistribution of antipsychotic drugs. Forensic Sci. Int. 222, 223−227, Erratum in: Forensic Sci. Int. 2013; 228, 94.

Schreinzer, D., Frey, R., Stimpfl, T., Vycudilik, W., Berzlanovich, A., Kasper, S., 2001. Different fatal toxicity of neuroleptics identified by autopsy. Eur. Neuropsychopharmacol. 11, 117−124.

Sheil, A.T., Collins, K.A., Schandl, C.A., Harley, R.A., 2007. Fatal neurotoxic response to neuroleptic medications: case report and review of the literature. Am. J. Forensic Med. Pathol. 28, 116−120.

Shrestha, M., Hendrickson, R.G., Henretig, F.M., 2001. Striking extrapyramidal movements seen in large olanzapine overdoses. Clin. Toxicol. 39, 282.

Singh, L.K., Praharaj, S.K., Sahu, M., 2012. Nonfatal suicidal overdose of olanzapine in an adolescent. Curr. Drug Saf. 7, 328−329.

Skopp, G., 2004. Preanalytic aspects in postmortem toxicology. Forensic Sci. Int. 142, 75−100.

Stanworth, D., Hunt, N.C., Flanagan, R.J., 2012. Clozapine—a dangerous drug in a clozapine-naïve subject. Forensic Sci. Int. 214, e23−e25.

Stephens, B.G., Coleman, D.E., Baselt, R.C., 1998. Olanzapine-related fatality. J. Forensic Sci. 43, 1252−1253.

Thierauf, A., Musshoff, F., Madea, B., 2009. Post-mortem biochemical investigations of vitreous humor. Forensic Sci. Int. 192, 78−82.

Thompson, C., 1994. The use of high-dose antipsychotic medication. Br. J. Psychiatry 164, 448−458.

Trenton, A., Currier, G., Zwemer, F., 2003. Fatalities associated with therapeutic use and overdose of atypical antipsychotics. CNS Drugs 17, 307−324.

Tse, G.H., Warner, M.H., Waring, W.S., 2008. Prolonged toxicity after massive olanzapine overdose: two cases with confirmatory laboratory data. J. Toxicol. Sci. 33, 363−365.

Vivek, S., 2004. No QT interval prolongation associated with quetiapine overdose. Am. J. Emerg. Med. 22, 330.

Witchel, H.J., Hancox, J.C., Nutt, D.J., 2003. Psychotropic drugs, cardiac arrhythmia, and sudden death. J. Clin. Psychopharmacol. 23, 58−77.

Wooltorton, E., 2002. Antipsychotic clozapine (Clozaril): myocarditis and cardiovascular toxicity. Can. Med. Assoc. J. 166, 1185−1186.

Guide to the Interpretation of the Results of Some Chemical Pathology Tests

General guide only. Reference ranges may vary with age, sex, and other factors. Many laboratories produce their own reference ranges. Special care is needed in the interpretation of enzyme activities such as acetylcholinesterase.

Analyte		Sample	Reference Range	Alternative Reference Range
Acetylcholinesterase		Red cell	10–20 MU mol Hb^{-1}	160–310 U g Hb^{-1a}
Alanine aminotransferase (ALT, SGPT)		Serum	<50 IU L^{-1}	–
Albumin		Serum	35–50 g L^{-1}	3.5–5 g dL^{-1}
Alkaline phosphatase		Serum	40–130 IU L^{-1}	–
Anion gap		[derived]^b	10–15 mmol L^{-1}	10–15 mEq L^{-1}
Aspartate aminotransferase (AST, SGOT)		Serum	<40 IU L^{-1}	–
Bicarbonate		Serum	20–30 mmol L^{-1}	20–30 mEq L^{-1}
Bilirubin ("direct" = unconjugated)		Serum	<5 μmol L^{-1}	<0.3 mg dL^{-1}
Bilirubin (total)		Serum	<25 μmol L^{-1}	<1.5 mg dL^{-1}
Calcium (total)^c		Serum	2.20–2.60 mmol L^{-1}	8.8–10.4 mg dL^{-1}
Chloride		Serum	100–110 mmol L^{-1}	350–390 mg dL^{-1}
Cholinesterase^d		Plasma	3–9 kU L^{-1}	–
C-reactive protein (CRP)		Serum	<10 mg L^{-1}	<1 mg dL^{-1}
Creatine kinase (CK)		Serum	<150 IU L^{-1}	–
Creatinine		Serum	50–135 μmol L^{-1}	0.6–1.5 mg dL^{-1}
Eosinophil count		Blood	0.4–0.6 nL^{-1}	0.4–0.6 × 10^9 L^{-1}
Erythrocyte count^e	Male	Blood	4.0–5.5 pL^{-1}	4.0–5.5 × 10^{12} L^{-1}
	Female	Blood	3.8–4.8 pL^{-1}	3.8–4.8 × 10^{12} L^{-1}

(Continued)

(Continued)

Analyte		Sample	Reference Range	Alternative Reference Range
Erythrocyte sedimentation rate (ESR)		Blood	$2-30^f$ mm h^{-1}	–
Globulin		Serum	$20-35$ g L^{-1}	$2.0-3.5$ g dL^{-1}
γ-Glutamyl transferase (GGT)		Serum	<55 IU L^{-1}	–
Glucose (fasting)		Plasma	$4-7$ mmol L^{-1}	$72-126$ mg dL^{-1}
Hematocrit (HCT)^g	Male	Blood	$0.38-0.48$	–
	Female	Blood	$0.33-0.43$	–
Hemoglobin	Male	Blood	$120-165$ g L^{-1}	$12.0-16.5$ g dL^{-1}
	Female	Blood	$115-150$ g L^{-1}	$11.5-15.0$ g dL^{-1}
Hydrogen ion concentration (H$^+$)		Blood	$36-44$ nmol L^{-1}	$36-44$ mEqL^{-1}
International normalized ratio (INR)		Blood	$0.8-1.2$	–
Iron		Serum	$8-30$ µmol L^{-1}	$45-168$ µg dL^{-1}
Lactate^h		Blood	$0.6-1.6$ mmol L^{-1}	$5.4-14.4$ mg dL^{-1}
Lactate dehydrogenase (LDH) (total^i)		Serum	<250 IU L^{-1}	–
Leukocyte count^j (adults)		Blood	$4-11$ nL^{-1}	$4-11 \times 10^9$ L^{-1}
Methemoglobin		Blood	$<1\%$ Hb^a	–
Osmolality		Serum	$280-295$ mmol kg^{-1}	$280-295$ mOsm kg^{-1}
Osmolar gap		[derived]^k	± 10 mmol L^{-1}	–
pCO$_2$		Blood	$4.5-6.1$ kPa	$34-46$ mm Hg
pH		Blood	$7.36-7.44$	–
Phosphate		Serum	$0.8-1.5$ mmol L^{-1}	$2.5-4.6$ mg dL^{-1}
pO$_2$		Blood	$12-15$ kPa	$90-113$ mm Hg
Potassium		Plasma	$3.5-5.0$ mmol L^{-1}	$14-20$ mg dL^{-1}
Protein (total)		Serum	$65-75$ g L^{-1}	$6.5-7.5$ g dL^{-1}
Prothrombin time		Blood	$10-15$ s	–
Sodium		Serum	$135-145$ mmol L^{-1}	$310-330$ mg dL^{-1}
Urate		Serum	$200-400$ µmol L^{-1}	$3.4-6.8$ mg dL^{-1}
Urea		Serum	$3-8$ mmol L^{-1}	$14-48$ mg dL^{-1}
Zinc protoporphyrin (ZPP)		Red cell	<0.64 µmol L^{-1}	<40 µg dL^{-1}

^{a}Hb, hemoglobin.
^{b}[Sodium] − ([Chloride] + [Bicarbonate]).
^{c}Affected by albumin concentration.
^{d}Pseudocholinesterase.
^{e}Red cell count (RBC).
^{f}Upper limit markedly age dependent.
^{g}Packed cell volume (PCV).
^{h}Special precautions in sample collection/storage.
^{i}Method dependent
^{j}White cell count (WBC).
^{k}Measured osmolality = (2Na$^+$ + K$^+$ + Glucose + Urea) (all mmol L^{-1}).

Index

Note: Page numbers followed by "*f*" and "*t*" refer to figures and tables, respectively.

Printed in the United States
By Bookmasters